Oxford Medical Publications

Assessing quality of life in clinical trials

Assessing quality of life in clinical trials
Methods and Practice

SECOND EDITION

Edited by

Peter Fayers

Professor of Medical Statistics
Department of Public Health
University of Aberdeen Medical School
Aberdeen
UK

and

Ron Hays

Professor of Medicine
UCLA School of Medicine
Division of General Internal Medicine and Health Services Research
Los Angeles, CA
USA

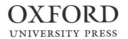

OXFORD
UNIVERSITY PRESS

OXFORD
UNIVERSITY PRESS

Great Clarendon Street, Oxford OX2 6DP

Oxford University Press is a department of the University of Oxford.
It furthers the University's objective of excellence in research, scholarship,
and education by publishing worldwide in

Oxford New York
Auckland Cape Town Dar es Salaam Hong Kong Karachi Kuala Lumpur Madrid Melbourne
Mexico City Nairobi New Delhi Taipei Toronto Shanghai

With offices in
Argentina Austria Brazil Chile Czech Republic France Greece Guatemala Hungary Italy Japan
South Korea Poland Portugal Singapore Switzerland Thailand Turkey Ukraine Vietnam

Oxford is a registered trade mark of Oxford University Press
in the UK and in certain other countries

Published in the United States
by Oxford University Press Inc., New York

A catalogue record for this title is available from the British Library
Data available

Library of Congress Cataloguing in Publication Data

ISBN 0-19-852769-1 (Hbk)

10 9 8 7 6 5 4 3 2 1

Typeset in Minion
by Cepha Imaging Pvt. Ltd., Bangalore, India
Printed in Great Britan
on acid-free paper by
Biddles Ltd, King's Lynn

Preface

Quality of life assessment has progressed considerably since 1998 when we and our many co-authors produced the book *Quality of Life Assessment in Clinical Trials: Methods and Practice*. Quality of life has now become a standard end point in many randomized clinical trials and other studies. Thus, it is timely to provide not just an update, but a completely new edition that reviews the current state of art and also discusses topical issues including areas where active research is in progress.

Although we have retained the title *Quality of Life*, many would argue that 'Health-related quality of life' (HRQoL) is more accurate, to emphasize that we are focusing on the effects of disease and its treatment. Equally, there is a shift towards preferring the generality of the term 'Patient-reported outcomes', which encompasses dimensions such as patient satisfaction with care as well as HRQoL. In accordance with current usage, irrespective of the semantic arguments about terminology, this book regards quality of life and HRQoL as similar and largely overlapping concepts.

Section 1 discusses the development and evaluation of generic and disease-targeted questionnaires (Chapter 1.1), and not only reviews the modern use of traditional psychometric methods in constructing these instruments (Chapters 1.3 and 1.4), but also covers the role of qualitative methods (Chapter 1.2) which have become considerably more advanced and with a stronger scientific basis over recent years – although developments in these methods remain under-utilized by many designers of instruments. This section also introduces Rasch models and item response theory, the use of which has grown appreciably over the past few years (Chapter 1.5).

Having decided the items that should be included in an instrument, there is next the problem of converting the items into their usable forms; this is the general thrust of Section 2. Chapter 2.1 discusses the problems of translating and ensuring the validity of a questionnaire in different languages. Two more chapters (2.2 and 2.3) expound the use of item response theory and illustrate how it is fundamentally changing the approach towards questionnaire design and development. Item response theory, together with the widespread use of computers, enables exciting new approaches such as computer adaptive testing (CAT) in which the most appropriate item for gathering information from a patient is dynamically selected on the basis of what is so far known about the patient. However, not all patients are able to use computers and it is not always possible to obtain valid information by self-assessment (e.g., cognitively impaired); instead, proxy assessment may be required. Long regarded with suspicion, recent investigations into proxy assessment shed light into when it may be appropriate and useful; current knowledge about potential bias arising from this and other context effects is outlined in Chapter 2.4.

Under analysis, the first three chapters (3.1–3.3) address the perennial problems of longitudinal data analysis and the methods of analysing studies with missing data. Advances in methods of statistical analysis, accompanied by newer facilities in statistical software, make possible techniques that provide better interpretation of results from studies that follow patients over time, and enable the impact – primarily, potential bias – of missing data to be explored. But as always prevention is better than cure (Chapter 3.2). Another analytical area of growing interest is the role of differential item functioning for assuring the validity of a questionnaire – can we identify items that perform inconsistently in particular subgroups, for example with respect to cultural differences or (as when translations are suboptimal) language differences (Chapter 3.4)? Finally in this section, Chapter 3.5 covers the importance of good reporting and communication of results from clinical trials.

Section 4 emphasizes the interpretation of results. Many critics of standard HRQoL instruments protest that only the patient can identify which issues they regard as most important, and only the patient can assign the corresponding weights to these issues. This has led to individualized measures, and Chapter 4.1 demonstrates that these methods yield useful data, and reports the increasing experience with such measures. Chapter 4.2 deals with the more general aspects of interpretation: what should a clinician understand when told that a patients' HRQoL is 54, or that a patient has changed by 13 units on a 100-point scale? Many approaches have been developed to resolve such questions. One proof of the importance of assessing HRQoL in clinical trials lies in the number of trials that have shown clinically important effects (or, conversely, convincingly demonstrated treatment equivalence). Chapter 4.3 comprehensively reviews 'successes' in HRQoL assessment. One problem with assessing HRQoL is that patients adapt in various ways over time – they may alter their views of 'worst imaginable quality of life', change their internal standards (recalibration), or alter their priorities. Response shift – Chapter 4.4 – covers a range of phenomena and can explain both the well-known coping or adaptation to illness as well as other changes that can make HRQoL data tricky to interpret. Finally, although the majority of HRQoL questionnaires have been developed for use in clinical trials, surveys or other assessments of groups of patients, there is now an awareness that perhaps these same questionnaires can provide a clinician with invaluable individual-patient data from which patient management decisions can be made (Chapter 4.5).

Section 5 starts by exploring the role of single-item questions about 'your overall health'. As Chapter 5.1 shows, these seemingly vague yet simple questions have repeatedly been found to be extremely highly predictive of clinical outcome and survival in many disease areas. The rest of this section explores particular groups of measures – generic adult measures (5.2), children and adolescents – for whom there are a number of very specific issues when developing measures (5.3), and neurological conditions, which also raise other difficulties of assessment (5.4).

Section 6 goes beyond the individual clinical trial. How can we use clinical trial and other data to make macro-decisions, as in health economics? These decisions may demand knowledge of values of the trade-off between HRQoL, cost and survival – but should those values come from the general public, patients, or others? Chapter 6.1 introduces the issues and indicates some of the logical problems that arise. Chapter 6.2 reviews performance-based measures, and Chapter 6.3 examines the powerful technique of discrete choice experiments, which are a recent introduction to medical research. The last chapter (6.4) looks at methods of combining the results from a group of clinical trials assessing the same treatment effect; systematic reviews and meta-analytic techniques have only recently begun to be applied to HRQoL outcomes in clinical trials.

Thus this book covers a wide range of topics, emphasizing new and innovative approaches that are of practical and clinical importance, reviewing the current state of the art and illustrating the benefits and potential of in HRQoL assessment in clinical trials. We thank the contributors to this volume for their diligence, perseverance, and creative products.

Peter Fayers and Ron Hays, January 2004

Contents

Contributors

Jakob Bue Bjorner, MD, PhD
QualityMetric, Inc.
Lincoln, RI
USA

David Cella, PhD
Professor and Director
Center on Outcomes Research and
Education
1001 University Place
Evanston, IL
USA

Stephen Joel Coons, PhD
Professor
Division of Social and Administrative
Sciences
University of Arizona College of Pharmacy
Tucson, AZ
USA

Diane L. Fairclough, PhD
University of Colorado Health Sciences
Center
Denver, CO
USA

Peter Fayers, PhD
Professor of Medical Statistics
Department of Public Health
University of Aberdeen Medical School
Aberdeen
UK

David Feeny, PhD
Professor of Economics and Public
Health Sciences
Edmonton, AB
Institute of Health Economics
University of Alberta
Canada

Karen Gerard, MSc
Health Care Research Unit
University of Southampton
Southampton General Hospital
Southampton
UK

Mogens Groenvold, MD, PhD
Bispebjerg Hospital
Department of Palliative Medicine
Copenhagen
Denmark

Ron Hays, PhD
Professor of Medicine
UCLA School of Medicine
Divison of General Internal Medicine
and Health Services Reasearch
Los Angeles, CA
USA

Stefan Höfer, PhD
Marie Curie Research Fellow
Department of Psychology
Medical School
Royal College of Surgeons in Ireland
Dublin
Ireland

Ellen Idler, Phd
Institute for Health, Healthcare Policy
and Aging Research
Rutgers University
New Brunswick, NJ
USA

Paul Kind, MSc, MPhil
Centre for Health Economics
University of York
Heslington
York
UK

Madeleine King, PhD
Centre for Health Economics, Research
and Evaluation (CHERE)
University of Technology
Sydney
Australia

Jeanne M. Landgraf, MA
Vice President and Chief Scientific Officer
HealthAct, Inc.
Boston, MA
USA

Patrick Marquis, PhD
Managing Director
MAPI Values USA
Boston, MA
USA

Elaine McColl, MSc
Director
Newcastle Clinical Trials Unit
Centre for Health Services Research
University of Newcastle upon Tyne
Newcastle upon Tyne
UK

Ciaran O'Boyle, PhD
Professor of Psychology
Medical School
Royal College of Surgeons in Ireland
Dublin
Ireland

David Osoba, MD
QOL Consulting
Vancouver
Canada

Morten Aagaard Petersen, MSc
Bispebjerg Hospital
Department of Palliative Medicine
Copenhagen
Denmark

Bryce B. Reeve, PhD
Outcomes Research Branch
Applied Research Program
Division of Cancer Control and
Population Sciences
National Cancer Institute
Bethesda, MD
USA

Dennis Revicki, PhD
Director and Senior Research Leader
Centre for Health Outcomes
Research
MEDTAP International, Inc.
Bethesda, MD
USA

Lena Ring, PhD
Marie Curie Research Fellow
Department of Psychology Medical
School
Royal College of Surgeons in Ireland
Dublin
Ireland

Mandy Ryan, PhD
Professor in Health Economics
Health Economics Research Unit
University of Aberdeen
Medical School
Aberdeen
UK

Carolyn Schwartz, ScD
QualityMetric, Inc.
Lincoln, RI
USA

Neil Scott, MA, MSc
Department of Public Health
University of Aberdeen Medical School
Aberdeen
UK

James W. Shaw, Phd, Pharm D, MPH
Tobacco Control Research Branch
Behavioural Research Program
Division of Cancer Control and
Population Sciences
National Cancer Institute
Bethesda, MD
USA

Mirjam A. G. Sprangers, PhD
Associate Professor
Department of Medical Psychology
Academic Medical Center
University of Amsterdam
Amsterdam
The Netherlands

Galina Velikova, MD, PhD
Cancer Research UK and University of
Leeds Cancer Med Research Unit,
St James' Hospital
Leeds
UK

Barbara G. Vickrey, MD, MPH
Professor of Neurology
Department of Neurology
UCLA School of Medicine
Los Angeles, CA
USA

John Ware, PhD
CEO and Chief Scientific Officer
Quality Metric Incorporated
Lincoln, NI
USA

Penny Wright, MSc
Cancer Research UK
Clinical Centre
St James's University Hospital
Leeds
UK

Section 1

Developing and evaluating questionnaires

Generic versus disease-targeted instruments

Ron D. Hays

Generic health-related quality of life (HRQoL) instruments are designed to be applicable across a wide range of populations and interventions. Disease-targeted measures, in contrast, are designed to be relevant to a particular disease, such as diabetes or lupus. This chapter compares and contrasts generic and disease-targeted HRQoL instruments, discussing the pros and cons of both kinds of measures.

Generic measures

Generic measures are designed to be relevant to anyone. They are analogous to intelligence tests in that different people can be compared to one another because they have taken the same test. Generic measures have two basic forms: (1) profile; and (2) preference-based. Profile measures are designed to yield scores on multiple aspects of HRQoL. Preference-based measures are designed to produce a single summary score that cuts across the multiple domains of HRQoL. For more information about preference measures see Kind (Chapter 6.1) and Feeny (Chapter 6.2).

The SF-36, a generic measure, is the most widely used HRQoL survey instrument in the world today. It comprises 36 items selected from a larger pool of items used in the RAND Medical Outcomes Study (MOS). Twenty of the items are administered using a past four weeks reporting interval. The SF-36 assesses eight health concepts using multi-item scales (35 items):

1. Physical functioning (10 items),
2. Role limitations caused by physical health problems (4 items),
3. Role limitations caused by emotional problems (3 items),
4. Social functioning (2 items),
5. Emotional well-being (5 items),
6. Energy/fatigue (4 items),
7. Pain (2 items), and
8. General health perceptions (5 items).

An additional single item assesses change in perceived health during the last 12 months.

Generic profile HRQoL measures such as the SF-36 are used to compare the relative burden of disease for different groups of patients. For example, the HRQoL of 2864 HIV-infected adults participating in the HIV Cost and Services Utilization Study, a probability sample of adults with HIV receiving health care in the United States, was compared with that of patients with other chronic diseases and to the general US population (Hays *et al.* 2000). SF-36 physical functioning scores were about the same for adults with asymptomatic HIV disease as for the US general population but were much worse for those with symptomatic HIV disease by 1 standard deviation (SD), and worse still, by another 1 SD, for those who met criteria for AIDS. Patients with AIDS had worse physical functioning that those with some of the other chronic diseases (epilepsy, gastroesophageal reflux disease, clinically localized prostate cancer, clinical depression, diabetes). SF-36 emotional well-being was comparable among patients with various stages of HIV disease, but was significantly worse than the general US population and patients with other chronic disease, with the exception of depression.

The SF-36 has also been used to assess HRQoL among patients with different diseases over time. For example, patients with hypertension, diabetes and depression in the MOS were compared at baseline and two years post-baseline (Hays *et al.* 1995).

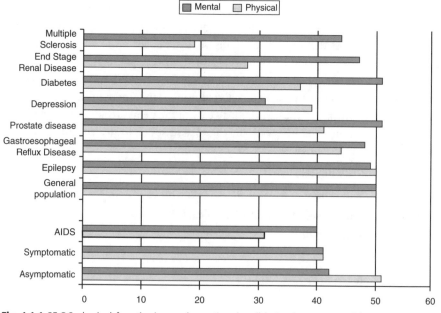

Fig. 1.1.1 SF-36 physical functioning and emotional well-being in persons with HIV. From Hays *et al.* (2003).

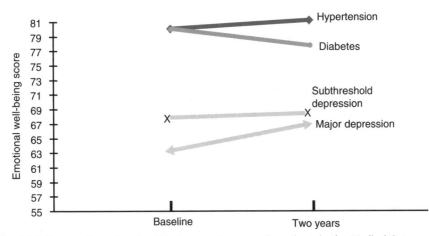

Fig. 1.1.2 Course of emotional well-being over two years in patients in the Medical Outcomes Study. From Hays *et al.* (1995).

As expected, patients with depression at baseline had substantially worse emotional well-being than patients with chronic medical illnesses (hypertension, diabetes) at baseline of the study. Would these differences persist over time? Figure 1.1.2 shows the course of emotional well-being from baseline to two years later. This picture indicates a relatively flat line for the chronic medical illnesses and positive gains in emotional well-being over time for the patients who were depressed at baseline, especially those with major depression. Nonetheless, patients depressed at baseline continued to demonstrate relatively poor emotional well-being two years later.

Meaningful and valid comparisons of different groups assume that the generic measure is equivalent in the different groups. This means that the HRQoL scales should have the same level of acceptability, reliability and validity in different segments of the population. In HRQoL studies, some attention has been paid to evaluating cross-group equivalence involving different language or race/ethnic subgroups. For example, Yu *et al.* (2003) compared the reliability and mean scores of the English and Chinese versions of the SF-36 in a sample of 309 Chinese nationals bilingual in Chinese and English living in the US. Similarly, the International Quality of Life Assessment Project evaluated the equivalence between the US English and translations of the SF-36 into multiple languages including Dutch, Spanish, German, Japanese, and Italian (Gandek *et al.* 1998).

Disease-targeted measures

Disease-targeted measures are constructed to fill the gaps in generic instruments by tapping aspects of HRQoL that are of particular relevance to people with the condition of interest. Rather than advocate using only one or the other, the most typical recommendation is to supplement a generic measure with disease-targeted items (Patrick and Deyo 1989). For example, the Kidney Disease Quality of Life (KDQOL™) Instrument (Hays *et al.* 1994) includes the SF-36 as the generic core plus items that assess symptoms and problems associated with kidney disease, the effects of kidney disease on daily activities, burden of kidney disease, work, quality of social interaction, sexual function, and sleep. It is important to note that several of these concepts could be included in a generic HRQoL measure (work, quality of social interaction, sexual function, sleep). They are included in the KDQOL™ because they are important for people with kidney disease but are not included in the generic core instrument. Hence, it is clear that disease-targeted items are tied to the generic core and are not necessarily disease-specific. Table 1.1.1 illustrates this point by listing concepts measured by a sample of six generic (SF-36, Sickness Impact Profile, WHO-QOL, Quality of Well-Being Scale, Health Utilities Index Mark 3, EQ-5D) and four targeted (MOS-HIV, KDQOL™, ESI-55, NEI-RQL) HRQoL instruments. Note that there is considerable overlap in the content, but there are also some unique concepts represented in the targeted measures.

Disease-targeted measures have the potential to be more sensitive to smaller differences and smaller change over time than generic measures, because they are selected to be particularly relevant to a given condition. For example, in a study of HRQoL in men treated for localized prostate cancer, there were no differences on the SF-36 between those treated with surgery, radiation, watchful waiting, or an age and zip-coded matched control group (Litwin *et al.* 1995). However, disease-targeted measures of sexual, urinary and bowel function and distress revealed worse HRQoL among the treatment groups (radiation, surgery).

A fundamental consideration in the evaluation of disease-targeted measures used in tandem with generic cores is demonstrating that the former capture unique information. Shahriar *et al.* (2003) noted that there is a paucity of evidence showing unique information in the MOS-HIV compared to the SF-36 in studies of patients with HIV. In contrast, the SF-36 PCS and MCS were found to have low correlations with most of the National Eye Institute Visual Functioning Questionnaire (NEI-VFQ) scales in a study of 598 persons with common chronic eye diseases (Mangione *et al.* 1998). Similarly, the National Eye Institute Refractive Error Quality of Life (NEI-RQL) multi-item scales were found to account for 29 per cent of the variance in a satisfaction with correction item beyond that explained by the SF-36 and the NEI-VFQ (Hays *et al.* 2003).

Summary

Generic and disease-targeted HRQoL measures provide complementary information and are, therefore, both important in clinical studies. Generic measures provide the basis of comparing different people, regardless of personal characteristics, with one another. Targeted measures provide the most relevant information for a given condition and

Table 1.1.1 Examples of generic and disease-targeted HRQoL measures

Instrument	Concepts	Type of Measure
SF-36	Physical functioning, role limitations – physical, pain, general health perceptions, emotional well-being, role limitations – emotional, energy, social functioning	Generic
Sickness Impact Profile	Ambulation, mobility, body care and movement, communication, alertness behaviour, emotional behaviour, social interaction, sleep and rest, eating, work, home management, recreation and pastimes	Generic
WHO-QOL	Physical domain, psychological domain, level of independence, social relationships, environment, spirituality/religion/personal beliefs	Generic
Quality of Well-Being Scale	Mobility, physical activity, social activity, symptom/problem complexes	Generic
Health Utilities Index III	Vision, hearing, speech, ambulation, dexterity, emotion, cognition, pain	Generic
EQ-5D	Mobility, self-care, usual activity, pain/discomfort, anxiety/depression	Generic
MOS-HIV	Physical functioning, role functioning, pain, social functioning, emotional well-being, energy/fatigue, cognitive functioning, general health, health distress, overall QOL	Targeted
KDQOL™	Burden of kidney disease, quality of social interaction, cognitive function, symptoms/problems, effects of kidney disease, sexual function, sleep, social support, work status, dialysis staff encouragement, patient satisfaction, overall health rating	Targeted
ESI-55	General health perceptions, energy/fatigue, overall QOL, social function, emotional well-being, cognitive functioning, physical functioning, pain, role limitations – emotional, role limitations – physical, role limitations – memory	Targeted
NEI-RQL	Clarity of vision, expectations about vision, near vision, far vision, diurnal fluctuations, activity limitations, glare, symptoms, dependence on correction, worry, suboptimal correction, appearance, satisfaction with correction	Targeted

help to round out a generic measure. It is recommended that generic and disease-targeted measures be used in tandem whenever possible to provide the strengths of both approaches.

Because of response burden, it is challenging to include items to tap both generic and disease-targeted HRQoL. To help with the trade-off between items for one purpose or another, it is recommended that the generic core be selected to contain the minimal number of items possible to provide the maximum possible coverage of the disease-targeted piece. For instance, when one is interested in knowing about the HRQoL of a group of people with a specific disease, it is worth considering using the SF-12 (Ware *et al.* 1996) rather than the SF-36 as the generic core. The savings of 24 items on the generic side will open up greater flexibility for exploring in detail the all-important targeted content side.

References

Gandek B., Ware J. E., Aaronson, N. K., Alonso, J., Apolone, G., Bjorner, J., Brazier, J., Bullinger, M., Fukuhara, S., Kaasa, S., Leplège, A., and Sullivan, M. (1998). Tests of data quality, scaling assumptions, and reliability of the SF-36 in eleven countries: Results from the IQOLA Project. *Journal of Clinical Epidemiology*, **51**, (11), 1149–1158.

Hays, R. D., Cunningham, W. E., Sherbourne, C. D., Wilson, I. B., Wu, A. W., Cleary, P. D., McCaffrey, D. F., Fleishman, J. A., Crystal, S. C., Collins, R., Eggan, F., Shapiro, M. F., and Bozzette, S. A. (2000). Health-related quality of life in patients with Human Immunodeficiency Virus Infection in the United States: Results from the HIV Cost and Services Utilization Study. *American Journal of Medicine*, **108**, 714–722.

Hays, R. D., Kallich, J. D., Mapes, D. L., Coons, S. J., and Carter, W. B. (1994). Development of the Kidney Disease Quality of Life (KDQOL) Instrument. *Quality of Life Research*, **3**, 329–338.

Hays, R. D., Mangione, C. M., Ellwein, L., Lindblad, A. S., Spritzer, K. L., and McDonnell, P. J. (2003). Psychometric properties of the National Eye Institute – Refractive Error Quality of Life (NEI-RQL) Instrument. *Ophthalmology*, **110**, 2292–2301.

Hays, R. D., Wells, K.B., Sherbourne, C. B., Rogers, W. H., and Spritzer, K. (1995). Functioning and well-being outcomes of patients with depression compared to chronic general medical illness. *Archives of General Psychiatry*, **52**, 11–19.

Litwin, M., Hays, R.D., Fink, A., Ganz, P. A., Leake, B., Leach, G. E., and Brook, R. H. (1995). Quality of life outcomes in men treated for localized prostate cancer. *Journal of the American Medical Association*, **273**, 129–135.

Mangione, C. M., Lee, P. P., Pitts, J., Gutierrez, P., Berry S., and Hays, R. D. (1998). Psychometric properties of the National Eye Institute Visual Function Questionnaire, the NEI-VFQ. *Archives of Ophthalmology*, **116**, 1496–1504.

Patrick, D. L. and Deyo, R. A. (1989). Generic and disease-specific measures in assessing health status and quality of life. *Medical Care* 27, (3 Suppl.), S217–S232.

Shahriar, J., Delate, T., Hays, R. D., and Coons, S. J. (2003). Commentary on using the SF-36 or MOS-HIV in studies of persons with HIV disease. *Health and Quality of Life Outcomes*, **1**, (25), Epub July 9 (7 pages).

Ware, JE Jr, Kosinski, M., and Keller, S. D. (1996). A 12-Item Short-Form Health Survey: Construction of scales and preliminary tests of reliability and validity. *Medical Care*, **34**, (3) 220–233.

Yu, J., Coons, S. J., Draugalis, J. R., Ren, X. S., and Hays, R. D. (2003). Equivalence of the Chinese version and the U.S.-English version of the SF-36 Health Survey. *Quality of Life Research*, **12**, 449–457.

Developing questionnaires

Elaine McColl

The focus of this chapter is how qualitative research methods and cognitive aspects of survey methodology can be applied in the development of a new quality of life instrument. The emphasis is on the stages of item generation and wording, the establishment of content and face validity, and the initial stages of instrument pre-testing.

Developing an instrument – the role of qualitative methods

In the past, many developers of quality of life measures adopted a 'top-down' approach to determining instrument content. The conceptualization and operationalization of 'impairment' or 'quality of life', and the choice of items to be included, was determined primarily by a review of the literature and of the content of existing instruments. 'Expert' input to the development process was generally confined to the views of clinicians and researchers, and lay persons' views were seldom considered (Bowling 1995). A risk of this top-down approach is that the resultant instrument will not fully reflect those aspects of health and quality of life most important to people experiencing a particular disease. This lack of patient-centredness may pose a threat to content validity and may mean that treatment outcomes of relevance to the patient are not included, thereby threatening responsiveness to change (Guyatt and Cook 1994).

To ensure greater relevance of instrument content to patients, Guyatt and colleagues have for several years incorporated patients' views in the development of their measures of quality of life for a wide range of chronic conditions (e.g. Guyatt *et al.* 1989; Juniper *et al.* 1992). Similarly, the WHOQOL group (Skevington *et al.* 1997; WHO-QOL Group 1998) consulted widely with lay persons across a wide range of cultures. This process of seeking lay input on the meaning of health and the impact on quality of life of living with an index condition is now becoming the norm. A further advantage of lay involvement is that the developer can gain a greater insight into the language and terminology used by the target respondents, and can thus ensure that the vocabulary used in the instrument is culturally appropriate.

Where lay people are to be involved in the item generation phase of instrument development, qualitative research methods are the key means of data collection. Two main approaches are used: individual interviews and focus groups.

In describing qualitative techniques for individual interviews, Britten (1995) distinguishes between three types of research interview – structured, semi-structured and unstructured. Structured interviews utilize predetermined, standardized questions, generally with fixed response options and presented in a pre-specified order. As such, they are best suited to the collection of quantitative data on a well-understood topic. For the exploratory research needed in instrument development, a more qualitative approach is required. The aim is to allow the respondents their own voice, to explore the issues must important to them and to avoid making unwarranted assumptions or imposing the perspective of a researcher or clinician. Both semi-structured and unstructured interviews can be used to this end, with most researchers favouring the former. Semi-structured interviews utilize open-ended questions and a loose structure or agenda, initially set by the researcher but flexible enough to allow issues important to the respondent to emerge. (By contrast, completely unstructured interviews largely follow the respondent's agenda and are more conversational in nature.) Interviews are normally tape-recorded, to ensure that questions and answers are captured verbatim and to minimize the need for the interviewer to take contemporaneous notes.

Semi-structured interviews generally utilize a topic guide, defining the general areas or health-related quality of life (HRQoL) issues to be explored. Commonly, the development of the initial topic guide is based on a review of the relevant literature and of the content of existing quality of life measures, and perhaps on the views of health professionals regarding the likely impact of the index condition. For example, the interviewer may start off with a very broad question, such as 'What is it like to live with (name of condition)?'. Assuming that the researcher conceptualises 'quality of life' as multidimensional, encompassing physical, social and psychological well-being, follow-up questions may ask more specifically about the impact of the condition on these aspects of life and on specific activities and roles – for instance 'How does (name of condition) affect your ability to move about?', 'How does it affect you at work?', 'How does it influence your relationship with family and friends?'. However, the wording and ordering of the topics may be varied from interview to interview, to allow issues of particular relevance to that respondent to be pursued in greater detail. Moreover, if respondents spontaneously mention issues that are not explicitly mentioned in the topic guide, the researcher should probe for more details on how the index condition affects these dimensions of quality of life. In all cases, it is important to use open questions, such as 'What … ?', 'How … ?', 'To what extent … ?', which do not presuppose a particular response. Closed questions – for example, 'Does your (name of condition) limit the work you can do?' – can result in acquiescence bias by implying to the respondent that a positive response is required.

Sampling for qualitative research

In qualitative research, both for individual interviews and for focus group discussions, sampling strategies are generally systematic but non-probabilistic. The aim is not statistical representativeness, but rather 'to identify specific groups of people who … possess characteristics … relevant to the phenomenon being studied' (Mays and Pope 1995; Pope and Mays 1995). Respondents are not selected at random but instead are purposively or theoretically sampled because they are expected to facilitate investigation of 'an aspect of behaviour relevant to the research' (Mays and Pope 1995); thus the sample may be deliberately constructed to ensure inclusion of respondents displaying different characteristics believed to be related to the phenomenon under investigation. For example, it is likely that age, gender, life-stage, duration and severity of illness may affect illness experiences. In identifying item content for a quality of life instrument, an adequate spread of respondents across these characteristics should be ensured.

There is no consensus about sample size for qualitative research and *a priori* power calculations are not made. Rather, data are analysed as they are gathered, and data collection is terminated once no new themes are emerging – this is termed the point of 'data saturation'. Although the exact sample size cannot be completely determined in advance, experience shows that six to eight respondents often suffice for a homogeneous sample (i.e. where experiences are broadly similar across respondents and the main focus is on commonality of issues – as is most likely to be the case in developing HRQoL measures), while from twelve to twenty may be needed when looking for 'disconfirming evidence' (Kuzel 1992) (i.e. where it is important to ensure that discordant and non-consensual views are also heard). Where illness experiences are expected to vary across subgroups of individuals, these numbers of respondents may be required within each subgroup. Guidelines from the European Organisation for Research and Treatment of Cancer (Blazeby *et al.* 2001) recommend interviewing five to ten respondents in each treatment group or disease stage in the development phase of a new module.

Focus groups

Either in parallel with individual semi-structured interviews or in their place, many researchers now choose to use focus group discussions in generating item content (e.g Litwin *et al.* 1999). A focus group is used to collect information by inviting a number of respondents to discuss a given topic as a group, under the guidance of a moderator.

Although exact recommendations regarding size of group vary, a focus group generally comprises between three and twelve respondents, a moderator and, optionally, a co-facilitator. The moderator has a key role in promoting group interaction, maximizing interaction between respondents and keeping the discussion focused around a topic guide. Where a co-facilitator is used, his/her role is to support the moderator, look after the recording equipment and take brief contemporaneous notes (e.g. details of who is speaking and of any non-verbal interaction). Most authorities (e.g. Fern 1982) recommend that each focus group should be relatively homogeneous and that members should be strangers to one another. A heterogeneous group can lead to inhibition in raising issues that do not seem to be shared by other respondents, while people who already know each other may rely on taken-for-granted assumptions regarding the very topics of interest to the researcher. Where marked heterogeneity is expected in the population of interest, conducting multiple focus groups, with each group being relatively homogenous in composition, is advisable.

Focus groups versus individual interviews

A number of advantages of focus groups over individual interviews have been postulated. It is suggested that the explicit use of group interaction in this form of qualitative data collection may lead to more and better quality information being generated (Lederman 1990). Issues may be raised which might never arise in individual interviews, as focus group members spark ideas off one another, and peer-group effects may provoke greater candour and provide a more emotionally charged atmosphere, leading to greater disclosure.

However, there is little empirical evidence to support this view. Thomas and colleagues (Thomas *et al.* 1995) used both methods in generating item content for a measure of satisfaction with nursing care. They found that certain topics were more likely to be raised in focus groups, but that there was no difference between the two approaches in respect of the depth of data generated; thus, relying on individual interviews alone would not have led to significant omissions in item content. They concluded that, while concepts could potentially be generated more rapidly through focus groups, there were significant logistical problems in assembling suitably homogenous groups of respondents. Although their experiences were in respect of individuals about to be or recently discharged from hospital, it is possible that similar difficulties might be experienced in assembling focus groups to generate item content for a quality of life measure. Individuals with more severe illness, or whose ability to get around outside the home is limited by their condition, may be less willing to participate; this could be a potential source of bias. Even when suitable groups can be assembled, there is a risk of the discussion being monopolized by the more vocal members, even though their experiences may not be shared by others. There is also the risk of acquiescence bias and 'forced compliance' whereby some respondents express agreement with the viewpoint of the moderator (also a risk with individual interviews), or with other more forceful group members, although this is not their actual view. These risks place great demands on moderators, who should be aware of these potential problems and must be able to counteract them.

Thus the choice between focus groups and individual semi-structured interviews for item generation is not clear-cut. The potential advantages and disadvantages of each method need to be weighed up in relation to the population of interest. A combination of both techniques may be required.

Analysis of qualitative data in instrument development

Analytic techniques for data generated through individual semi-structured interviews and focus group discussions are broadly similar. The first step is to transcribe the tape-recorded interview or discussion. A verbatim transcription, rather than para-phrasing, is the norm. However, there is usually no need to employ special conventions of punctuation to indicate the length of pauses or the nature of speech hesitancies. Each interview should be transcribed as soon as possible after its completion, and the transcript should be reviewed, and amended as required, by the interviewer or moderator.

In contrast to quantitative research, where most of the analysis is carried out when all the data have been collected, data collection and analysis proceed in parallel in qualitative research. Ongoing review and analysis of each completed transcript is required to identify whether any modifications to the topic guide are required (e.g. to explore an issue raised in one interview with subsequent respondents to see whether this is a common experience) and to inform the theoretical sampling of further respondents. Once no qualitatively different themes emerge, the point of 'data saturation' has been reached and data collection should be terminated.

Where qualitative research is being undertaken as an end in itself, a grounded theory approach to analysis (Strauss and Corbin 1994) is generally advocated. By 'grounded theory', Strauss and Corbin (1994) mean 'theory derived from data, systematically gathered and analysed through the research process' (1994 p. 12). They argue that, in theory at least, a researcher should not generally start out with a preconceived notion or model in mind, but rather should allow the concepts and theories to emerge from the data (i.e. be 'grounded' in the data). To this end, they recommend an elaborate system of coding and comparisons in the analysis of qualitative data.

In identifying item content for a quality of life instrument, however, qualitative research is a means to an end, rather than an end in itself. Moreover, although the researcher is open and receptive to new issues being raised by the respondents, instrument development is also likely to be informed by existing theories and conceptual frameworks about what constitutes 'quality of life'. For that reason, although some researchers have claimed to have adopted a 'grounded theory' approach (e.g. Fitzsimmons *et al.* 1999), the majority of instrument developers do not adhere strictly to the intensive coding procedures espoused by Strauss and Corbin (1994). A simplified approach, such as the Framework technique (Ritchie and Spencer 1994), involving identifying, abstracting, charting and matching themes which are recurrent across the data set, will generally suffice. The key steps in this technique are summarized in Box 1.

Pre-testing an instrument – the role of cognitive methods

The term 'Cognitive Aspects of Survey Methodology' (CASM) is applied to the growing interdisciplinary effort – including survey methodologists, cognitive and social psychologists, and sociolinguists – to investigate and understand the cognitive processes employed by respondents in reading, comprehending and interpreting the questions or declarative statements used to elicit information in a questionnaire, and in formulating and providing answers to those stimuli (Barofsky 1996; Jobe 2003).

> **Box 1 Key steps in the Framework technique for qualitative analysis**
>
> 1. **Familiarization** – gaining an overview of the material gathered (e.g. through reading transcripts)
> 2. **Identifying a thematic framework** – drawing upon *a priori* themes from topic guide, emergent themes from interviews, analytical themes from repeated issues
> 3. **Indexing** – applying the thematic framework systematically to the body of data by coding each fragment/section of interview transcript
> 4. **Charting** – building up a picture of the data as a whole; rearranging the data according to themes
> 5. **Mapping and interpretation** – aggregating patterns of data; weighing up importance and dynamics of issues; searching for an overall structure in the data; synthesising the findings.

Cognitive models of survey response

Jobe (2003) identifies seven models of the cognitive processes involved in survey response. The best known is that of Tourangeau and colleagues (Tourangeau *et al.* 2000), who have proposed a four-stage model of the question response process: comprehension; retrieval; judgement; response. First, the respondent must perceive and attend to the question, infer its meaning and thus identify the nature of the information sought by the researcher. There is scope here for misunderstanding what the researcher is asking, with a consequent threat to measurement validity and reliability. In the retrieval stage, the respondent has to: develop a strategy and a set of cues for retrieving the relevant material from long-term memory; retrieve that information and fill in any gaps in memory through inference or the use of short-cuts (heuristics). Again, characteristics both of the question (and its associated response categories) and of the recalled material can affect the accuracy and comprehensiveness of this process (Jobe *et al.* 1993). Retrieval, however, does not necessarily yield a direct answer to the question posed. Respondents may need to synthesize, supplement or otherwise process the information retrieved into a single overall judgement; they may also need to adjust an initial judgement to allow for omissions in retrieval (Tourangeau *et al.* 2000). The type of question – for example, the length of the recall period – may influence these judgement tasks and processes. The final stage in the model involves 'mapping' the initially adjudged response on to one of the response categories offered. This is not necessarily straightforward. The response categories offered may involve 'vague quantifiers' (Sudman *et al.* 1996), posing respondents with difficulties in choosing the most appropriate option; the wording and physical orientation of response categories may also influence respondents. Respondents may 'satisfice' (Krosnick 2000), choosing the response that requires the least cognitive effort; for example, in self-completion questionnaires, primacy effects – a tendency to choose the first listed option that appears relevant – have been demonstrated. Moreover, having made an initial choice of response category, respondents may consciously or subconsciously edit their response, in the interests of self-presentation, consistency or other criteria (Tourangeau *et al.* 2000).

Clearly, this model is applicable to questions about health status and quality of life (Schechter *et al.* 1999). Quality of life assessments typically require respondents to understand complex questions which deal with abstract concepts; effectively retrieve information from long-term memory; aggregate that information; apply frequency judgements, magnitude estimation and decision heuristics in selecting which response category to endorse.

Principles of CASM, in particular psychological theories of perception and cognition, can also inform user-friendly design and formatting of questionnaires. Jenkins and Dillman have expounded a useful framework for instrument design (Jenkins and Dillman, 1997) while Mullin and colleagues (Mullin *et al.* 2000) and Meadows and co-workers (Meadows *et al.* 2000) have reviewed and employed these principles in the assessment of HRQoL.

Cognitive pre-testing techniques

Cognitive pre-testing methods (Collins 2003) are useful in indicating how respondents interpret questions, response categories and instructions and how they go about formulating their answers. However, with few exceptions (e.g. Barofsky, 1996; Schechter *et al.* 1999; Mallinson, 2002), little has been published about the application of these techniques in the assessment of HRQoL.

Willis and colleagues (Willis *et al.* 1991) distinguish between evaluative and experimental techniques in cognitive testing. The former generally yield qualitative data, while the latter are hypothesis-driven and generally yield quantitative data. In developing a new instrument, the qualitative, evaluative techniques are the more appropriate in the earlier phases of development (for example, to identify the range and types of problems that may arise in answering the question), while the experimental techniques can be applied in the subsequent testing and validation phases (for example, to validate self-reports of consultation behaviour, or time off work or school, against documentary records, or to test hypotheses regarding whether the identified problems are more likely to occur in certain subgroups of the population).

The non-experimental methods can be conveniently subdivided into those involving expert review of a draft instrument (described below), and those involving direct interaction between a researcher, or specially trained interviewer, and test respondents; the latter include focus group discussions (discussed above) and individual cognitive interviews (also described below). Experimental methods can be divided into two broad categories. One is the 'field experiment' (Jobe 2003) in which a questionnaire that has been designed or refined using CASM principles is tested against a 'standard' or original questionnaire, and the responses from the two approaches compared, ideally against an external validation standard (such as documentary sources, or a more intensive method of data collection such as a contemporaneous symptom diary). The other is the experiment embedded in a field survey (Jobe 2003) where respondents are randomly allocated in an appropriately powered experimental design, to different approaches to data collection or to posing the question and/or response categories. The choice of interventions is determined by CASM theories or empirical evidence in the general survey literature; examples of such experiments from the health-related field are comparisons of the relative placement of generic and condition-specific HRQoL instruments (McColl *et al.* 2003) and of instructions to respondents about the order of recall of visits to healthcare providers (Jobe *et al.* 1991).

Expert reviews

This approach involves an expert appraisal (generally structured, and often based on best practice in question design – such as the avoidance of double-barrelled questions) of a draft questionnaire, to pinpoint vocabulary or other aspects of the question, and its associated response categories and instructions, that may be unduly cognitively demanding (Forsyth and Lessler 1991; Lessler and Forsyth 1996).

One tool for this type of appraisal is the computerized system Questionnaire Understanding Aid (QUAID *http://mnemosyne.csl.psyc.memphis.edu/QUAID/ quaidindex.html*) (Graesser *et al.* 2000). A user name and password is required, but there is, at the time of writing, no charge for the use of the software. Each item in the questionnaire can be individually entered into this appraisal system, which analyses that item in terms of five categories: unfamiliar technical terms; imprecise or vague relative terms; vague or ambiguous noun-phrases; complex syntax; working memory overload. However, the items are analysed in isolation; in practice, a self-completion questionnaire is viewed in its entirety by respondents and meaning can thus be derived from context.

Forsyth and Lessler (1991; Lessler and Forsyth, 1996) have produced a formal coding system based on Tourangeau's four-stage model of the survey response process. Willis and Lessler (1999) have built on this system to produce the Questionnaire Appraisal Scheme (QAS-99), a paper-based instrument for evaluating draft questionnaires prior to going into the field. The QAS-99, including full instructions on its use is, at the time of writing, in the public domain at *http://www.appliedresearch.cancer.gov/areas/ cognitive/qas99.pdf.*

Cognitive interviewing

Cognitive interviewing (Willis 1994) is a technique in which a trained interviewer seeks to elicit the cognitive processes employed by a respondent in answering survey questions.

Respondents are asked to give feedback on their understanding of the question and associated response categories and instructions, and to verbalize how they have gone about producing their answers, with particular emphasis on retrieval from memory and subsequent judgements and decisions.

One approach to providing this feedback is concurrent 'think aloud', in which respondents are asked to verbalize their reactions and thought processes as they go through the required steps, while the interviewer takes notes or tape-records these comments.

However, not all test respondents can cope with verbalizing their thought processes as they go along. An alternative approach is respondent debriefing, using concurrent or retrospective probes. In this approach, the respondent answers the questions in self-completion mode, and the interviewer asks explicitly about the cognitive processes employed, using directive probes, such as:

♦ What kind of information did you think this question was asking for?

♦ Did you happen to notice this instruction before the question?

♦ What did you think you needed to do to answer this question?

♦ What sorts of things were you thinking about when you answered this question?

♦ I see that you selected (label for chosen response category)? What does (label for chosen response category) mean to you? What does (label for adjacent response category) mean to you? In what circumstances would you have chosen that answer?

♦ I noticed that you hesitated before you answered that question. Why was that? How confident are you about the response you gave?

As with the think-aloud approach, the interviewer takes notes of or tape-records the responses to these probing questions. Probing may be conducted as each question is answered (concurrent probes), or after the question or whole questionnaire has been self-completed (retrospective probes). Probes can be standardized (all respondents are asked about the same cognitive processes, using identical probing questions) or ad hoc (probes vary from respondent to respondent and depend on the answer(s) given to the question under review and to responses to initial probes).

Each approach has its advantages and disadvantages, as summarized in Boxes 2 and 3.

Complementary techniques include paraphrasing (getting the respondent to rephrase the question in their own words), card sorting (in which respondents are asked to group like items together, to inform assessments of the dimensionality of the instrument) and elicitation of ratings and rankings, for example, indicating the relative placement of response categories, a technique employed in determining the verbal descriptors for the response categories of the WHOQOL (Skevington and Tucker 2001).

As with qualitative interviews, and in contrast to the random probability sampling procedures used in later stages of instrument validation, samples for cognitive interviews are purposively selected to ensure representation of groups who may have different

Box 2 Comparison of different approaches to cognitive interviewing

Concurrent think-aloud

Advantages	*Disadvantages*
Concurrent reporting, so hindsight biases are minimized	Too demanding for some respondents
Respondent driven, so avoids imposing the questionnaire designer's or researcher's perspective	Respondents may wander 'off-topic'. Interview process may be 'reactive' – asking respondent to think carefully about how they are producing their answers may actually change the question–answer process, and respondents may consciously or subconsciously reconstruct reality
Lower interviewer burden, so interviewer is more free to listen and observe, and risk of interviewer bias is reduced	

Respondent de-briefing (concurrent and retrospective probing)

Advantages	*Disadvantages*
Less demanding on respondents than concurrent 'think-aloud'	Respondents may not be able to explain their cognitive processes, even with the assistance of probes
Driven by the interviewer, so can focus on anticipated problems or areas of specific interest to researcher	Likely only to find out about issues which the researcher chooses to ask about
	As for concurrent 'think-aloud', the interview process may be reactive

problems with responding (e.g. to ensure a good spread of age groups, levels of education and literacy). The test respondents should, however, be drawn from the same population in which the instrument will be used in practice. There is no hard-and-fast rule about sample size; samples are usually relatively small (usually not more than 25, across multiple rounds of pre-testing).

Cognitive interviewing can take place in the respondents' own homes or at a central 'cognitive laboratory', with special facilities such as video-recorders and one-way mirrors. A small fee and/or travel expenses are usually paid to respondents, because a significant effort is required of them. Willis (1994) suggests that one-hour interviews are optimal, longer sessions being overly demanding on respondents. Respondents need assurances that it is the instrument, not they, that is under scrutiny, and that there are no right or wrong answers. The interviewer also needs to 'train' the respondent in

Box 3 Comparison of different approaches to probing

Concurrent probing

Advantages

Immediacy of response, so minimizes recall bias, hindsight bias and effects of question order and framing

Disadvantages

Artificiality – breaks up the normal flow of responding to the instrument

Switching of tasks can be distracting

Retrospective probing

Advantages

No interruption to normal flow of responding to the instrument, so especially appropriate in testing self-completion questionnaires

Potentially less reactive, especially if debriefing takes place after entire questionnaire has been answered, as there is less chance that probes to earlier questions will influence the respondent's approach to answering later items

Disadvantages

Long gap between answering question and responding to probes about the answer process

Greater risk of recall errors and biases

Greater risk of hindsight effects

Standardized probes

Advantages

Ensure equivalence of stimulus across respondents

Do not rely on judgement of interviewer about what to probe

Ensure that the issues of interest to the researcher are covered

Disadvantages

Can be very time-consuming to probe all aspects of response process for all items in the instrument (therefore it may be necessary to 'sample' questions to be probed)

Some probes may be irrelevant to some respondents (because they have spontaneously provided the required information)

Ad hoc probes

Advantages

Can capture unanticipated approaches and processes in responding to the question

Can pursue issues and problems specific to that respondent

Disadvantages

Relies on skills and insights of interviewer

what is required of them, particularly if the concurrent 'think aloud' approach is adopted. Demonstration and practice of the techniques are advisable, before commencing the cognitive interview proper.

Analysis of data from cognitive pre-testing

In cognitive interviews, the interviewer generally makes structured contemporaneous notes of specific problems identified through the cognitive interviewing process. In contrast to the analysis of qualitative interviews as described above, it is seldom necessary to transcribe in full a cognitive interview. Instead, the interviewer can simply review the tape by listening to it, and adding to the contemporaneous notes of problems identified. Aggregating comments, both within and across interviews, allows complete review of that draft of the instrument. Feedback from other forms of cognitive pre-testing, such as expert appraisal, can also be incorporated.

As in the analysis of in-depth interviews and focus group discussions, there is little need for quantitative analysis. Rather, the focus should be on identifying dominant trends (problems that appear to occur repeatedly) across interviews and other appraisals, and key 'discoveries' (problems that may only be identified through a single interview, but nonetheless have the potential to cause serious problems albeit in a minority of respondents in real life, or which might be expected to be reasonably common in the population as a whole) (Willis 1994).

As with qualitative data analysis, review and analysis of findings from cognitive interviews should be conducted as soon as possible after the interview. There is no point in carrying out several interviews if the instrument is manifestly and grossly flawed. If major problems are identified, it is better to make the revisions indicated by the review of a few interviews, and then continue with pre-testing this revised version.

Multiple rounds of pre-testing are often needed. For example, output from an expert appraisal might inform the construction of probes for subsequent cognitive interviewing. Having revised a draft instrument following a first round of cognitive interviews, it will be necessary to conduct further pre-tests, to ensure that the problems have in fact been rectified and that no new problems have been introduced. Willis (1994) recognizes that pre-testing could go on forever and that there is no such thing as a perfect question; nonetheless, he recognises diminishing returns from repeated rounds of interviews and suggests a maximum of three to four rounds, before proceeding to more formal validation and reliability testing or to instrument administration.

Conclusions

In summary, the optimal approach to item generation and wording, the establishment of content and face validity, and the initial stages of instrument pre-testing in developing a new quality of life instrument involves qualitative research (for content generation) and the application of CASM principles and techniques (to test and refine the instrument).

Both individual interviews and focus group discussions have their merits and problems, and either or both may be deployed depending on the nature of the study population and resource availability. Theories of the cognitive processes involved in the response process (Tourangeau *et al.* 2000; Jenkins and Dillman 1997) should be used in designing the questionnaire – both in wording and presenting questions and their associated response categories and in formatting the instrument. The next step should be an expert appraisal of the draft instrument, ideally using one or more structured approaches (Willis and Lessler 1999; Graesser *et al.* 2000). The results from this appraisal should be inform subsequent rounds of cognitive interviewing (Willis 1994), instrument refinement and re-testing, prior to formal psychometric evaluation of the refined instrument. Evaluative cognitive techniques, informed by theories of survey respondent behaviour, may also be deployed to advantage in subsequent field surveys, to extend the evidence base regarding effects of question wording and sequencing, mode of administration etc.

References

Barofsky, I. (1996). Cognitive aspects of quality of life assessment. In Spilker B. (ed.) *Quality of Life and Pharmacoeconomics,* 2nd edn, pp. 107–115. Philadelphia: Lippincott-Raven Publishers.

Blazeby, J., Sprangers, M., Cull, A., Groenvold, M., and Bottomley, A. (2001). *EORTC Quality of Life Group: Guidelines for Developing Questionnaire Modules,* 3rd edn. Brussels: EORTC.

Bowling, A. (1995) *Measuring Disease.* Buckingham: Open University Press.

Britten, N. (1985). Qualitative interviews in medical research. *BMJ,* **311** (6999), 251–253.

Collins, D. (2003). Pretesting survey instruments: An overview of cognitive methods. *Quality of Life Research,* **12,** 229–238.

Fern, E. F. (1982). The use of focus groups for idea generation: the effects of group size, acquaintanceship, and moderation on response quantity and quality. *Journal of Marketing Research,* **19,** 1–13.

Fitzsimmons, D., Johnson, C. D., George, S., Payne, S., Sandberg, A. A., Bassi, C., Beger, H. G., Birk, D., Buchler, M. W., Dervenis, C., Fernandez, C. L., Friess, H., Grahm, A. L., Jeekel, J., Laugier, R., Meyer, D., Singer, M. W., and Tihanyi, T. (1999). Development of a disease specific quality of life (QoL) questionnaire module to supplement the EORTC core cancer QoL questionnaire, the QLQ-C30 in patients with pancreatic cancer. EORTC Study Group on Quality of Life. *European Journal of Cancer,* **35,** 939–941.

Forsyth, B. H. and Lessler, J. T. (1991). Cognitive laboratory methods: a taxonomy. In Biemer, P. P., Groves, R. M., Lyberg, L. E., Mathiowetz, N. A. and Sudman, S. (eds) *Measurement Errors in Surveys,* 1st edn, pp. 167–183. New York: Wiley.

Graesser, A. C., Wiemer-Hastings, K., Kreuz, R., Wiemer-Hastings, P., and Marquis, K. (2000). QUAID: a questionnaire evaluation aid for survey methodologists. *Behavior Research Methods, Instruments and Computers,* **32,** 254–262.

Guyatt, G., Mitchell, A., Irvine, E. J., Singer, J., Williams, N., Goodacre, R., and Tompkins, C. (1989). A new measure of health status for clinical trials in inflammatory bowel disease. *Gastroenterology,* **96,** 804–810.

Guyatt, G.H. and Cook, D.J. (1994). Health status, quality of life, and the individual. *JAMA,* **272** (8), 630–631.

Jenkins, C. R. and Dillman, D. A. (1997). Towards a theory of self-administered questionnaire design. In Lyberg, L., Biemer, P., Collins, M., de Leeuw, E., Dippo, C., Schwarz, N. and Trewin, D. (eds) *Survey Measurement and Process Quality*, pp. 165–196. New York: John Wiley & Sons Inc.

Jobe, J. B. (2003). Cognitive psychology and self-reports: models and methods. *Quality of Life Research*, **12**, 219–227.

Jobe, J. B., Tourangeau, R., and Smith, A. F. (1993). Contributions of survey research to the understanding of memory. *Applied Cognitive Psychology*, **7**, 567–584.

Jobe, J. B., White, A. A., Kelley, C. L., Mingay, D. J., Sanchez, M. J., and Loftus, E. F. (1991). Recall strategies and memory for healthcare visits. *Milbank Quarterly*, **68**, 171–189.

Juniper, E. F., Guyatt, G. H., Epstein, R. S., Ferrie, P. J., Jaeschke, R., and Hiller, T. K. (1992). Evaluation of impairment of health related quality of life in asthma: development of a questionnaire for use in clinical trials. *Thorax*, **47**, 76–83.

Krosnick, J. A. (2000). The threat of satisficing in surveys: the shortcuts respondents take in answering questions. *Survey Methods Centre Newsletter*, **20**, 4–8.

Kuzel, A. J. (1992). Sampling in Qualitative Inquiry. In Crabtree B. F. and Miller W. I. (eds) *Doing Qualitative Research*, pp. 33–45. Newbury Park: Sage Publications.

Lederman, L. C. (1990). Assessing educational effectiveness: the focus group interview as a technique for data collection. *Communication Education*, **38**, 117–127.

Lessler, J. T. and Forsyth, B. H. (1996). A coding system for appraising questionnaires. In Schwarz, N. and Sudman, S. (eds) *Answering Questions: Methodology for determining cognitive and communicative processes in survey research*, pp. 259–291. San Francisco: Jossey-Bass.

Litwin, M. S., McNaughton-Collins, M., Fowler, F. J. Jr., Nickel, J. C., Calhoun, E. A., Pontari, M. A., Alexander, R. B., Farrar, J. T., and O'Leary, M. P. (1999). The National Institutes of Health chronic prostatitis symptom index: development and validation of a new outcome measure. Chronic Prostatitis Collaborative Research Network. *Journal of Urology*, **162**, 369–375.

Mallinson, S. (2002). Listening to respondents: a qualitative assessment of the Short-Form 36 Health Status Questionnaire. *Social Science and Medicine*, **54**, 11–21.

Mays, N. and Pope, C. (1995). Rigour and qualitative research. *BMJ*, **311**, 109–111.

McColl, E., Eccles, M. P., Rousseau, N. R., Steen, I. N., Parkin, D. W., and Grimshaw, J. M. (2003). From the generic to the condition-specific? Instrument order effects in quality of life assessment. *Medical Care*, **41**, 777–790.

Meadows, K. A., Greene, T., Foster, L., and Beer, S. (2000). The impact of different response alternatives on responders' reporting of health-related behaviour in a postal survey. *Quality of Life Research*, **9**, 385–391.

Mullin, P. A., Lohr, K. N., Bresnahan, B. W., and McNulty, P. (2000). Applying cognitive design principles to formatting HRQoL instruments. *Quality of Life Research*, **9**, 13–27.

Pope, C. and Mays, N. (1995). Reaching the parts other methods cannot reach: an introduction to qualitative methods in health and health services. *BMJ*, **311**, 42–45.

Ritchie, J. and Spencer, L. (1994). Qualitative data analysis for applied policy research. In Bryman, A. and Burgess, R. G. (eds) *Analyzing Qualitative Data*, pp. 173–194. London: Routledge.

Schechter, S., Beatty, P., and Willis, G. B. (1999). Asking survey respondents about health status: judgment and response issues. In Schwarz, N., Park, D., Knauper, B. and Sudman, S. (eds) *Cognition, Aging, and Self-Reports*, 1st edn, pp. 265–283. Philadelphia, PA: Psychology Press.

Skevington, S. M., Mac Arthur, P., and Somerset, M. (1997). Developing items for the WHOQOL: an investigation of contemporary beliefs about quality of life related to health in britain. *British Journal of Health Psychology*, **2**, 55–72.

Skevington, S. M. and Tucker, C. (2001). Designing response scales for cross-cultural use in health care: data from the development of the UK WHOQoL. *British Journal of Medical Psychology,* **72,** 51–61.

Strauss, A. L. and Corbin, J. (1994). *Grounded Theory Methodology: An overview. Handbook of qualitative research.* Thousand Oaks, CA: Sage.

Sudman, S., Bradburn, N. M., and Schwarz, N. (1996). *Thinking About Answers. The application of cognitive processes to survey methodology,* 1st edn. San Francisco, CA: Jossey-Bass Inc.

Thomas, L., McMillan, J., McColl, E., Hale, C., and Bond, S. (1995). Comparison of focus group and individual interview methodology in examining patient satisfaction with nursing care. *Social Sciences in Health,* **1,** 206–220.

Tourangeau, R., Rips, L. J., and Rasinski, K. (2000). *The Psychology of Survey Response,* 1st edn. Cambridge: Cambridge University Press.

WHOQOL Group (1998). The World Health Organization quality of life assessment (WHOQOL): development and general psychometric properties. *Social Science and Medicine,* **46,** 1569–1585.

Willis, G. B. (1994). *Cognitive Interviewing and Questionnaire Design: A training manual* (Working Paper No. 7). Hyattsville: National Center for Health Statistics.

Willis, G. B. and Lessler, J. T. (1999). *Questionnaire Appraisal Scheme QAS-99.* Rockville, MD.: Research Triangle Institute.

Willis, G. B., Royston, P., and Bercini, D. (1991). The use of verbal report methods in the development and testing of survey questionnaires. *Applied Cognitive Psychology,* **5,** 251–267.

Further recommended reading

Qualitative methods

Crabtree, B. F. and Miller, W. I. (eds) *Doing Qualitative Research.* Newbury Park: Sage Publications.

Maykut, P. and Morehouse, R. (1994). *Beginning Qualitative Research: A philosophical and practical guide.* London: Falmer Press.

Morgan, D. L. and Krueger, R. A. (1997). *The Focus Group Kit.* London: Sage Publications.

Pope, C. and Mays, N. (1999). *Qualitative Research in Health Care,* 2nd edn. London: BMJ Books.

Silverman, D. (2000). *Doing Qualitative Research: A practical handbook.* London: Sage Publications.

CASM theories and methods

Schwarz, N. and Sudman, S. E. (eds) (1996). *Answering questions. Methodology for determining cognitive and communicative processes in survey research.* San Francisco, CA: Jossey-Bass Inc.

Schwarz, N., Park, D., Knauper, B., and Sudman, S. E. (eds) (1999). *Cognition, Aging, and Self-reports.* Philadelphia, PA: Psychology Press.

Stone, A. A., Turkkan, J. S., and Bachrach, C. E. (eds) (1999). *The Science of Self-report: Implications for research and practice.* Mahwah, NJ: Lawrence Erlbaum Associates.

Sudman, S., Bradburn, N. M., and Schwarz, N. (1996). *Thinking About Answers. The application of cognitive processes to survey methodology,* 1st edn. San Francisco, CA: Jossey-Bass Inc.

Tourangeau, R., Rips, L. J., and Rasinski, K. (2000). *The Psychology of Survey Response,* 1st edn. Cambridge: Cambridge University Press.

Reliability and validity (including responsiveness)

Ron D. Hays and Dennis Revicki

An understanding of the reliability and validity of health-related quality of life (HRQoL) measurement is needed to develop or select the best HRQoL measures for any given application. This chapter summarizes reliability and validity, and how these properties are used to evaluate HRQoL survey instruments.

Reliability

Reliability refers to the extent to which a measure yields the same number or score each time it is administered, all other things being equal (i.e., true change has not occurred in the attribute being measured). Classical test theory regards observed responses as consisting of the sum of true score and error. True score for an individual is assumed to be invariant on repeated measurements. However, two parallel measurements will yield non-identical observed scores as a result of random error of measurement. Because random errors are normally distributed, the true score will be located at the mean of the distribution of parallel measures. Observed HRQoL scores actually include a true score component, a systematic error component, and a random error component. If no random error is present the reliability is 1.0. Reliability approaches zero as the relative amount of random error increases.

Both the true score component and systematic error contribute to the reliability of the measure, because they drive the observed score for an individual towards a consistent value. However, systematic error leads to bias in measurement, because it causes the score to be consistently too high or too low relative to the true score. Systematic errors include social desirability responding (reporting in such a way as to minimize the presentation of undesirable and maximize the presentation of desirable characteristics), acquiescent responding (agreement with statement regardless of content), and observation bias (such as halo effects whereby a single positive feature colours the general impression and ratings of another).

Reliability assessment involves examining agreement between two or more measures of the same thing. There are four basic categories of reliability estimation, each reflecting somewhat different ways by which random error of measurement is estimated: inter-rater, equivalent forms, test–retest, and internal consistency reliability.

Inter-rater reliability

Inter-rater reliability refers to a comparison of scores assigned to the same target (either patient or other stimuli) by two or more raters (Marshall *et al.* 1994). Both rater selection and intra-individual response variability influence random error in this case.

The kappa statistic can be used if one is interested in estimating exact agreement between raters for a variable measured on a nominal, ordinal or interval-level scale (it is also possible to provide partial credit for non-exact agreement using a weighted kappa (Cohen 1968). Kappa is known as a quality index, because it compares observed agreement with agreement expected by chance. The general formula for kappa is

$$K = \frac{\text{observed proportion agreement} - \text{chance expected proportion agreement}}{1 - \text{chance expected proportion agreement}}$$

Agreement expected by chance is determined by assuming each rater made their ratings randomly but with probabilities equal to the overall proportions or marginal frequencies. The chance proportion is the proportion of pairs that would be expected to end up by chance in the diagonal representing agreement between one rater and another. The proportion of agreement expected by chance is computed just as are expected cell frequencies in chi-square based on the marginals from the two-way cross-tabulation of ratings.

Rules of thumb for interpreting the magnitude of kappa have been provided by Fleiss (1981) and Landis and Koch (1977). The limitations and extent to which kappa depends on the degree of the balance and symmetry of marginals is discussed elsewhere (Feinstein and Cicchetti 1990; Cicchetti and Feinstein 1990). The observed kappa can be divided by the maximum possible kappa given the marginals (calculated by summing up the minimum for each pair of column and row marginals and dividing by the number of pairs) to produce an adjusted kappa. For nominal data, kappa is mathematically equivalent to the intraclass correlation. For ordinal and interval-level data, weighted kappa and the intraclass correlation are equivalent under certain conditions (Fleiss and Cohen 1973).

Data from ratings provided from seven North American experts provide an example of estimating inter-rater reliability for interval-level variables. The experts were told the HRQoL was to be assessed using a generic HRQoL profile measure (such as the SF-36) in a longitudinal study with the possibility of noteworthy attrition over time. In addition, they were told that the study team was interested in deriving an overall summary HRQoL score. In providing their ratings, they were instructed that the study was facing severe time constraints in assessing HRQoL because of competing study needs. Experts were asked to rate each of eight approaches for deriving an overall HRQoL score (standard gamble, time trade-off, Health Utilities Index, EuroQoL, Quality of Well-Being Scale, global categorical rating/visual analogue, factor analysis, regression weights) on a 0–100 scale, with 0 representing the most inadequate and 100 representing

Table 1.3.1 Ratings of eight approaches to summarizing health-related quality of life by seven North American experts

Approach	Rater							Mean	SD
	1	2	3	4	5	6	7		
1	90	00	50	95	30	60	50	53.57	33.00
2	90	00	70	100	60	55	80	65.00	32.79
3	90	51	40	90	25	100	85	68.71	29.44
4	30	52	05	30	–	10	40	27.93	17.78
5	80	50	80	60	80	50	100	71.43	18.64
6	30	100	05	50	50	40	40	45.00	28.72
7	20	70	00	20	10	00	01	17.29	24.86
8	20	90	00	00	00	00	01	16.57	33.18

Note: Ratings were made on a 0–100 scale.
– represents missing data.

the most adequate approach. The ratings given by each of the seven raters for eight different approaches are provided in Table 1.3.1 along with the mean and standard deviation for each approach. The dash for one entry in the table represents a missing data point.

An ANOVA table summarizing the sources of variance of these ratings is given in Table 1.3.2. Reliability and intraclass correlation estimates are provided in Table 1.3.3. The reliability coefficients in Table 1.3.3 estimate the reliability for the average of multiple assessments (seven ratings) whereas the intraclass correlations estimate the corresponding reliability for a single assessment (one rater). In inter-rater reliability

Table 1.3.2 Sources of variance in North American experts' ratings of eight approaches to summarizing health-related quality of life

Source	Degrees of Freedom	Mean Square	Label for Mean Square
Ratees (N–1)	7	3608.69	BMS
Within	47	789.68	WMS
Raters (K–1)	6	825.72	JMS
Raters × ratees	41	784.40	EMS
Total	54		

Table 1.3.3 Reliability and intraclass correlation estimates for experts' ratings of eight approaches to summarizing health-related quality of life

Model	Reliability	Intraclass correlation
One-way	0.781	0.338
Two-way		
Fixed effects	0.783	0.340
Random effects	0.782	0.338

evaluations such as this example, one is most probably interested in the reliability of multiple ratings. The intraclass correlation would be of interest if the reliability of a single rater were of concern.

The one-way model separates the targets being rated (the eight approaches in the example) as the between-group variance and the remaining variance is assigned to the within-error term (Shrout and Fleiss 1979). The estimated reliabilities for the average rating and single rating (intraclass correlation) under the one-way model are 0.78 and 0.34, respectively (see Table 1.3.3).

If the number of assessments (raters) is the same across respondents, it is also possible to estimate the main effect of raters (i.e., mean differences). The two-way mixed (fixed rater effect) effects model estimates the reliability of the average of the multiple assessments by subtracting the mean square error from the mean square between, then dividing by the mean square between. The mean square error is estimated by the interaction between respondents and the multiple assessments (the main effect of multiple assessments is excluded from the error term). For this example, the estimated reliabilities of the average rating and single rating under this model, respectively, are 0.78 and 0.34 (see Table 1.3.3).

The two-way random effects model assumes that the different assessments (e.g., raters) are randomly selected. In this model, the main effect of multiple assessments is incorporated into the estimate of total variability. For the example, the estimated reliabilities of the average rating and single rating under this model are 0.78 and 0.34, respectively (see Table 1.3.3).

Shrout and Fleiss (1979) note that the one-way model will tend to yield smaller values than the two-way models and the random effects model will tend to yield lower values than the fixed effects model. (In the example summarized in Table 1.3.3, the estimates are all equivalent.) The fixed effects model is described as assessing consistency of raters because rater variance is ignored. The random effects model, in contrast, provides an estimate of agreement because it assesses whether raters are interchangeable. The formulae for each of these models are provided in Table 1.3.4.

The mean square within term in Table 1.3.2 is 789.68 and therefore the estimated common within-subject standard deviation is 28.10 (Bland and Altman 1996).

Table 1.3.4 Intraclass correlation and reliability formulae

Model	Reliability	Intraclass correlation
One-way	$\dfrac{MS_{BMS}-MS_{WMS}}{MS_{BMS}}$	$\dfrac{MS_{BMS}-MS_{WMS}}{MS_{BMS}+(K-1)MS_{WMS}}$
Two-way, fixed	$\dfrac{MS_{BMS}-MS_{EMS}}{MS_{BMS}}$	$\dfrac{MS_{BMS}-MS_{EMS}}{MS_{BMS}+(K-1)MS_{EMS}}$
Two-way, random	$\dfrac{N(MS_{BMS}-MS_{EMS})}{NMS_{BMS}+MS_{JMS}-MS_{EMS}}$	$\dfrac{MS_{BMS}-MS_{EMS}}{MS_{BMS}+(K-1)MS_{EMS}+K(MS_{JMS}-MS_{EMS})/N}$

MS = mean square; N = number of ratees; K = number of replications (e.g., raters).
Subscripts are defined in Table 1.3.2

This value is an estimate of the measurement error. We can check for the assumption that the error is not related to the magnitude of the ratings by correlating the means and standard deviations in Table 1.3.2. The Spearman rank order correlation between mean and standard deviation is not statistically significant ($rho = -0.17$, $P = 0.69$) for these data. The difference between the mean value for each approach and the true value is expected to be less than 1.96 times the measurement error 95 per cent of the time. The difference between two ratings for the same approach is expected to be less than 2.77 times the measurement error for 95 per cent of pairs of observations (2.77 times the measurement error is referred to as the repeatability).

Equivalent forms reliability

Equivalent forms reliability refers to the agreement between an individual's score on two or more measures designed to measure the same attribute. Both item selection and intra-individual response variability contribute to random error in this method of estimating reliability. If the forms are truly equivalent in terms of item content, then the correlation between scores provides a good estimate of their reliability. However, it is difficult to devise equivalent forms and intervening events or practice effects can distort the results from this method of reliability assessment. The same formula used for inter-rater reliability can be used to estimate equivalent forms reliability, with the different forms substituted for multiple raters.

Test–retest reliability

Test–retest reliability is the relationship between scores obtained by the same person on two or more separate occasions. Intra-individual response variability is used to estimate random error in test–retest assessments. The approach described above for inter-rater reliability is the same one used for test–retest reliability, with multiple times of assessment substituted for multiple raters. Several factors may influence the reliability of a measure between test dates, such as the conditions of administration, testing effects, specific factors affecting the participants in their daily lives, or the length of time between administration. The assessment of reliability is further complicated by the fact that changes in the attribute being measured may have occurred between administrations. For example, scores may change notably for patients assessed initially during a doctor's office visit (when they were symptomatic) and subsequently when their symptoms have gone away. A low test–retest correlation may therefore not accurately reflect the reliability of the test. Thus, test–retest assessments become less useful to the extent that real changes occur from the first to the second assessment of the attribute being measured.

Internal consistency reliability

Internal consistency reliability for a scale is a function of the number of items and their covariation. Random error due to item selection is modeled in this type of reliability estimate. Cronbach's (1951) alpha is the coefficient commonly used to estimate the reliability of instruments based on internal consistency. Cronbach's alpha is calculated using the two-way fixed effects model described for inter-rater reliability with items substituting for the rater effects. Generally, one is most interested in the reliability of the average of the items (rather than the intraclass correlation, or estimated reliability of a single item). Formulae for computing the significance of difference between alpha coefficients are provided elsewhere (Feldt *et al.* 1987).

For each reliability model, the intraclass correlation can be derived from the estimated reliability for multiple assessments using a variant of the Spearman-Brown prophecy formula (Clark 1935), where

$$R_{ii} = \frac{R_{tt}}{K + (1-K)R_{tt}}$$

Likewise, the reliability of the multiple assessments can be obtained from the intraclass correlation using the formula

$$R_{tt} = \frac{KR_{ii}}{1 + (K-1)R_{ii}}$$

Standards for reliability

For applications with group-level comparisons such as much of the HRQoL research, the standard for reliability of measures is less stringent than it is for individual assessment. Because different groups of people (e.g., HIV patients who receive or do not receive AZT treatment before the onset of AIDS) are compared rather than individuals, a 0.70 standard is appropriate for clinical trials and other group comparisons (Nunnally 1978). However, some people have presented arguments that the standard should be higher – for example, 0.80 has been suggested.

A reliability level of 0.90 was advocated by Nunnally (1978) as a minimum standard for measurement that is designed for interpretation of scores at the individual level. This recommendation stems from the fact that standard error of measurement is about one-third of the measure's standard deviation if it has a reliability of 0.90 (standard error of measurement is estimated by the product of the measure's standard deviation and the square root of the difference between the reliability of the measure and 1.0: $SD*(1-\text{reliability})^{1/2}$). Confidence intervals around and individual's estimated true score are wide at reliabilities below this recommended cut-off point.

In practice, even the 0.90 reliability threshold for individual assessment may be too stringent as an absolute standard. To achieve this level of reliability requires several items per scale. Many highly regarded instruments fail to meet these standards. For example, only two of the eight subscales (physical functioning and emotional well-being) in the SF-36 satisfied the 0.90 reliability standard in the Medical Outcomes Study (MOS) (Ware and Sherbourne 1992; Hays et al. 1993). Test–retest reliabilities (24 hour) for blood pressure and diastolic blood pressure reliabilities have been reported below this threshold as well – 0.87 and 0.67, respectively (Prisant et al. 1992).

Even if measures fall short of the 0.90 reliability level, obtaining this information is preferred to not doing so. Although the confidence interval around an individual patient's score is wider than one might like, the interval is still tighter than that based on no information at all. Clinicians need to be aware of the extent of unreliability in all of their measures and interpret them with appropriate caution. However, as noted above, reliabilities exceeding 0.70 are acceptable for group comparisons in randomized clinical trials and other clinical studies.

A Guttman scale is a special case of internal consistency

Large correlations among items in a multi-item scale contribute to internal consistency reliability. In HRQoL research, physical functioning scales have been shown frequently to exhibit a special type of internal consistency embodied in Guttman scales. Guttman scales consist of dichotomized items that adhere to a strict deterministic response model related to the prevalence of item endorsement. If observed data fit the Guttman scale model, then individuals with the same total scale score also tend to exhibit the same pattern of responses to each item in the scale. Thus, by knowing a person's scale score it is possible to predict with good accuracy their answer to every item in a Guttman scale. In general, the number of possible response patterns is two raised to a power equal to the number of items, but the number of response patterns consistent with a Guttman scale equals the number of items plus one.

To determine if a scale is consistent with the Guttman model, observed patterns of responses are compared with the patterns predicted for a Guttman scale, examining the degree to which observed response patterns deviate from the expected response patterns. The coefficient of reproducibility (CR) for Guttman scales is defined as the proportion of error (i.e. proportion of differences between observed and expected responses) subtracted from unity. A CR value of 0.90 or higher is considered acceptable (Menzel 1953). In addition, an index of reproducibility is typically computed by determining how well item modes reproduce the observed response patterns. Errors are counted as differences between each observed item response for an individual and the modal response for that item across all respondents (Goodenough 1944). This index, the minimum marginal reproducibility (MR), is used to calculate the coefficient of scalability (CS) defined as $(CR - MR)/(1 - MR)$. A CS of 0.60 has been recommended as a minimum standard for acceptability (Menzel 1953). The standard error of reproducibility for Goodenough scoring can be estimated by the square root of $[(1 + CR)(1 - CR)/NK]$ (Ellickson *et al.* 1992). Cunningham *et al.* (1995) provide an example application of Guttman scalogram analysis with HRQoL data. For recent methods of analysis that go beyond the traditional Guttman model, see the item response theory chapters.

Validity

Validity is the degree to which the measure reflects what it is supposed to measure rather than something else. The distinction between reliability and validity is important because a measure may be reliable (i.e., always yield the same score for the same patient), but it may be consistently measuring the wrong thing (i.e., not what it is supposed to measure).

Demonstrating reliability in measurement is essentially accumulating evidence indicative of the existence of a stable property over repeated measurement. Validity, in contrast, is an estimation of the extent to which an instrument measures what it was intended to measure. Reliability is necessary, but not sufficient for valid measurement. If an HRQoL measure does not yield a similar or identical number when an individual has not changed in health status (measured using some other method), it must not be providing a valid reading of the individual's HRQoL (i.e., both of the inconsistent numbers cannot be correct). The process of evaluating the validity of measures involves accumulating evidence of many different types which indicate the degree to which the measures denote what they were intended to represent. Usually, the evaluation of validity involves the formulation and testing of hypotheses about expected relationships between the target measure and other health-related variables. The following kinds of evidence are generally used to infer validity of measurement.

Content validity

Content validity is the extent to which a measure samples a representative range of the content under study. In interpreting content validity, questions regarding item sufficiency and patient population should be addressed carefully. For example, the range of items needed adequately to assess physical functioning in arthritic patients may be too gross for application to many coronary heart disease samples. Also, one or two aspects of depression, such as somatic complaints, dominate some self-report depression questionnaires. A clear idea of what aspects of a concept are to be measured is essential in assessing content validity. Content validity evaluations tend to be fairly subjective, but ideally include systematic comparison of a measure with existing standards, well-accepted theoretical definitions, expert opinions, and interviews with individuals for whom the measure is targeted (Stewart *et al.* 1992). Often in the development of a new scale a content map is created and items are constructed to cover the dimensions of interest.

Criterion validity

Criterion validity can be viewed as a special case of construct validity in which stronger hypotheses are made possible by the availability of a criterion or 'gold standard' measure. For example, a thermometer might serve as a gold standard against which self-reported temperature might be compared. There are no true gold standard HRQoL measures. Hence, HRQoL assessment is really largely based on content and construct validity assessment (see below).

Construct validity

To evaluate construct validity one hypothesizes how measures should 'behave' and confirms or disconfirms these hypotheses (Cronbach and Meehl 1955). Hypotheses are stated regarding the direction (and sometimes the strength) of relationships that might be expected, and validity is supported when the associations are consistent with hypotheses. Construct validation is iterative by its nature with empirical results feeding into revision of measures, retesting, and further revisions, if necessary. Over time, and repeated studies, we become more confident in the validity of the measure and its application in different populations.

For example, a HRQoL scale should reflect the impact of the disease by yielding scores for that group that differ in hypothesized ways from that of other groups. This 'know groups' strategy typically involves evaluating an instrument in relation to clinical measures of disease status (Stewart *et al.* 1992). Relative validity calculations (between group ANOVA F ratios) can be used to evaluate the sensitivity of different HRQoL measures to known groups differences. Relative validities are determined by dividing the F-statistic for each measure by the F ratio of a designed reference measure. The relative validity of the reference measure is thereby set to 1, by definition (Liang *et al.* 1985). These relative validities are equivalent to the ratio of sample sizes that would be required to detect the known group difference using one measure versus the other.

When a dichotomous criterion is used, it is possible to perform standard contingency table analysis, examining sensitivity and specificity of the HRQoL measure at designated cut-off points. To minimize the effects of a specific cut-off point, receiver operator characteristic (ROC) methods can be employed. Hanley and McNeil (1982) reported a practical method of estimating the area under an ROC curve using the Wilcoxon statistic. They also developed a non-parametric method for comparing ROC curves from the same sample (Hanley and McNeil 1983). The areas under ROC curves, their standard errors, and the significance of difference between areas for different measures can be calculated.

Convergent and discriminant validity are two fundamental aspects of construct validity. Convergent validity refers to the extent to which different ways of measuring the same trait intercorrelate with one another. For example, a performance-based measure of walking should be positively correlated with self-reported ability to walk a block (Siu *et al.* 1993*a*). Similarly, performance-based measures of daily activities, such as fastening buttons and preparing and boiling a pot of water, should be associated positively with self-reported activities of daily living.

Discriminant validity involves demonstrating that a measure does not correlate too strongly with measures that are intended to measure different traits. When two or more constructs (traits) are assessed using more than one method of assessment, convergent and discriminant validity can be assessed using multitrait-multi-method (MTMM) analytic methods (Campbell and Fiske 1959).

Procedures for implementing the MTMM methodology have been developed based on zero-order correlations among measures (Hayashi and Hays 1987) and confirmatory factor analysis (Kenny and Kashy 1992). The zero-order correlation method is generally easier to implement than confirmatory factor analysis. Some HRQoL studies have employed this approach (Nelson *et al.* 1990; Hadorn and Hays 1991; Siu *et al.* 1993a). Interpretation of MTMM data can be problematic if only zero-order correlations are examined (Cole 1987). Confirmatory factor analysis allows for explicit separation of trait, method, and unique variance, but ill-defined solutions and interpretation of method effects are a source of concern (Marsh 1989). See Chapter 1.4 for more information about factor analysis.

Responsiveness to change

The validity of a measure may be supported by cross-sectional analyses; however, the measure may not perform well at detecting small, but meaningful, changes over time. A final indicator of validity is responsiveness (Guyatt *et al.* 1987). Responsiveness refers to the ability of a measure to reflect underlying change (Hays and Hadorn 1992). Although reliability and cross-sectional validity studies have been conducted on the widely used HRQoL measures, there is relatively little information about their responsiveness.

HRQoL changes can be compared to change in clinical status, intervening health events, interventions of known or expected efficacy, and direct reports of change by patients or providers (MacKenzie *et al.* 1986; Chambers *et al.* 1987; Guyatt *et al.* 1987;

Guyatt *et al.* 2002). Responsiveness to change is most frequently evaluated using the effect size (ES) (Kazis *et al.* 1989), standardized response mean (SRM) (Liang, Fossel, and Larson 1990) and/or the responsiveness statistic (RS) (Guyatt *et al.* 1987). These indices are ratios of signal to noise. For all three indices, the numerator is the mean change and the denominators are the standard deviation at baseline (ES), the standard deviation of change for the sample (SRM), and the standard deviation of change for people who are deemed to not change (RS). ES provides a measure of the magnitude of change in response to the intervention; according to guidelines provided by Cohen (1992); 0.2 represents a small change, 0.5 a medium change, and 0.8 a large change. In addition, relative validity can be estimated using the ratio of the F-statistics.

The ES statistic ignores variation in change entirely, the SRM ignores information about variation in scores for clinically stable respondents, and the RS ignores information about variation in scores for clinically unstable respondents. When the results of a clinical trial comparing an intervention of known clinical efficacy with a control group are available, a useful measure of responsiveness is a between group *t*-statistic for change scores (see below). This *t*-statistic allows for direct determination of the sample size needed to detect a given clinical effect for a particular HRQoL measure. So, for a between group *t*-statistic for change,

$$\text{t-statistic} = (D_1 - D_2)/SE$$

Where D_1 = raw score change for intervention group; D_2 = raw score change for control group; SE = standard error of the difference between group means.

Examples of studies examining responsiveness include the evaluation of a symptom severity index in a sample of 169 gastroparesis patients who were receiving treatment (Revicki *et al.* 2003). This study found significant ($P < 0.0001$) changes in Gastroparesis Cardinal Symptom Index total scores for patients rated by clinicians as having improved (0.75 point decrease) compared to patients who were unchanged or worsening (0.06 point decrease). Siu *et al.* (1993b) provided three responsiveness statistics in an analysis of 120 older persons entering a residential care facility. They found that the physical function scale from the Medical Outcomes Study 20-item short-form health survey was more sensitive to decrements in physical performance than were the Darthmouth Cooperative (COOP) Group physical function chart, the Katz activities of daily living scale, and the Lawton-Brody instrumental activities of daily living scale. None of the measures were very sensitive to improvement in performance based physical function. Beusterien *et al.* (1996) found that the introduction of recombinant human erythropoietin to dialysis patients increased scores on the SF-36 energy scale by 9.3 points (about one-half a standard deviation) from baseline to follow-up (average of 99 days). In addition, significant improvements were observed on physical functioning, social functioning, and emotional well-being.

The standard error of measurement (SEM) has been suggested as another approach to assessing responsiveness (Wyrwich *et al.* 1999a; Wyrwich *et al.* 1999b; Guyatt *et al.* 2002).

The SEM is defined as the variability between an individual's observed score and true score, and is calculated as the baseline standard deviation multiplied by the square root of 1 minus the reliability of the measure. Research has indicated that a 1 SEM is roughly equivalent to the minimal important difference, determined using anchor-based methods (Wyrwich *et al.* 1999a; Wyrwich *et al.* 1999b).

Additional work is needed to relate the different responsiveness statistics to one another. If one statistic suggests one conclusion about relative scale performance and a second statistic suggests a different conclusion, which one is to be believed? For example, Smith (1997) has argued that the traditional indicators of responsiveness are inadequate and that a more appropriate indicator is the correlation between prospective changes and retrospective reports of change. It is also important to put the different responsiveness statistics on a common metric. For example, Kim *et al.* (2003) calibrated different indices by deriving regression equations from one to another in a sample of adults enrolled in an antiepileptic drug trial.

A final caveat is that there is a tendency to focus only on the size of the responsiveness statistic, without considering the size difference one should expect theoretically. In the quest to show that an instrument is responsive to change, instrument developers may fail to note that the degree of change should vary depending on whether the consequence of the intervention or perturbation in status is minor (getting bumped by a pedestrian) or major (getting hit by a truck). The estimation of the minimally importance difference is an example in which the change is hypothesized to be relatively small because the intervention is by definition minimal (see Chapter 4.2).

Summary

It is important to evaluate the reliability of HRQoL measures before widespread use in clinical trials and health outcome studies. A number of techniques are available for evaluating the inter-rater reliability, equivalent forms reliability, internal consistency reliability, and test–retest reliability of scales. The main methods for determining the reliability of a scale are introduced in this chapter. Reliability is a necessary measurement characteristic of a scale, and provides evidence of its stability over different repeated measurement. However, a scale may be reliable, but not valid – that is, it does not measure what it is intended to measure.

Validity of a scale reflects how well it measures what is intended to measure. For the developer and users of an HRQoL scale, the accumulation of evidence of the scale's validity is continuous. The key question for validity evidence is whether the scale is valid for a particular application in a specific population. The assessment of validity normally begins with an assessment of content validity and then evaluates the construct validity (including responsiveness of the scale to clinically meaningful changes). Reliability and validity are key psychometric criteria for measures used in clinical trials. Ongoing accumulation of research evidence regarding a scale's validity is important for demonstrating the scale's usefulness in a wide variety of research applications and patient populations.

References

Buesterien, K. M., Nissenson, A. R., Port, F. K., Kelly, M., Steinwald, B., and Ware, J. E. (1996). The effects of human erythropoeitin on functional health and well-being in chronic dialysis patients. *Journal of American Society of Nephrology*, 7, 163–173.

Bland, J. M. and Altman, D. G. (1996). Measurement error. *British Medical Journal*, 312, 1654.

Campbell, D. T. and Fiske, D. W. (1959). Convergent and discriminant validation by the multitrait-multimethod matrix. *Psychological Bulletin*, 56, 81–105.

Chambers, L. W., Haight, M., Norman, G., and MacDonald, L. (1987). Sensitivity to change and the effect of the mode of administration on health status measurement. *Medical Care*, 25, 470–480.

Cicchetti, D. V. and Feinstein, A. R. (1990). High agreement but low kappa: II. Resolving the paradoxes. *Journal of Clinical Epidemiology*, 43, 551–558.

Clark, E. L. (1935). Spearman-Brown formula applied to ratings of personality traits. *Journal of Educational Psychology*, 26, 552–555.

Cohen, J. (1968). Weighted kappa: nominal scale agreement with provision for scaled disagreement or partial credit. *Psychological Bulletin*, 70, 213–220.

Cohen, J. (1992). A power primer. *Psychological Bulletin*, 112, 155–159.

Cole, D. A. (1987). Utility of confirmatory factor analysis in test validation research. *Journal of Consulting and Clinical Psychology*, 55, 584–594.

Cronbach, L. J. (1951). Coefficient alpha and the internal structure of tests. *Psychometrika*, 16, 297–334.

Cronbach, L. J. and Meehl, P. E. (1955). Construct validity in psychological tests. *Psychological Bulletin*, 52, 281–302.

Cunningham, W. E., Bozzette, S. A., Hays, R. D., Kanouse, D. E., and Shapiro, M. F. (1995). Comparison of health-related quality of life in clinical trial and non-clinical trial human immunodeficiency virus-infected cohorts. *Medical Care*, 33, AS15–25.

Ellickson, P. L., Hays, R. D., and Bell, R. M. (1992). Stepping through the drug use sequence: longitudinal scalogram analysis of initiation and heavy use. *Journal of Abnormal Psychology*, 101, 441–451.

Feinstein, A. R. and Cicchetti, D. V. (1990). High agreement but low kappa: I. The problems of two paradoxes. *Journal of Clinical Epidemiology*, 43, 543–549.

Feldt, L. S., Woodruff, K. J., and Salih, F. A. (1987). Statistical inference for coefficient alpha. *Applied Psychological Measurement*, 11, 93–103.

Fleiss, J. L. (1981). *Statistical Methods for Rates and Proportions*, 2nd edn. New York: Wiley.

Fleiss J. L. and Cohen, J. (1973). The equivalence of weighted kappa and the intraclass correlation coefficient as measures of reliability. *Educational and Psychological Measurement*, 33, 613–619.

Goodenough, W. H. (1944). A technique for scale analysis. *Educational and Psychological Measurement*, 4, 179–190.

Guyatt, G., Walter, S., and Norman, G. (1987). Measuring change over time: assessing the usefulness of evaluative instruments. *Journal of Chronic Disease*, 40, 171–178.

Guyatt, G., Osoba, D., Wu, A. W., Wyrwich, K. W., and Norman, G. R. (2002). Methods to explain the clinical significance of health status measures. *Mayo Clinic Proceedings*, 77, 371–383.

Hadorn, D. C. and Hays, R. D. (1991). Multitrait-multimethod analysis of health-related quality of life preferences. *Medical Care*, 29, 829–840.

Hanley, J. A. and McNeil, B. J. (1982). The meaning and use of the area under a receiver operating characteristic (ROC) curve. *Radiology*, 143, 29–36.

Hanley, J. A. and McNeil, B. J. (1983). A method of comparing the areas under receiver operating characteristic curves derived from the same cases. *Radiology*, **148**, 839–843.

Hayashi, T. and Hays, R. D. (1987). A microcomputer program for analyzing multitrait-multimethod matrices. *Behavior Research Methods, Instruments, and Computers*, **19**, 345–348.

Hays, R. and Hadorn, D. (1992). Responsiveness to change: an aspect of validity, not a separate dimension. *Quality of Life Research*, **1**,73–75.

Hays, R. D., Sherbourne, C. D., and Mazel, R. M. (1993). The RAND 36-item health survey 1.0. *Health Economics*, **2**, 217–227.

Kazis, L. E., Anderson, J. J., and Meenan, R. F. (1989). Effect sizes for interpreting changes in health status. *Medical Care*, **27**, S178–189.

Kenny, D. A. and Kashy, D. A. (1992). Analysis of the multitrait-multimethod matrix by confirmatory factor analysis. *Psychological Bulletin*, **112**, 165–172.

Kim, S., Hays, R. D., Birbeck, G. L., and Vickrey, B. G. (2003). Responsiveness of the quality of life in epilepsy inventory (QOLIE-89) in an antiepileptic drug trial. *Quality of Life Research*, **12**, 147–155.

Landis, J. R. and Koch, G. G. (1977). The measurement of observer agreement for categorical data. *Biometrics*, **33**, 159–174.

Liang, M. J., Larson, M. G., Cullen, K. E., and Schwartz, J. A. (1985). Comparative measurement efficiency and sensitivity of five health status instruments for arthritis research. *Arthritis and Rheumatology*, **28**, 545–547.

Liang, M. J., Fossel, A. H., and Larson, M. G. (1990). Comparisons of five health status instruments for orthopedic evaluation. *Medical Care*, **28**, 632–642.

MacKenzie, C. R., Charlson, M. E., DiGioia, D., and Kelley, K. (1986). Can the sickness impact profile measure change? An example of scale assessment. *Journal of Chronic Disease*, **39**, 429–438.

Marsh, H. W. (1989). Confirmatory factor analyses of multitrait-multimethod data: many problems and few solutions. *Applied Psychological Measurement*, **13**, 335–361.

Marshall, G. N., Hays, R. D., and Nicholas, R. (1994). Evaluating agreement between clinical assessment methods. *International Journal of Methods in Psychiatric Research*, **4**, 249–257.

Menzel, H. (1953). A new coefficient for scalogram analysis. *Public Opinion Quarterly*, **17**, 268–280.

Nelson, E. C., Landgraf, J. M., Hays, R. D., Wasson. J. H., and Kirk, J. W. (1990). The functional status of patients: how can it be measured in physicians' offices? *Medical Care*, **28**, 1111–1126.

Nunnally, J. (1978). *Psychometric Theory*, 2nd edn. New York: McGraw-Hill.

Prisant, L. M., Carr, A. A., Bottini, P. B., Thompson, W. O., and Rhoades, R. B. (1992). Repeatability of automated ambulatory blood pressure measurements. *Journal of Family Practice*, **34**, 569–574.

Revicki, D. A., Rentz, A. M., Dubois, D., Kahrilias, P., Stanghellini, V., Talley, N. J., and Tack, J. (2003). Development and validation of a patient-assessed gastroparesis symptom severity measure: the Gastroparesis Cardinal Symptom Index. *Alimentary and Pharmacological Therapy*, **18**, 141–150.

Shrout, P. E. and Fleiss, J. L. (1979). Intraclass correlations: uses in assessing rater reliability. *Psychological Bulletin*, **86**, 420–428.

Siu, A. L., Hays, R. D., Ouslander, J. G., Osterweil, D., Krynski, M., and Gross, A. (1993a). Measuring functioning and health in the very old. *Journal of Gerontology: Medical Sciences*, **48**, M10–14.

Siu, A. L., Ouslander, J. G., Osterweil, D., Reuben, D. B., and Hays, R. D. (1993b). Change in self-reported functioning in older persons entering a residential care facility. *Journal of Clinical Epidemiology*, **46**, 1093–1102.

Smith, K. W. (1997). Measuring responsiveness in quality of life research. Paper presented at the meeting of the Drug Information Association, Scottsdale, Arizona, 13 January 1997.

Stewart, A. L., Hays, R. D., and Ware, J. (1992). Methods of validating MOS health measures. In Stewart A. L. and Ware J. E. (eds) *Measuring Functioning and Well-being: The Medical Outcomes Study approach.* Durham, NC: Duke University Press.

Ware, J. E. and Sherbourne, C. D. (1992). The MOS 36-item short-form health survey (SF-36): I. Conceptual framework and item selection. *Medical Care,* **30,** 473–483.

Wyrwich, K. W., Nienaber, N. A., Tierney, W. M., and Wolinsky, F. D. (1999a). Linking clinical relevance and statistical significance in evaluating intra-individual changes in health-related quality of life. *Medical Care,* **37,** 469–478.

Wyrwich, K. W., Tierney, W. M., and Wolinsky, F. D. (1999b). Further evidence supporting an SEM-based criterion for identifying meaningful intra-individual changes in health-related quality of life. *Journal of Clinical Epidemiology,* **52,** 861–873.

Evaluating multi-item scales

Ron D. Hays and Peter Fayers

Assessing the extent to which items in multi-item scales represent hypothesized concepts is a fundamental component of the development and evaluation of QoL measures. Multitrait scaling analysis and confirmatory factor analysis are two methods of assessment that are commonly used to determine the extent to which data confirm a priori expectations about survey items. In contrast, exploratory factor analysis is a technique that can be used to help identify clusters of items not necessarily hypothesized in advance. This chapter provides an overview of the use of each of these techniques in the evaluation of multi-item scales.

Multitrait scaling

Construct validity evaluation involves accumulating evidence of many different types that indicate the degree to which QoL measures represent what they were intended to represent. Thus, we examine the extent to which different 'traits' behave in the way that we would expect them to – where, in QoL terminology, traits are often called dimensions, subscales or constructs. Hypotheses are stated regarding the direction (and sometimes the strength) of a relationship that might be expected, and validity is supported when the associations are consistent with hypotheses. Convergent and discriminant validity are two fundamental aspects of construct validity. Convergent validity refers to the extent to which different ways of measuring the same trait intercorrelate with on another. Discriminant validity involves demonstrating that a measure does *not* correlate too strongly with measures that are intended to indicate different traits than that measure. For example, the correlation between a measure of loneliness and a measure of health locus of control would not be expected to be very large (Hays and DiMatteo 1987). When more than one method of data collection or scale construction has been used, convergent and discriminant validity can be assessed using multitrait–multimethod (MTMM) analytic methods. When multiple traits are assessed using a single method, the MTMM analytic strategy is not applicable. However, the general principles of convergent and discriminant validity can be applied.

A widely used practice in QoL research is to evaluate the internal consistency reliability (item convergence) of multi-item scales by estimating Cronbach's (1951) alpha coefficient. Alpha provides an indication of the degree of convergence between different items

Table 1.4.1 Synthetic multitrait/multi-item correlation matrix

	Trait 1	Trait 2	Trait 3
Item 1	0.80*	0.20	0.20
Item 2	0.80*	0.20	0.20
Item 3	0.80*	0.20	0.20
Item 4	0.20	0.80*	0.20
Item 5	0.20	0.80*	0.20
Item 6	0.20	0.80*	0.20
Item 7	0.20	0.20	0.80*
Item 8	0.20	0.20	0.80*
Item 9	0.20	0.20	0.80*

* Item-scale correlation, corrected for overlap.

hypothesized to represent the same construct or trait. Multitrait scaling goes beyond internal consistency by evaluating item discrimination, or the extent to which items correlate more highly with their hypothesized scale than they do with other scales.

Item-scale correlations are the fundamental elements of multitrait scaling (Ware *et al.* 1983) and constitute the multitrait/multi-item (MTMI) correlation matrix. A synthetic MTMI matrix is shown in Table 1.4.1. Three different traits are defined by three items each: Trait 1 (Items 1–3), Trait 2 (Items 4–6), and Trait 3 (Items 7–9). Each row of the MTMI matrix contains correlations between scores for one item and all hypothesized traits (defined by the sum of items comprising each trait). Each column contains correlations between the scores for one trait and all items in the analysis, including those hypothesized to be part of that trait and those hypothesized to be part of other traits. Correlations between items hypothesized to define a given trait and the trait itself need to be 'corrected for overlap' so that estimates of the item–trait relationships are not spuriously inflated.[1]

Item convergence is supported if an item correlates substantially (corrected correlation of 0.30 or above) with the scale it is hypothesized to represent. This is the traditional internal-consistency criterion. For scales that have a previous history of development, and for which analyses are intended to refine and add finishing touches rather than develop from scratch, a more stringent convergence criterion (i.e., larger correlation) can be applied. Each of the indicators shown in the synthetic example in Table 1.4.1 demonstrates convergence, correlating 0.80 with the hypothesized trait (items corrected for overlap are marked with an asterisk).

[1] A variable X is obviously correlated with the scale score $S = \text{sum}(X + \textit{other variables})$ because X is in both terms; if S comprises n random independent variables, the expected correlation is $1/\sqrt{n}$.

Therefore to examine the correlation of X with the scale, S must first be recalculated without X.

Item discrimination is supported if the highest correlation in a row of the MTMI matrix is the correlation between the item and the trait it is hypothesized to measure, and this correlation is significantly larger than the other correlations in the row. The significance of the difference of these correlations can be evaluated using Steiger's (1980) *t*-test for dependent correlations. Item discrimination is shown for all nine items given in Table 1.4.1. Each item-convergent correlation is significantly larger than the other correlations in the same row. The correlations between traits are also evaluated in multitrait scaling: zero-order (i.e., simple, unadjusted) correlations between scales and correlations adjusted for unreliability of measurement (Guilford 1954). These correlations should be appreciably less than unity to support the distinctiveness of the traits. The adjusted correlations will be higher than the raw correlations and approximate unity if the traits are not distinct. The adjusted correlations provide supplemental information, but should be interpreted with caution because they can be poor estimates of the true correlation and actually exceed the 1.0 upper correlation bound.

Confirmatory factor analysis

In confirmatory factor analysis, one must first hypothesize a model to explain the observed interrelationships among items. The degree of fit between a confirmatory factor model and data can then be evaluated. Parameter estimates indicating the relations between each item and the hypothesized traits and estimates of the unique variance associated with each item are products of confirmatory factor analysis. Confirmatory factor analysis is a form of structural equation modelling (measurement model), and the technique is extensively described in introductory texts such as Byrne (1994).

The chi-square statistic indicates whether the patterns of relations among variables generated by the hypothesized model are significantly divergent from those in the observed sample data. If chi-square is statistically significant, the relationships generated by the model are significantly different from the observed data and, thus, the model is not entirely consistent with the data. Statistical *non-significance* implies that a model provides an adequate representation of the data. However, the likelihood of rejecting a model based on chi-square is dependent upon sample size. If the sample size is large enough, essentially all models are statistically rejectable because they are all simplified approximations of complex constructs. Conversely, with a small enough sample size, only grossly misfitting models become statistically rejectable. That is, models that explain essentially all of the relevant information in a set of data based on a very large sample size may still be rejectable on statistical grounds. In contrast, too many models may appear to provide adequate fit to data from small samples if statistical significance only is relied upon.

To complement the chi-square statistic, measures of practical fit can be calculated. Rho (non-normed), delta (normed), and the comparative fit index provide measures of practical significance because they represent the proportion of statistical information in the data that is accounted for by a model. To calculate these measures of fit, the hypothesized model is compared against a 'null' model.[2] A null model is one that hypothesizes zero correlations (i.e., no covariation) among the measures in the analysis. The null model is the most restricted model possible and thus provides a maximum chi square to which other models can be compared. Models with practical fit values less than 0.90 should not be accepted, because such models can often be easily and substantially improved.

To evaluate multi-item scales using confirmatory factor analysis, one begins by specifying a confirmatory factor analysis model with hypothesized factor loadings and factor correlations. The statistical significance and size of the factor loadings can be used to evaluate item convergence.

Item discrimination is evaluated in two ways. First, it is assessed by determining whether or not freeing up (i.e., estimating) factor loadings currently fixed at zero in the model will improve the level of model fit. Examining modification indexes facilitates the identification of fixed parameters that, if estimated, will improve model fit. Lagrange multiplier modification indexes (see, e.g., Bentler 1995 or Byrne 1994) are useful for this purpose. The need to add these parameters may suggest a lack of discrimination at the item level. Unidimensional construct definition is violated when indicators load on multiple constructs (Anderson and Gerbing 1988).

Second, the discrimination between traits defined in the confirmatory factor analytic model can be examined by inspecting the correlations between factors. Large correlations indicate a lack of discrimination between traits. To determine if a pair of traits is indistinguishable, a confirmatory factor model, in which a factor correlation is fixed at unity, can be compared to a model in which the correlation is freely estimated. If the more restricted model (fixed correlation at unity) fits the data as well as the less restricted model (correlation freely estimated), then it is reasonable to conclude that the traits are indistinguishable.

Example application of multitrait scaling and confirmatory factor analysis

Data from the Medical Outcomes Study (MOS) are analyzed to illustrate the multitrait scaling methodology. In the MOS, patient satisfaction with medical care was measured

[2] Delta is the difference in the chi-square statistic between the null model and the substantive model, divided by chi-square for the null model. The numerator of rho is calculated by dividing the chi-square statistic for the null model and the substantive model by the degrees of freedom for these models and computing the difference. The denominator of rho is the chi-square statistic divided by the degrees of freedom for the null model minus one. The comparative fit index is calculated by subtracting from unity the ratio of the chi-square for the substantive model minus its degrees of freedom divided by the result of subtracting the degrees of freedom for the null model from the chi-square of the null model. It is linearly related to rho.

every six months using a periodic satisfaction survey, the PSQ-III (Marshall *et al.* 1993). The PSQ-III consists of 50 items that assess general satisfaction and satisfaction with six specific dimensions of medical care: technical quality, interpersonal quality, communication, financial aspects, time spent with provider, and access/availability/ convenience.

Patient satisfaction ratings obtained at baseline of the MOS from 1192 patients of medical providers were analyzed here. For this analysis, ratings of satisfaction with the provider's *technical quality* (6 items), *interpersonal manner* (6 items) and *communication skills* (5 items), and satisfaction with *financial arrangements* (8 items) were examined. Each of these four aspects of care was hypothesized to be distinct based on prior research (Ware *et al.* 1983).

Multitrait scaling was conducted using the Multitrait Analysis Program (MAP) (Hays and Hayashi 1990). From raw data input, MAP yields item frequencies, item and scale descriptive statistics (e.g., mean, standard deviation, variance), scale internal consistency estimates, item-scale correlations, and correlations among scales. Confirmatory factor analysis was performed using the EQS program (Bentler 1995).

Multitrait scaling analysis results

Table 1.4.2 provides the MTMI correlation matrix for the 25 patient satisfaction items hypothesized to represent the four dimensions of satisfaction with medical care. Item–scale correlations for hypothesized traits are corrected for item overlap and are designated with an asterisk. These item convergence coefficients are reasonably large, ranging from 0.48 to 0.73. Internal consistency reliability, as estimated by Cronbach's alpha coefficient, was 0.80 or higher for each scale. Thus, the items representing the four traits are internally consistent and exhibit item convergence.

Item discrimination is examined by comparing the convergent correlations with the other correlations in the same row of the MTMI matrix. Correlations within two standard errors of the corresponding convergent correlations (denoted by @) are indicative of lack of item discrimination. It is important to note that because the standard error decreases, the likelihood of supporting item discrimination increases with a larger sample size. In the example, each of the items hypothesized to measure satisfaction with technical quality correlates with satisfaction with communication about as high (within two standard errors) as it correlates with the sum of the other items measuring technical quality. Similarly, all of the satisfaction with communication items correlates about as highly with the technical quality and interpersonal aspects scales as they do with the other communication items. In summary, items hypothesized to assess technical quality, interpersonal aspects and communication lack discrimination.

The correlations between the scales formed by summing items designed to measure each of the four dimensions of care are presented in Table 1.4.3. These correlations provide further indication of the lack of discrimination (at the level of the traits)

Table 1.4.2 Multitrait/multi-item correlation matrix for patient satisfaction ratings

	Technical	Interpersonal	Communication	Financial
Technical				
1	0.66*	0.63@	0.67@	0.28
2	0.55*	0.54@	0.50@	0.25
3	0.48*	0.41	0.44@	0.26
4	0.59*	0.53	0.56@	0.26
5	0.55*	0.60@	0.56@	0.16
6	0.59*	0.58@	0.57@	0.23
Interpersonal				
1	0.58	0.68*	0.63@	0.24
2	0.59@	0.58*	0.61@	0.18
3	0.62@	0.65*	0.67@	0.19
4	0.53@	0.57*	0.60@	0.32
5	0.54	0.62*	0.58@	0.18
6	0.48@	0.48*	0.46@	0.24
Communication				
1	0.58@	0.59@	0.61*	0.26
2	0.47@	0.50@	0.50*	0.25
3	0.58@	0.66@	0.63*	0.23
4	0.66@	0.66@	0.67*	0.25
5	0.66@	0.71@	0.70*	0.25
Financial				
1	0.35	0.35	0.35	0.72*
2	0.17	0.14	0.15	0.65*
3	0.25	0.23	0.23	0.61*
4	0.18	0.15	0.16	0.67*
5	0.31	0.27	0.29	0.70*
6	0.24	0.23	0.22	0.73*
7	0.25	0.23	0.25	0.55*
8	0.34	0.31	0.31	0.64*
Cronbach's alpha	0.80	0.82	0.82	0.88

Note: Standard error of correlation is 0.03.

Technical = satisfaction with technical quality; Interpersonal = satisfaction with interpersonal aspects; Communication = satisfaction with communication; Financial = satisfaction with financial arrangements.

@ Correlation is within two standard errors of the correlation of the item with its hypothesized scale.

* Item-scale correlation, corrected for overlap.

Table 1.4.3 Correlations between patient satisfaction scales

	Technical	Interpersonal	Communication	Financial
Technical	1.00	0.75	0.76	0.34
Interpersonal	0.93	1.00	0.80	0.31
Communication	0.94	0.98	1.00	0.32
Financial	0.41	0.36	0.38	1.00

Note: Zero-order correlations are provided above the diagonal; correlations adjusting for unreliability of measurement are given below the diagonal.

between technical quality, interpersonal aspects and communication; adjusted correlations (for unreliability of measurement) between scales were 0.93 or higher.

Confirmatory factor analysis results

First, the hypothesized confirmatory factor model was estimated. Although this model was statistically rejectable, indicating that there is some evidence that it is not a perfect model, it fit the data fairly well according to practical fit criteria (delta = 0.88, rho = 0.88, CFI = 0.89). The standardized parameter estimates for this initial model are given in Table 1.4.4. Goodness of fit results for this model and subsequent models are reported in Table 1.4.5. All of the parameter estimates were statistically significant and in the hypothesized direction. The correlations between the technical quality, interpersonal aspects and communication latent variables were 0.93 or greater.

Next, a model was estimated fixing the correlation between satisfaction with interpersonal aspects and satisfaction with communication, the most strongly intercorrelated traits, at 1.00. This model fit the data significantly less well than the initial model (λ^2 (1), N = 1192 = 13.11, $P < 0.01$), indicating that ratings of interpersonal aspects of care and communication are not entirely synonymous. Despite the statistically significant chi-square difference test, practical fit for these two models was identical (Δ delta = 0.00, Δ rho = 0.00, Δ CFI = 0.00). Thus, the interpersonal and communication scales are, for practical purposes, indistinguishable.

Lagrange multiplier tests were examined to identify factor loadings that, if estimated, would improve model fit. The need to add these loadings is indicative of problems with item discrimination. A total of 25 factor loadings were identified that would lead to a univariate improvement in model fit and a substantively reasonable parameter change (i.e., suppression effects were disallowed). Fourteen of these loadings were identified as providing a significant multivariate improvement in fit (after dependencies among multiplier tests were considered). These loadings are noted by footnotes in Table 1.4.4. Four additional loadings for interpersonal and financial items and three additional loadings for the technical and communication items were suggested. Adding these

Table 1.4.4 Standardized parameter estimates for confirmatory factor analytic model

Factor Loadings

	Technical	Interpersonal	Communication	Financial	Unique
Technical					
1	0.77	—	a,b	—	0.64
2	0.60	—	—	—	0.80
3	0.53	—	—	a,b	0.85
4	0.63	—	—	—	0.77
5	0.66	a,b	a	—	0.75
6	0.67	—	—	—	0.74
Interpersonal					
1	—	0.72	—	—	0.69
2	a,b	0.69	a	—	0.72
3	—	0.77	—	—	0.64
4	—	0.64	a,b	a,b	0.76
5	—	0.68	—	—	0.73
6	a	0.52	—	a,b	0.86
Communication					
1	—	—	0.69	—	0.73
2	—	—	0.54	a,b	0.84
3	—	a,b	0.73	—	0.69
4	a,b	—	0.76	—	0.66
5	—	—	0.82	—	0.58
Financial					
1	a	a,b	a	0.77	0.64
2	—	—	—	0.69	0.72
3	—	—	—	0.66	0.76
4	—	—	—	0.72	0.70
5	a	a	a,b	0.75	0.66
6	—	—	—	0.77	0.63
7	a	a	a,b	0.59	0.80
8	a,b	a	a	0.70	0.72

	Technical	Interpersonal	Communication	Financial
Technical	1.00			
Interpersonal	0.93	1.00		
Communication	0.94	0.97	1.00	
Financial	0.40	0.34	0.36	1.00

a – Factor loading that would lead to a significant improvement in fit according to Lagrange multiplier tests, univariate.

b – Factor loading that would lead to a significant improvement in fit according to Lagrange multiplier tests, multivariate.

Table 1.4.5 Goodness-of-fit indexes for confirmatory factor analysis models

Model	df	chi-square	delta	rho	CFI
Null	300	15038.37	—	—	—
Hypothesized four-factor model	269	1864.41	0.88	0.88	0.89
Three-factor model, fixing correlation at 1.0	270	1877.52	0.88	0.88	0.89
Modified four-factor model, adding 14 factor loadings	255	1558.31	0.90	0.90	0.91

Note: All models were statistically rejectable, $P < 0.01$.

14 loadings results in a model that was statistically rejectable, but the model fit the data well according to practical criteria (delta = 0.90, rho = 0.90, CFI = 0.91).

Exploratory factor analysis

Exploratory factor analysis can be a useful aid to identify item clusters that were not hypothesized in advance, because it summarizes the intercorrelations among items in terms of underlying dimensions or factors. Items that correlate more highly with one another than with other items will tend to load together on the same factor. There are two main components of exploratory factor analysis: (1) estimating the number of underlying dimensions; and (2) rotating the number of factors to identify which items cluster together on the same factor. We use an analysis of the SF-12 health survey in a random sample of 6565 adult enrollees that received managed care from a group practice association (Hays *et al.* 1998) as an example of an exploratory factor analysis.

Number of factors decision

There are several number of factors criteria that can be useful in helping to identify the number of dimensions underlying the covariances among the items. The most commonly applied criterion is the Kaiser 'eigenvalue greater than one' rule of thumb. The criterion is based on the logic that you should only include a factor if its eigenvalue exceeds 1.0, the variance of a standardized item. For the SF-12 items in the sample of managed care enrollees, 2 of the 12 eigenvalues exceeded 1.0: 4.85, 1.69, 0.93, 0.86, 0.76, 0.60, 0.50, 0.46, 0.39, 0.37, 0.32 and 0.29.

A nice supplemental criterion to employ along with the eigenvalue greater than one rule of thumb is 'parallel analysis'. Parallel analysis involves estimating eigenvalues using squared multiple correlations and comparing the resulting eigenvalues with those expected by chance alone. Factors should only be retained if their eigenvalues are larger than what one would expect by chance. In the example, parallel analysis indicated

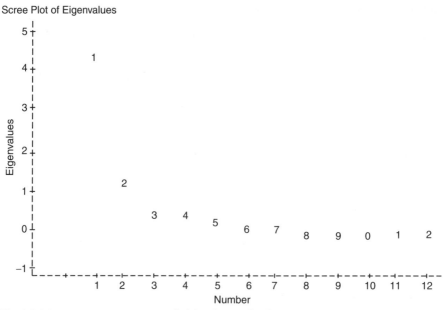

Fig. 1.4.1 Scree test suggests two underlying factors for the SF-12.

that no more than five factors should be rotated. As in this example, parallel analysis often provides an upper bound for the number of factors rather than an estimate of the right number of factors to rotate.

The scree test is an important adjunct to the first two criteria. The eigenvalues subjected to the parallel analysis can be plotted on the y-axis as a function of number of factor on the x-axis. The scree is identified by the place where the curve connecting adjacent eigenvalues flattens out or forms an elbow. The number of points in the curve above the scree indicates the number of factors. In the example dataset, the scree test suggests two underlying factors.

A final criterion worth considering is practical fit as indexed by Tucker and Lewis reliability coefficient using maximum likelihood (ML) analysis. As with confirmatory factor analysis, a delta of at least 0.90 is needed and experience suggests that coefficients closer to 0.95 are desirable. ML also produces a statistical test of fit, but it is typically rejectable for any reasonable sample size. In the example, the Tucker and Lewis reliability coefficient was 0.81, 0.86 and 0.95 for 2, 3 and 4 factors, respectively.

Factor rotation

After determining the number of dimensions underlying the data, it is then possible to rotate factors to produce a solution for interpretation. It is not uncommon for the number-of-factors criteria to suggest a range of possible number of factors rather than to narrow it down to a specific number of dimensions. Hence, it is common to rotate different number of factors within the identified range and to examine the rotated solutions to determine which produce a more reasonable substantive summary of the intercorrelations among items.

Factors can be rotated by assuming that they are either uncorrelated (orthogonal rotation) or correlated (oblique rotation). The most common orthogonal rotation is Varimax. There are a number of oblique rotations, but one of the more commonly performed rotations is Promax. An oblique rotation is often a good idea because it provides an opportunity to estimate the associations between factors, rather than assume that they are uncorrelated. With either rotation, one needs to specify how communalities for the items will be estimated. The two most common methods of communality estimation are to insert 1's in the diagonal of the matrix or squared multiple correlations (SMCs).

Table 1.4.6 provides an example of a Promax rotated two-factor solution (SMC communalities) for the SF-12 items. The first factor represents physical health and the second factor mental health. The physical functioning, pain, role limitations due to physical health, and general health rating items load moderately to highly on the physical health factor. The emotional well-being and role limitations due to emotional problems items load highly on the mental health factor. The energy and social functioning items load on both factors about equally. The estimated correlation between the physical and mental health factors was 0.48 in this sample.

Note that for illustration we analyzed the SF-12 items using a factor analysis procedure that assumes the items are normally distributed. However, the most appropriate

Table 1.4.6 Promax rotated two-factor solution (standardized regression coefficients)

	Physical	Mental
i2	0.78061	−0.12742 moderate activities
i5	0.77352	−0.02502 limited in kind of work (physical)
i3	0.75218	−0.09453 climbing stairs
ri8	0.64928	0.14712 pain interference
i4	0.64186	0.14610 accomplished less (physical)
ri1	0.49601	0.20243 general health rating
i11	−0.05387	0.70397 downhearted
ri9	−0.03593	0.68568 calm and peaceful
i6	0.02810	0.65594 accomplished less (emotional)
i7	0.03694	0.60838 less carefully (emotional)
ri10	0.36979	0.44360 lot of energy
i12	0.24047	0.21564 social function

Estimated correlation between physical and mental health factors is 0.48.

model for these items would be a categorical factor analysis model that models the observed variables as arising from an underlying continuum (Muthén 1984).

Adequacy of factor models

All the methods described so far are predicated on the assumption that the multi-item scales contain items that reflect the underlying level of the hypothesized trait. For many dimensions of HRQoL this may be a reasonable assumption. However, disease-targeted instruments may contain a number of items representing disease-related symptoms or the side-effects of treatment. These items are likely to be correlated with each other because of characteristics of the disease or treatment, and the correlations may therefore not indicate anything about HRQoL constructs. However, assessment of such items may be very important. In terms of HRQoL, these items are 'causal variables' that affect quality of life, unlike the items in psychometric scales that are chosen specifically because they are 'indicator variables'. For example, Fayers and Hand (2002) reviewed a number of publications about the Rotterdam symptom checklist, in which researchers had proposed a variety of inconsistent factor solutions. They described a clinical trial for colorectal cancer that used the same questionnaire and for which an exploratory factor analysis produced yet another seemingly strange combination of symptoms in one factor – lack of appetite, decreased sexual interest, and dry mouth. But all these symptoms are side-effects of one of the treatment arms in that trial – interferon. Thus the factor merely reflected the correlations between the symptoms – causal variables – and did not indicate anything about the hypothesized QoL constructs. This also explained why the other publications had claimed to find so many different factors structures.

Another example is that Juniper *et al.* (1997) described the development of an asthma HRQoL instrument and the confusing results that they obtained when comparing factor analysis against patients' opinions of item importance/impact, and commented 'we believe that all items of functional impairment that are important to patients, irrespective of their association with each other, should be included in a disease-specific quality-of-life instrument' (p. 237). Fayers *et al.* (1998) commented that these results could be fully explained by the distinction between causal variables and indicator variables.

In many cases, clinicians may find it convenient to group symptoms and side effects into summary scores or indexes. But although these clinical summaries can be useful, frequently they will violate the psychometric assumptions of multi-item scales. Items representing causal variables may exhibit correlations unrelated to HRQoL traits. Scales including those items are not amenable to the application of simple correlation-based analyses, including multi-trait scaling and exploratory factor analysis, although it is possible to use methods such as structural equation modelling.

Summary

Multitrait scaling is a straightforward approach to scale analysis that focuses on items as the unit of analysis and utilizes the logic of convergent and discriminant validity. This methodology incorporates item discrimination evaluation in addition to internal consistency as a standard aspect of scale analysis. Although confirmatory factor analysis is more sophisticated than multitrait scaling, it is more difficult, time-consuming, and expensive to use in practice. Multitrait scaling may be sufficient for evaluations of multi-item scales in many applications of QoL scales.

References

Anderson, J. C. and Gerbing, D. W. (1988). Structural equation modeling in practice; A review and recommended two-step approach. *Psychological Bulletin*, **103**, 411–423.

Bentler, P. M. (1995). *EQS Structural Equations Program Manual*. Encino, CA: Multivariate Software, Inc.

Byrne, B. (1994). *Structural Equation Modelling with EQS and EQS/Windows: Basic concepts, applications and programming*. Thousand Oaks, CA: Sage Publications.

Cronbach, L. J. (1951). Coefficient alpha and the internal structure of tests. *Psychometrika*, **16**, 297–334.

Fayers, P. M. and Hand D. J. (2002). Causal variables, indicator variables and measurement scales: an example from quality of life. *J. R. Statistic. Soc. A*, **165**, 233–261.

Fayers, P. M., Groenvold, M., Hand, D. J., and Bjordal, K. (1998). Clinical impact versus factor analysis for quality of life questionnaire construction. *J. Clin. Epidem.*, **51**, 285–286.

Guilford, J. P. (1954). *Psychometric Methods*. New York: McGraw-Hill.

Hays, R. D., Brown, J. A., Spritzer, K. L., Dixon, W. J., and Brook, R. H. (1998). Satisfaction with health care provided by 48 physician groups. *Archives of Internal Medicine*, **158**, 785–790.

Hays, R. D. and DiMatteo, M. R. (1987). A short measure of loneliness. *Journal of Personality Assessment*, **51**, 69–81.

Hays, R. D. and Hayashi, T. (1990). Beyond internal consistency reliability: Rationale and User's Guide for Multitrait Scaling Analysis Program on the microcomputer. *Behavior Research Methods, Instruments and Computers*, **22**, 167–175.

Juniper, E. F., Guyatt, G. H., Streiner, D. L., and King, D. R. (1997). Clinical impact versus factor analysis for quality of life questionnaire construction. *J. Clin. Epidem.*, **50**, 233–238.

Marshall, G. N., Hays, R. D., Sherbourne, C., and Wells, K. B. (1993). The structure of patient ratings of outpatient medical care. *Psychological Assessment*, **5**, 477–483.

Muthén, B. (1984). A general structural equation model with dichotomous, ordered categorical, and continuous latent variable indicators. *Psychometrika*, **49**, 115–132.

Steiger, J. H. (1980). Tests for comparing elements of a correlation matrix. *Psychological Bulletin*, **87**, 245–251.

Ware, J. E., Snyder, M. R., Wright, R., and Davies, A. R. (1983). Defining and measuring patient satisfaction with medical care. *Evaluation and Program Planning*, **6**, 247–263.

Applying item response theory modelling for evaluating questionnaire item and scale properties

Bryce B. Reeve and Peter Fayers

Developing a health-related quality of life (HRQoL) questionnaire that is psychometrically sound and captures the full burden of disease or treatment upon a person, requires a thorough questionnaire development process that integrates survey development tools from the qualitative sciences, cognitive aspects of survey methodology, and the field of psychometrics. This chapter describes the role of item response theory (IRT) models in questionnaire evaluation and development. For multi-item scales, IRT models provide a clear picture of the performance of each item (question) in the scale and how the scale functions overall for measuring the construct of interest in the study population. IRT methods can lead to short reliable questionnaires that are tailored to the population of interest.

Item response theory models

IRT refers to a set of mathematical models that describe, in probabilistic terms, the relationship between a person's response to a survey question and his or her level of the 'latent variable' being measured by the scale. This latent variable is usually a hypothetical construct, trait, domain, or ability, which is postulated to exist but cannot be directly measured by a single observable variable or item. Instead, it is indirectly measured using multiple items or questions in a multi-item scale. The underlying latent variable, expressed mathematically by the Greek letter theta (θ), may be any measurable construct, such as mental health, fatigue, or physical functioning. The person's level on this construct is assumed to be the only factor that accounts for their response to each item in a scale. For example, a person with high levels of depression will have a high probability of responding that 'most of the time' they 'felt downhearted and blue'. Someone with hardly any depression is more likely to respond 'little of the time' or 'none of the time'. Provided as a reference guide, Table 1.5.1 summarizes the terminology used in this and other chapters.

Table 1.5.1 Key terms and definitions

Term	Definition
Category response curve (CRC)	See item characteristic curve (ICC).
Classical test theory (CTT)	Traditional psychometric methods such as factor analysis and Cronbach's α, in contrast to IRT.
Dichotomous (binary) response categories	An item having two response categories such as yes/no, true/false, or agree/disagree.
Discrimination parameter (a, α) – slope	IRT model item parameter that indicates the strength of the relationship between an item and the measured construct. Also, the parameter indicates how well an item discriminates between respondents below and above the item threshold parameter, as indicated by the slope of the ICCs.
Information function/curve	Indicates the range over θ for which an item or scale is most useful (reliable) for measuring persons' levels.
Item	A question in a scale.
Item characteristic curve (ICC)	Models the probabilistic relationship between a person's response to each category for an item and their level on the underlying construct (θ). Also called category response curve (CRC).
Item-total correlation	Measure of the relationship between an item and the total score from the set of items within the scale. Higher correlations indicate a stronger relationship between the item and scale score.
Local independence assumption	Once you control for the dominant factor influencing a person's response to an item, there should be no significant association among the item responses.
Polytomous response categories	An item having two or more response categories. For example, a 5-point Likert type scale.
Scale	Consists of multiple items that measure a single domain such as fatigue.
Standard error of measurement (SEM)	Describes an expected observed score fluctuation due to error in the measurement tool. Standard deviation of error about an estimated score.
Theta (θ)	Unobservable construct (or latent variable) being measured by a scale.
Threshold parameter (b, β) – difficulty, location	IRT model item parameter that indicates the severity or difficulty of an item response. The location along the θ-continuum of the item response categories.
Unidimensionality assumption	Assumes that one underlying (or dominant) factor accounts for a person's response to a question within a scale.

Traditional approaches to measurement scales (i.e., classical test theory) are based on *averages* or *simple summation* of the multiple items. In contrast, IRT models are founded on the *probability* that a person will make a particular response according to their level of the underlying latent variable. Thus IRT is analogous to logistic regression, which is widely used in medical statistics. The objective is to model each item by estimating the properties describing its performance. The relationship between a person's response to an item and the latent variable is expressed by 'item characteristic curves' (ICCs), also called category response curves (CRCs).

Figure 1.5.1 presents ICCs for the dichotomous item: 'As a result of any emotional problems, have you accomplished less than you would like?' This question was taken from the role-emotional subscale of the RAND-36/SF-36 instrument (Hays and Morales 2001; Ware and Sherbourne 1992) and combined with the other items in the scale along with items in the vitality, social functioning, and mental health subscales to form a 14-item "mental health" scale. Response data collected from 888 breast cancer survivors approximately 24 months after breast cancer diagnosis were used for the illustrations in this chapter. The latent variable "mental health" is represented by θ along the horizontal x-axis. Individuals with poor mental health are to the left on this axis, while people with good mental health are to the right. Numbers on the θ-axis are expressed in standardized units, and in our examples the population mental health has been standardized to have zero mean and standard deviation of one. Thus a mental health score of $\hat{\theta} = -2.0$ indicates that the person lies two standard deviations below the population mean. The vertical axis indicates the probability that a person will select one of the item's response categories. The two ICCs in Figure 1.5.1 indicate that the

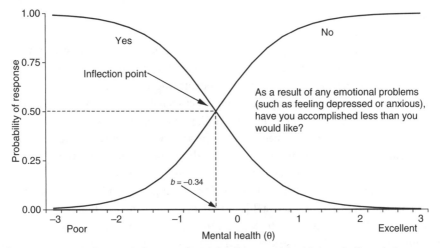

Fig. 1.5.1 IRT item characteristic curves (ICCs) for the mental health item indicated above. The ICC models the probability of a person to endorse one of the response categories (Yes or No) conditional on their mental health level. The difficulty parameter (*b*) indicates the level of mental health necessary for a person to have a 50% for endorsing the response category.

probability of responding 'yes' or 'no' to the item asking 'have you accomplished less than you would like?' depends on the respondent's level of mental health. Poor mental health leads to a high probability of selecting 'yes,' and high mental health to 'no'.

The ICCs in Figure 1 are represented by logistic curves that model the probability P that

$$P(X_i = 1 \mid \theta, a_i, b_i) = \frac{1}{1 + e^{-a_i(\theta - b_i)}} \qquad \text{(Equation 1)}$$

a person will respond 'no' (for the curve labelled 'no') to this item. This is a function of the respondent's level of mental health (θ), the relationship (a) of the item to the measured construct, and the severity or 'threshold' (b) of the item in the scale. In IRT, a and b are commonly referred to as item discrimination and item difficulty (or threshold) parameters, respectively. Since P in Equation 1 is the probability of responding 'no', the equation for the responding 'yes' is just $1-P$, as illustrated by the curve labelled 'yes' in Figure 1.5.1.

The item threshold (difficulty, or severity level), b, is the point on the latent scale where a person has a 50 percent chance of responding 'no' to the item. In Figure 1.5.1, the item's threshold value is $b = -0.34$, which is close to 0.0, indicating that people with mental health levels near the population mean ($\theta = 0$) are equally likely to respond 'no' or 'yes' to this question. The intersection point of the ICCs, identified by the threshold parameter, locates where an item is optimal for differentiating respondents' mental health levels around that point. An item with low threshold parameters is optimal for differentiating among persons with poor mental health functioning and vice versa. The threshold parameter varies for each item in a scale, and estimated parameters can be compared to select items to measure different parts of the mental health continuum.

The discrimination or slope parameter (a) in Equation 1 describes the strength of an item's ability to differentiate among people at different levels along the trait continuum. An item optimally discriminates among respondents who are near the item's threshold b. The discrimination parameter typically ranges between 0.5 and 2.5 in value. The slope is measured at the steepest point (the inflection point), and is $a = 1.82$ in Figure 1.5.1. The larger the a parameter, the steeper the slope and the more effective the item. Steep slopes, where the ICC increases relatively rapidly, indicate that small changes in the latent variable lead to large changes in item-endorsement probabilities. Items with large a parameters contribute most to determining a person's $\hat{\theta}$ score. For example, 'Did you feel tired?' had a higher discrimination parameter ($a = 2.19$) and item-total correlation ($r = 0.68$) than the item 'Have you been a very nervous person?' ($a = 1.05$, $r = 0.48$, respectively). Thus the slope of the ICC for the 'tired' item will be steeper than the slope of the 'nervous' item, thus 'tired' has better discrimination. A slope of zero represents a horizontal ICC, indicating that irrespective of the person's level there is always a 50:50 chance of responding 'yes' or 'no' – an entirely uninformative item.

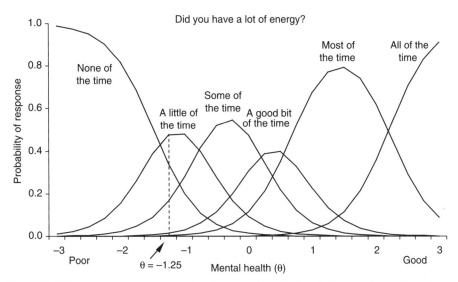

Fig. 1.5.2 IRT category response curves for the mental health item indicated above. There is a curve for each of the item's response options. The vertical dashed line indicates the probability for person 1.25 standard deviations below the population mean to respond to each of the six response categories.

IRT can also model items with more than two response options. The item 'Did you have a lot of energy?' has six response categories, and the ICCs are presented in Figure 1.5.2. Several IRT models are available for 'polytomous' responses, and the Graded Response Model (Samejima 1969) chosen for this data analysis estimated one item discrimination parameter and five threshold parameters (the number of categories minus one) to represent the location along the θ-scale where the probability exceeds 50 per cent that the response is in the associated category or higher category. In Figure 1.5.2, people with very poor mental health (e.g. θ < −2) have a high probability of answering 'none of the time'. A person at θ = −1.25 (indicated by a vertical dashed line) has a 34 per cent probability of endorsing high energy 'none of the time', 48 per cent probability of 'little of the time', 17 per cent probability of 'some of the time', and is unlikely to respond 'a good bit of the time', 'most of the time' or 'all the time'. Moving to the right along the θ-axis, people with better mental health will endorse response categories associated with better health.

Information functions

Information functions indicate the range over θ where an item or scale is best at discriminating among individuals. Higher information denotes more precision (or reliability). The shape of an *item* information function is defined by the item discrimination, *a*, and threshold, *b*, parameters. The threshold determines the location of the information function on the horizontal θ-axis. Thus threshold parameters evaluate how well a particular item matches levels of the construct being studied;

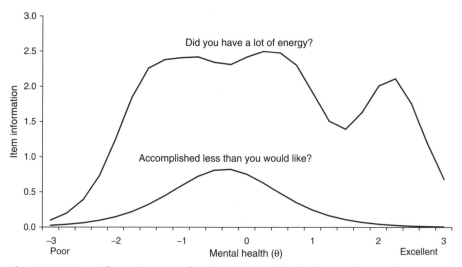

Fig. 1.5.3 IRT item information curves for the two mental health items indicated above. Each curve describes the range over θ for which the item is most useful (precise) for measuring persons' mental health levels.

ideally items should be well spaced across the continuum. Information magnitude is indicated on the vertical axis, and items with high discrimination have the most peaked information function because higher discrimination means the item can better differentiate among individuals who lie near the threshold value. Figure 1.5.3 presents item information functions for the two items of Figures 1.5.1 and 1.5.2. The information function for the 6-category 'energy' item is broader than that for the two-category 'accomplished less' item, because the greater number of response categories allows broader coverage of the continuum. Also, 'energy' is more peaked than 'accomplished less', indicating that the 'energy' item contributes more precision to the measurement of mental health.

Item information functions can identify items that perform well or poorly. Low information for one item may indicate that the item: (1) measures something different from other items in the scale, (2) is poorly worded and needs to be rewritten, (3) is too complex for the respondents, or (4) is placed out of context in the questionnaire.

The individual item information functions can be summed across all items in the scale to form the 'scale information function'. Figure 1.5.4 shows this for the 14-item RAND-36 Mental Health scale. Information magnitude and the associated reliability ($r = 1-1/information$) are shown. The scale is reliable ($r > 0.80$) for measuring mental health across the full continuum. The function is peaked at the lower end of the scale, indicating that poor mental health is measured with most precision. Reliability decreases when measuring excellent mental health.

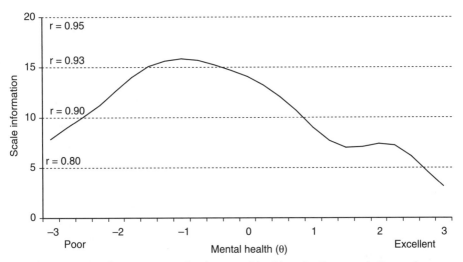

Fig. 1.5.4 IRT scale information curve for the mental health scale. The curve indicates the range over θ for which the scale is most informative (precise) for measuring persons' mental health levels. Horizontal dashed lines indicate the approximate level of reliability associated with different information magnitudes.

The standard error of measurement is $SEM = 1/\sqrt{information}$, and varies according to θ. For a person at θ = 1.5 (a person 1.5 standard deviations above the mean score) the information is 7, and thus the reliability is 0.86 and the SEM is 0.38.

Common IRT models

IRT models can handle unidimensional or multidimensional data, binary or polytomous responses, and ordered or unordered responses. Table 1.5.2 presents the models most frequently used in HRQoL assessment. Two of these are for dichotomous items (e.g. yes/no or agree/disagree), whereas the remainder are polytomous models suitable for more than two response categories. All these models are unidimensional and designed to measure a single construct.

The so-called Rasch models are identified with asterisks in Table 1.5.1. Non-Rasch models (also called two-parameter models) estimate a discrimination (slope) parameter for each item, suggesting that items be differentially weighted with regard to the underlying construct, whereas Rasch models assume equal discrimination. Equation 1 represents the two-parameter logistic IRT model for dichotomous response data, with discrimination parameter a_i that varies from item to item as indicated by the subscript i. The simple Rasch model is obtained if all a_i are constrained to be equal.

The simplicity of the Rasch model confers several advantages. Any two items' threshold parameters can be compared, independent of the group of subjects being surveyed (specific objectivity), and any two persons' scores can be compared irrespective of the particular subset of items being administered. Also, fitting Rasch models is possible

Table 1.5.2 Commonly-used item response theory (IRT) models in HRQoL assessment

IRT Model	Item Response Format	Model Characteristics
Rasch Model*/One Parameter Logistic Model	Dichotomous	Discrimination power equal across all items. Threshold varies across items.
Two Parameter Logistic Model	Dichotomous	Discrimination and threshold parameters vary across items.
Graded Response Model	Polytomous	Ordered responses. Discrimination varies across items.
Nominal Model	Polytomous	No prespecified item response order. Discrimination varies across items.
Partial Credit Model*	Polytomous	Discrimination power constrained to be equal across items.
Rating Scale Model*	Polytomous	Discrimination equal across items. Distance between item threshold steps equal across items.
Generalized Partial Credit Model	Polytomous	Generalization of the Partial Credit Model that allows discrimination to vary across items.

* Models belonging to the family of Rasch models.

with smaller sample sizes. However, these properties only hold if the model fits the data adequately, and frequently the simple Rasch model is unrealistic.

IRT model assumptions

The parametric, unidimensional IRT models described above make three key assumptions about the data: (1) unidimensionality, (2) local independence, and (3) that the IRT model fits the data. It is important that these assumptions be evaluated. However, IRT models are robust to minor violations and no real data ever meet the assumptions perfectly.

Unidimensionality posits that the set of items measure a single continuous latent construct θ. In other words, a person's level on this single construct gives rise to that person's item responses. This assumption does not preclude a set of items from having a number of minor dimensions (subscales), but does assume that one dominant dimension suffices to explain the underlying structure. Scale dimensionality can be evaluated by factor analysis of the item responses. If multidimensionality is indicated by factor analysis and supported by clinical theory, it may be appropriate to divide the scale into subscales. Multidimensional IRT models do exist, but are complex.

Local independence means that if θ is held constant there should be no association among the item responses. Violation of this assumption may result in biased parameter estimates, leading to erroneous decisions when selecting items for scale construction. Local independence can be evaluated by examining the residual correlation matrices to look for systematic error among item clusters that may indicate a violation of the assumption. The impact of local dependence can be explored by observing how the IRT item parameters and person scores change when one of the locally dependent items are dropped.

Model fit can be examined at both the item and person level, to determine whether the estimated item and person parameters can reproduce the observed item responses (Reise in press). Graphical and empirical approaches can evaluate item fit (e.g., Hambleton *et al.* 2000; Orlando and Thissen 2000) and person fit (Embretson and Reise 2000). Currently, no standard set of fit indices is universally accepted, and a number of different indices are reported by IRT software. Since IRT models are probabilistic models, most fit indices measure deviations between the predicted and observed response-frequencies. The citations above describe many types of residual analyses that can be used to evaluate model fit.

Applying IRT to evaluate item and scale properties and to suggest scale improvement

Item threshold levels and discrimination can be plotted as ICCs and information curves, to show the contribution of each question to the scale. This enables evaluation of how well an item performs in terms of its relevance or contribution for measuring the underlying construct, the level of the underlying construct targeted by the question, the possible redundancy of the item relative to other items in the scale, and the appropriateness of the response categories. Item-level information can be combined to provide pictures of how well the scale performs in terms of breadth and depth of coverage across the construct. IRT models provide a powerful tool for development of scales that are short, reliable, and targeted towards their study population.

Relevance and difficulty of the item content

Multi-item scales may measure latent constructs such as mental health, fatigue or patient satisfaction with medical care. In such scales not all items will be equally strongly associated with the underlying factor. The stronger the relationship, the better that item is for estimating a person's score. There are a number of ways to evaluate the relevance of items. Applying classical test theory (CTT), one would look at an item-score's correlation with the total scale score. In IRT, an item's relationship with the underlying construct is reflected in the discrimination parameter.

Table 1.5.3 presents CTT statistics and IRT parameter estimates for the 14 items making up the Mental Health Summary Scale. The column labelled 'item-total correlation' shows the different item-weights on the mental health construct. Questions such as 'Did you have a lot of energy?' and 'Have you felt downhearted and blue?' have high

Table 1.5.3 Mental health item properties

Mental Health Questions	CTT Statistics			IRT Model Item Properties					
	Mean (SD)	Item-total correlation	Alpha if item deleted	a	$b1$	$b2$	$b3$	$b4$	$b5$
Did you feel full of pep?	3.50 (1.32)	0.71	0.89	2.67	-1.64	-0.89	0.06	0.63	2.31
Did you have a lot of energy?	3.41 (1.35)	0.73	0.89	2.90	-1.48	-0.74	0.11	0.70	2.20
Did you feel worn out?	4.29 (1.24)	0.67	0.89	2.04	-2.62	-1.58	-1.01	0.04	1.35
Did you feel tired?	3.92 (1.20)	0.68	0.89	2.19	-2.29	-1.35	-0.65	0.49	2.03
What extent have your physical/emotional problems interfered with social activities?	4.25 (1.03)	0.64	0.89	2.11	-2.8	-1.79	-1.03	-0.22	
How much time have physical/emotional problems interfered with social activities?	4.18 (1.04)	0.65	0.89	2.04	-2.85	-1.90	-0.85	-0.09	
Cut down the amount of time you spent on work or other activities?	1.80 (0.40)	0.53	0.90	1.96	-1.08				
Accomplished less than you would like?	1.60 (0.49)	0.55	0.90	1.82	-0.34				
Didn't do work or other activities as carefully as usual?	1.76 (0.43)	0.50	0.90	1.65	-0.98				
Have you been a very nervous person?	4.97 (1.13)	0.48	0.90	1.05	-4.89	-3.31	-2.53	-1.03	0.48
Have you felt so down in the dumps that nothing could cheer you up?	5.40 (1.00)	0.61	0.90	1.71	-3.43	-2.87	-2.46	-1.41	-0.49
Have you felt calm and peaceful?	3.93 (1.25)	0.63	0.89	1.72	-2.56	-1.49	-0.52	0.24	2.51
Have you felt downhearted and blue?	4.97 (1.10)	0.67	0.89	1.73	-3.31	-2.51	-1.91	-0.78	0.43
Have you been a happy person?	4.48 (1.10)	0.59	0.90	1.62	-3.55	-2.33	-1.17	-0.44	1.69

Note: Some of the item wordings have been cut to minimize table space. IRT item parameter estimates (a = discrimination parameter, b = threshold parameter) were generated using Samejima's (1969) Graded Response Model and using the IRT software MULTILOG (Thissen 1991). All items have been scored (or reverse-scored) so higher scores reflect better mental health.

item-total correlations ($r = 0.73$ and $r = 0.67$, respectively), and are helpful in defining the underlying construct. The question, 'Have you been a very nervous person?' has the lowest item-total correlation ($r = 0.48$). This same pattern of relationships can be observed in Table 1.5.3 when looking at the IRT discrimination (a) parameters estimated by Samejima's (1969) Graded Response Model. These relationships appear intuitively plausible given the phrasing of the items.

Not only is the relevance or discrimination of the item important, but also its *difficulty* or *location*. 'Difficulty' is borrowed from educational assessment, where the goal is to match item difficulty with student ability. For example, nothing is learned about six-grade students' math ability if they are given an easy math question that all can answer, or a difficult math problem that none can solve. Likewise, one learns little about a healthy person's mental state with a question like 'Do you have suicidal thoughts?' because most people would answer 'no'. However, that question becomes informative for people with high levels of depression.

In CTT, item difficulty is measured by mean scores. Table 1.5.3 presents mean scores for the 14 mental health items. These indicate item 'severity', with low means, indicating poor mental health. The question 'Have you felt so down in the dumps that nothing could cheer you up?' has a high mean score (5.40) corresponding to the response categories 'none-' or 'a little' of the time, which indicates the sample is mentally healthy. In IRT, item difficulty is reflected by the threshold parameters (b); this item has six response levels and thus five difficulty-parameters $b1$ to $b5$. The threshold parameters for this item are all negative, from -3.43 to -0.49, indicating that the item functions best when measuring people with poor mental health. Figure 1.5.5 summarizes this clearly – the dashed information curve shows 'down in the dumps' to be informative when measuring people with poor mental health, but uninformative for others.

Both item relevance (discrimination) and location (difficulty) are important features in determining the best items for a particular study population. Figure 1.5.5 provides two other item-information curves. To measure a person with poor mental health, the 'down in the dumps' question is most informative. To measure someone with average levels of mental health, the question, 'Have you accomplished less than you would like?' is the optimal choice. For someone with good to excellent mental health, the first two items are not appropriate but the question 'Have you been a happy person?' is the best choice. IRT modelling facilitates the task of picking questions that match items to the study population.

Evaluating appropriateness of response categories

One decision when developing a questionnaire is the choice of the item response options, from a simple dichotomous 'yes' or 'no' to a seven-point or more response scale. If pilot or other prior data are available, CTT and IRT can provide helpful information. In CTT, one can check response frequencies for under or over utilized categories, although this may lead to erroneous decisions. For example, the response categories and associated response frequencies for the question, 'Did you feel worn out?' were: 'all the time' 24; 'most of the time' 74; 'a good bit of the time' 89; 'some of the time' 266; 'a little of the time' 304; and

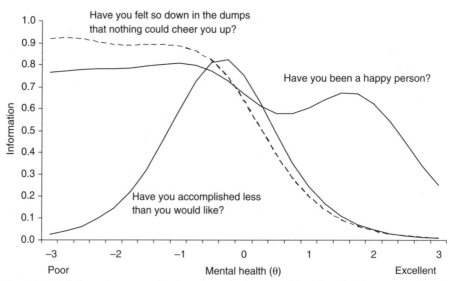

Fig. 1.5.5 IRT information curves for three items in the mental health scale. The 'accomplished less' question has two response options (note the narrow curve), and the other two items have six response categories, thus a broader curve.

'none of the time' 131. One might conclude that 'all of the time' and 'most of the time' were the less informative categories, but let's look at the IRT results.

In contrast to Figure 1.5.2 which showed an ideal picture of a well functioning item with spread out response categories, Figure 1.5.6 presents the ICCs for 'feeling worn out'. The category 'a good bit of the time' is overshadowed by 'most of the time' and 'some of the time'; nowhere along the mental health continuum was this response category more likely to be chosen than other options. Thus 'a good bit of the time' could be dropped. The first two response categories should be retained, despite the results from CTT analysis, because they measure poor mental health functioning.

Finally, ICCs for the question, 'Have you felt so down in the dumps that nothing could cheer you up?' are presented in Figure 1.5.7. The ICCs show that only 'some of the time', 'a little of the time' and 'none of the time' are utilized by this sample. When an ICC shows one response category covering a large area of the θ-continuum, additional categories may be desirable.

Evaluating item redundancy

CTT attempts to increase reliability by lengthening multi-item scales. Often this results in questionnaires with items that are redundant in content but different in phrasing. For example, the first four items in Table 1.5.3 belong to the Vitality subscale. Not surprisingly, the items for 'pep', 'energy', (not) 'worn out' and (not) 'tired' are highly correlated and have very high internal consistency (α-reliability = 0.89). However, short questionnaires are strongly preferred for health outcomes populations.

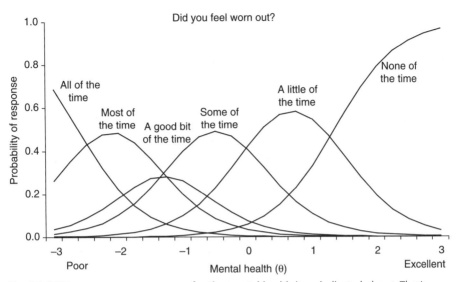

Fig. 1.5.6 IRT category response curves for the mental health item indicated above. The 'a good bit of the time' response is overshadowed by its neighbor categories suggesting this option may need to be considered to be dropped in future revisions of the scale.

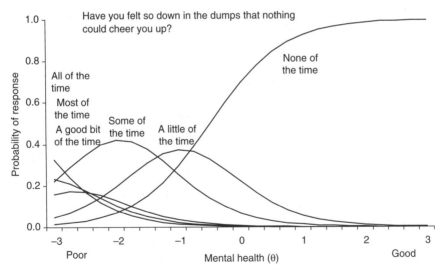

Fig. 1.5.7 IRT category response curves for the mental health item indicated above. Most respondents endorse 'none of the time' for this 'down in the dumps' question. Responses to the other five response categories suggest poor mental health.

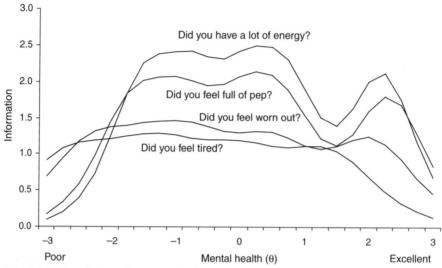

Fig. 1.5.8 IRT item information curves for four vitality questions in the mental health scale.

The item information curves, in Figure 1.5.8, indicate content redundancy for these two item pairs. The pair of curves for the 'energy' and 'pep' have identical patterns, as do those for the 'tired' and 'worn out'; they provide redundant information. Little content information is lost if the questionnaire is shortened by deleting the 'pep' and 'worn out' items. While the redundancy among these items is also apparent from reading the item content, there are times when two or more seemingly very different items can still occupy the same informational space, and the developer may wish to remove one of them to shorten the questionnaire.

Evaluating content equivalence – differential item functioning

Questions should be equally applicable to all targeted populations. Thus a lot of care is taken when instruments are translated to other languages. However, despite linguistic equivalence, populations may give culturally different responses. In a depression questionnaire, Azocar *et al.* (2001) found that a Latino population endorsed 'I feel like crying' more than an Anglo population, because Latinos regard crying as socially acceptable behaviour. This resulted in Latinos receiving a higher average depression score than Anglos. This is known as differential item functioning (DIF).

DIF occurs whenever one group consistently responds differently to an item than another group. In other words, respondents with similar levels of θ have different probability of responding to an item according to their population membership. Scales containing such items have reduced validity for between-group comparisons because their scores are influenced by a variety of attributes other than those intended.

IRT provides an attractive framework for identifying items with DIF. Item characteristic curves (ICCs) can be estimated separately for each group. Differences between the ICCs indicate that the probabilities of item endorsement vary according to group membership.

DIF detection and interpretation is discussed in greater detail in the chapter by Groenvold and Petersen. DIF analysis has been used to detect item equivalence across racial, gender, cultural, and treatment groups; and between two administration modes (e.g. telephone versus self-administered) and two translated language versions (Azocar *et al.* 2001; Morales *et al.* 2000; Teresi 2001; Fleishman *et al.* 2002; Orlando and Marshall 2002).

Scale analysis using IRT models

IRT scale analysis consists of evaluating scale information/reliability and the standard error of measurement (SEM), as in Figure 1.5.4. In contrast, CTT estimates a single reliability coefficient for all score values (usually Cronbach's α). Cronbach's α-reliability for the 14-item MH scale was 0.90, which implies that the scale is adequate. It is more likely, however, that the reliability varies, depending on who is being measured. Figure 1.5.4 shows that reliability is very high ($r > 0.90$) for individuals with low to middle levels of mental health (i.e., $-2.5 < \theta < 1$), and less precise, although still adequate, outside this range. The SEM for moderate to low mental health scores can be calculated to be approximately $1/\sqrt{11} = 0.3$, whereas for higher scores it rises to $1/\sqrt{3} = 0.58$. In CTT, the SEM for all score levels was 0.31.

The IRT scale information, and equivalently the SEM curve, evaluates the performance of an instrument. A developer wishing to shorten the instrument can delete an item and recalculate the new scale information curve to see the consequences. Information curves can also indicate areas for improvement. In our example, the curve suggests adding more items that discriminate among people who have good or excellent mental health.

Key methodological considerations for IRT modelling

Should I use CTT or IRT methods?

Applying IRT models does not imply abandoning CTT. Rather, IRT complements CTT to provide thorough analysis of an instrument. A researcher skilled in CTT could have found similar psychometric issues in the MH Summary scale to those we demonstrated. However, the ability of IRT models to describe item functioning along a continuum cannot be easily achieved with CTT. Major benefits of IRT are its comprehensive representation of content, and its ability to determine the optimal number of response categories for individual items.

Other sound and appealing features of IRT modelling are discussed in Embretson and Reise (2000) and Reeve (2003). One essential feature is that item properties are invariant with respect to the sample of respondents. This means that the threshold and discrimination parameters remain stable even when the items are administered to different groups of people. It is this item-parameter invariance that makes IRT ideal for evaluating DIF across groups. It also enables 'test-equating', which is the linking onto a common metric of two or more questionnaires that measure the same domain. Furthermore, person scores are also invariant with respect to the set of questions used in an IRT-based scale. This provides the basis for computerized adaptive testing, where respondents receive different sets of questions but their scores can be compared.

Which IRT model should I use?

This is a difficult question and there is no single answer to it; we offer one perspective. Several key factors are involved in deciding which model to use: (1) the number of item response categories; (2) the construct being measured; (3) the purpose of the study; and (4) the sample size (discussed in the next section). First, the number of response categories limits the choice of IRT models, as described in Table 1.5.2.

Second, the nature of the construct being measured will affect the choice of model. Models in Table 1.5.2 assume that a single domain is the only factor affecting a person's responses to the items in the scale. However, complete unidimensionality, especially in HRQoL assessment, is rare, and the researcher must decide how much this assumption can be relaxed. While IRT models are robust to minor violations of the unidimensionality assumption, the greater the departure from this, the less satisfactory the model. Non-Rasch two-parameter models, which allow discrimination to vary from item to item, are more robust to departures from unidimensionality than Rasch models which assume equal loading of each item on the underlying construct. Rasch models may be a good choice for measuring constructs like mobility, where questions such as 'Can you walk a short distance?' and 'Can you run a mile?' have an obvious hierarchical ordering of difficulty. Many HRQoL domains are multifaceted and items in such a scale will have different relationships (correlations) with the underlying construct. Non-Rasch models may then be the more appropriate choice for reflecting item properties. However, there is a divide between those psychometricians who will only use Rasch models because of their strong statistical properties, and those who will use any IRT model (including Rasch) to find the best fit and the best interpretation.

The choice of model relates also to the purpose of the study. Non-Rasch models may be better for capturing the nature of the questions and the respondents' behaviour to the questions, and may be better for evaluating the psychometric properties of a questionnaire if data have been collected on an existing instrument. However, Rasch models may be appropriate for defining behaviour according to well-understood mathematical rules. It may also be possible to revise a questionnaire, selecting only items that meet the strict assumptions of this model, especially when choosing items from a large pool.

Other models exist. Multi-dimensional IRT models (Wilson in press) can improve the measurement of each domain by using information from other correlated domains. The added information improves reliability, especially for scales with few items. Non-parametric IRT models (Ramsay 1997) are helpful when sampling distributions are skewed, when respondent behaviour to items does not form a monotonically increasing item characteristic curve across the θ continuum, or when one needs an initial estimate for an exploratory look at the response data.

For a more complete discussion of IRT models, see Embretson and Reise (2000), Thissen and Wainer (2001), and van der Linden and Hambleton (1997).

What sample size does one need for IRT analysis?

There are many issues involved, and no definitive answer. We briefly address the main issues. First, the choice of IRT model affects the required sample sizes: Rasch models estimate fewest parameters, and thus smaller sample sizes are adequate for stable parameter estimates – perhaps as few as 100 (Linacre 1994, suggests 50 for the simplest Rasch model). This makes Rasch models attractive to health outcomes researchers, as large samples are often unavailable. For non-Rasch models, it has been shown that the Graded Response IRT Model can be estimated with 250 respondents, but around 500 are recommended for accurate parameter estimates (Embretson and Reise 2000). Non-Rasch software typically employs maximum-likelihood routines to estimate IRT parameters, and requires larger sample sizes for estimation.

Study purpose can affect the sample size. To evaluate questionnaire properties, one does not need large sample sizes for a clear picture of response behaviour, although it is important to have a heterogeneous sample that accurately reflects the range of population characteristics. But if the purpose is to generate accurate IRT scores for a questionnaire, or to calibrate items in an item bank for CAT, sample sizes over 500 are required.

Another important consideration is the sampling distribution of the patients. Ideally, patients should be spread fairly uniformly over the range of interest. Items at extreme ends of the construct will have higher standard errors associated with their estimated parameters if fewer people are located there. The size of standard error that is acceptable will depend on the researcher's measurement goals.

The better the item response data meet the IRT assumptions of unidimensionality, conditional independence, and hierarchical ordering by difficulty, the smaller the sample size need be. Also, the relationship between the items and the measured construct is important, as poorly related items may require larger sample sizes (Thissen 2003). Increasing the number of response categories also increases the need for larger samples, as more item parameters must be estimated. The ideal is to have respondents in each cell of all possible response patterns for a set of items; however, this is rarely achieved. At the least, it is important to have some people respond to each of the categories for every item to allow the IRT model to be fully estimated.

Conclusion

The main goal of this introductory IRT chapter was to demonstrate the wealth of information that can be gained by using these models. IRT is invaluable for evaluating the psychometric properties of both new and existing scales, and for revising questionnaires based on these findings. We have shown how item-characteristic curves can evaluate the response categories for items, and how this helps questionnaire developers determine whether more or fewer response categories are needed. We have illustrated how information curves enable developers to evaluate item and scale functioning over the range of the underlying construct, allowing developers to tailor their instrument for maximum precision when measuring study populations.

The real attraction of IRT models to the health outcomes community is the application of computer adaptive tests (CAT), which integrate the powerful features of IRT with the advances in computer technology. CAT delivers dynamic measures that tailor each questionnaire for each individual, based on information provided by their responses to previous questions. Therefore each person receives a different set of questions, yet their scores can be combined or compared with others because the items have been calibrated by IRT models. CAT offers shorter yet more reliable questionnaires that can for example be administered over Internet or personal handheld devices. The chapter by Bjorner and Ware provides details of CAT.

If IRT provides so many useful tools for evaluating and developing instruments, why is its use not more widespread? Several obstacles limit the use of IRT. First, most researchers have been trained in CTT statistics, are comfortable interpreting these statistics, and can easily generate from readily available software the familiar summary statistics such as Cronbach's α. In contrast, IRT models require advanced knowledge of measurement theory to understand their mathematical complexity, to check that assumptions are met, and to choose the appropriate model. In addition, supporting software and literature are not well adapted for researchers outside the field of educational measurement.

Despite the conceptual and computational challenges, the many potential advantages of IRT models should not be ignored. Knowledge of IRT is spreading within the academic disciplines of psychology, education, and public health. More books and tutorials are being written on the subject, and user-friendly software is being developed. Research that applies IRT models is appearing more frequently in health outcomes literature. A better understanding of the models and applications of IRT is emerging, and this will result in health outcomes instruments that are shorter, more reliable, and better targeted toward the populations of interest.

References

Azocar, F., Arean, P., Miranda, J., and Munoz, R. F. (2001). Differential item functioning in a Spanish translation of the Beck Depression Inventory. *Journal of Clinical Psychology*, **57** (3), 355–365.

Embretson, S. E. and Reise, S. P. (2000). *Item Response Theory for Psychologists*. Mahwah, NJ: Lawrence Erlbaum Associates.

Fleishman, J. A., Spector, W. D., and Altman, B. M. (2002). Impact of differential item functioning on age and gender differences in functional disability. *Journal of Gerontology: Social Sciences*, **57B** (5), S275–S284.

Hambleton, R. K., Robin, F., and Xing, D. (2000). Item response models for the analysis of educational and psychological test data. In H. Tinsley and S. Brown S. (eds), *Handbook of Applied Multivariate Statistics and Mathematical Modeling*, pp. 553–585. San Diego, CA: Academic Press.

Hays, R. D. and Morales, L. S. (2001). The RAND-36 measure of health-related quality of life. *Annals of Medicine*, **33**, 350–357.

Linacre, J. M. (1994). Sample size and item calibration stability. *Rasch Measurement Transactions*, **7**, 4, 328.

Morales, L. S., Reise, S. P., and Hays, R. D. (2000). Evaluating the equivalence of health care ratings by whites and Hispanics. *Medical Care*, **38** (5), 517–527.

Orlando, M. and Marshall, G. N. (2002). Differential item functioning in a Spanish translation of the PTSD checklist: detection and evaluation of impact. *Psychological Assessment*, **14** (1), 50–59.

Orlando, M. and Thissen, D. (2000). Likelihood-based item-fit indices for dichotomous item response theory models. *Applied Psychological Measurement*, **24**, 50–64.

Ramsay, J. O. (1997). A functional approach to modeling test data. In W. J. van der Linder and R. K. Hambleton (eds) *Handbook of Modern Item Response Theory*, pp. 381–394. New York: Springer.

Reeve, B. B. (2003). Item response theory modeling in health outcomes measurement. *Expert Review of Pharmacoeconomics and Outcomes Research*, **3** (2), 131–145.

Reise, S. P. (in press). Item response theory and its applications for cancer outcomes measurement, In J. Lipscomb, C. Gotay and C. Snyder (eds), *Outcomes Assessment in Cancer*. Cambridge: Cambridge University Press.

Samejima, F. (1969). Estimation of latent ability using a response pattern of graded scores, *Psychometrika Monographs*, **34** (4) Pt. **2**, Whole No. 17.

Teresi, J. A. (2001). Statistical methods for examination of differential item functioning (DIF) with applications to cross-cultural measurement of functional, physical and mental health, *Journal of Mental Health and Aging*, **7** (1), 31–40.

Thissen, D. (1991). *MULTILOG User's Guide, Version 6.3*. Chicago, IL: Scientific Software.

Thissen, D. (2003). Estimation in Multilog. In M. du Toit (ed.) *IRT from SSI: Bilog-MG, Multilog, Parscale, Testfact*. Lincolnwood, IL: Scientific Software International.

Thissen, D. and Wainer, H. (eds) (2001). *Test Scoring*. Mahwah, NJ: Lawrence Erlbaum Associates.

van der Linden, W. J., and Hambleton, R. K. (eds) (1997). *Handbook of Modern Item Response Theory*. New York, NY: Springer-Verlag.

Ware J.E. and Sherbourne, C. D. (1992). The MOS 36-Item Short-Form Health Survey (SF-36): I. Conceptual framework and item selection. *Medical Care*, **30**, 473–83.

Wilson, M. (in press). Subscales and summary scales: issues in health-related outcomes. In J. Lipscomb, C. Gotay, and C. Snyder (eds) *Outcomes Assessment in Cancer*. Cambridge: Cambridge University Press.

Section 2

Adapting and using questionnaires

Translating and evaluating questionnaires: cultural issues for international research

Patrick Marquis, Dorothy Keininger, Catherine Acquadro and Christine de la Loge

Introduction

Advances in new technologies (Schieber *et al.* 1993; Gold *et al.* 1996) and changes in lifestyles have resulted in a shift from acute life-threatening illnesses to an increased prevalence of chronic and long-term illnesses (CDC 1994, 2002) in an ageing population (Fieldstein 1993). To better understand the consequences of chronic conditions on patients' lives and to evaluate the benefit of new treatments, researchers are developing more meaningful end points based on patients' perceptions. Therefore, Patient Reported Outcomes (PRO) questionnaires, including quality of life questionnaires, are being developed, evaluated and used in clinical research with increasing frequency. PROs inform patient management and are utilized in policy decisions (Guyatt *et al.* 1993; Schipper *et al.* 1996; Apolone *et al.* 2001; Burke 2001). They are also used as criteria for licensing and promoting new medicines. For example, a recent survey conducted by the FDA shows that one-third of all newly registered medicines between 1997 and 2002 were approved with a PRO claim on the label (Burke 2003).

Due to the international nature of clinical research, the globalization of the market and cost constraints (Schieber *et al.* 1993; Gold *et al.* 1996), the need for cross-culturally valid PRO questionnaires has grown considerably. However, linguistic and cultural differences present unique challenges in the development and evaluation of PROs. Although one can argue that those challenges have been the focus of cross-cultural psychology for many years and are not unique (Berry *et al.* 1992), it is important to note the distinction between cross-cultural psychological and clinical research (Table 2.1.1). Cross-cultural psychological research has historically focused on identifying and quantifying cultural differences and involves the comparison of cultures, whereas international clinical researchers are interested in the effects of treatments on the outcomes measured in different cultures. Moreover, when measuring outcomes in different cultures, clinical researchers strive to minimize bias and other confounding

Table 2.1.1 Characteristics of questionnaires for use in cross-cultural psychology versus cross-cultural clinical research

	Cross-cultural psychology research	**Cross-cultural clinical research**
Main objective	Comparison of cultures	Comparison of treatment effect across cultures
Key property	Ability to discriminate	Responsiveness over time
Role of culture questionnaire outcomes in the model	The culture is the dependant variable The outcomes measured by the questionnaire are independent variables	The outcomes measured by the questionnaire is the dependant variable The culture is an independent confounding variable
Data aggregation across languages	Not needed	Mandatory to reach sufficient power for the analysis of treatment effect
Equivalence required	Construct equivalence Scalar equivalence	Concept equivalence Construct equivalence Metric equivalence

factors related to cultures and languages. Indeed, clinical researchers typically strive to obtain equivalence across cultures in their outcomes assessments in order to validate the aggregation of data from multiple cultures for analysis. Therefore, the requirements for developing, translating and evaluating PRO questionnaires for use in international clinical programs are specific; in particular, possible bias related to cross-cultural issues should be minimized. The critical question for cross-cultural clinical research is under which conditions data from a multi-language trial may be aggregated for a meaningful and valid treatment analysis.

Before reviewing translation, it is important to understand the objectives of translation and any potential factors that may interfere with achieving these objectives fully.

Objectives of translation

In international clinical programs, the primary objective of translations for measuring PROs is to develop a cross-culturally equivalent questionnaire. In other words, the goal for the translated versions is to elicit responses from patients equal to those obtained through the original questionnaire version, in a population with the same clinical status and the same general characteristics, such as age and gender, as the original culture.

Unquestionably, a simple translation is insufficient for achieving this objective. Rather, a process involving two stages, linguistic and psychometric, must be conducted. The linguistic stage focuses on translating the concepts measured by the original version of the questionnaire into equivalent concepts in other languages (i.e., other cultures). The second stage is the psychometric testing of the questionnaire. This stage is fundamental, because equivalence is a measurement characteristic that can be demonstrated only through the analysis of measurement properties and their consistency with the original questionnaire performances. The initial linguistic stage should be viewed only as a means for achieving equivalence and as a way to properly handle the possible bias resulting from the process of adapting a questionnaire into another language. This entire process is often referred to as linguistic validation, even though this term is ambiguous in its meaning.

Bias and equivalence in cross-cultural research

Bias or differential item functioning

Systematic differences or bias, such as a tendency for one cultural group to score an item systematically too high or too low, threaten the validity of cross-cultural comparisons. The literature refers more and more to the term differential item functioning (DIF) rather than 'bias'. Typically, three types of bias are considered in cross-cultural research: method bias, item bias and construct bias. Method bias refers to characteristics of the instrument or its administration. For example, in relation to instrument characteristics, Hui and Triandis (1989) found that Hispanics tended to choose extremes on a five-point scale more often than Caucasian Americans. Differences in physical conditions during administration can also lead to method bias. Such differences include a noisy environment, the presence of other people or communication problems between the examiner and interviewer. Item bias refers to measurement error at the item level due to inadequate translation or inappropriate item formulation, including inappropriate translation of the response scale. Finally, construct bias occurs when the construct measured is not identical across the cultural groups. The construct, also referred to as the domain, is comprised of the aggregation of all concepts (represented by each item) relevant for the construct. For example, the four items assessing the different aspects of fatigue and energy (full of pep, lot of energy, worn out, tired) have been gathered under the construct 'vitality' in the SF-36. A construct may demonstrate poor content validity after translation into another language because some concepts important in the original culture are not relevant in the new culture, or because additional concepts should be measured in the new culture to obtain satisfactory content validity for the construct.

These biases may be related to cultural differences regarding the concepts of health and illness, levels of literacy, concordance between written and spoken versions of language, taboo subjects and social desirability effects. Furthermore, idioms, which abound in some PRO questionnaires, are very difficult to translate. Table 2.1.2 describes the causes of different types of bias and assesses the ability of a thorough translation process for addressing these issues.

It is obvious that a literal or simple translation of items into other languages cannot prevent pitfalls and cultural issues. Although a thorough translation process should be

Table 2.1.2 Types and causes of bias and ability to address them through thorough translation

		Ability of a thorough translation to address the bias
Item bias	Poor item translation	Yes
	Inadequate item formulation or inappropriateness of the item content	Yes
	Additional traits or abilities held by the item	Yes
Method bias	Differential in social desirability	No
	Differential in response style such as extreme choices or acquiescence	No
	Differential in the familiarity with item content	No in most cases
Construct bias	Lack of overlap in the definition of the construct (i.e., domain)	No
	Lack of appropriateness of the content of the construct	No in most cases
	Incomplete coverage of the construct (i.e., domain)	No

able to address most of the issues related to translation quality and the relevance of concepts, it will not solve issues related to the cultural compatibility of the constructs measured and their exhaustiveness (content validity) in other cultures.

In fact, regardless of the quality of the translation process, situations will arise in which a questionnaire or a particular question is not applicable for some cultures. Adapting a question that is highly specific to a given culture will be impossible if the underlying concept measured is not relevant or salient for the target culture. In these cases, the translation should not be 'forced' by trying to obtain a translation for a question. Rather, it may be concluded that the item is culture-specific and should therefore be excluded from a cross-cultural instrument.

Equivalence

To date, there has been no consensus in the PRO field as to the minimum requirements for establishing that translations of a questionnaire are cross-culturally equivalent to the original and appropriate for aggregation of data. Indeed, there is a lack of clarity in the PRO literature as to which types of equivalence are defined. Herdman *et al.* (1998) clearly illustrate the need for providing lucidity in this area, when they indicate that there are at least 19 different types of 'equivalence' used by different authors and when they explain that the term 'conceptual equivalence' is used in numerous ways.

Hui and Triandis (1985) proposed four types of equivalence in cross-cultural psychology: conceptual or functional equivalence (i.e., equivalence of the construct), equivalence in the operationalization of the construct (i.e., construct operationalized or measured with the same procedure), item equivalence (i.e., the same questionnaire with the same items carrying the same meaning) and scalar equivalence (same metric). This comprehensive approach is difficult to apply in the PRO field because, in the vast majority of cases, the foreign versions of a questionnaire are obtained through translations performed from an original version developed in one culture. This method, called sequential (see below), does not integrate the analysis of the different concepts composing the construct in each country. Therefore, the equivalence of the theoretical construct is not assessed. Instead translation concentrates on item equivalence. Each item must have identical meaning (must measure the same concept) within each culture. If an item has a different meaning in any of the various languages, then in effect two different concepts are being evaluated and any combining of data or comparisons of scores across those cultures are inappropriate. However, the PRO field appears to have adopted a pragmatic approach, demonstrated by the fact that the majority of translation guidelines assume that constructs are relevant and equivalent across cultures. These guidelines do not require an initial investigation of the relevance and content validity of the theoretical constructs measured by a questionnaire in other cultures.

Van de Vijver and Leung (1997) proposed a simple version of cross-cultural equivalence based on three types: construct (or structure) equivalence, measurement unit equivalence (identical measurement unit, but different origins of the scales) and scalar equivalence (ratio level). This classification helps PRO researchers better understand the level of equivalence that can be claimed for a questionnaire targeted to cross-cultural research. However, the level of equivalence which can be claimed across cultures depends on the method used to obtain the versions in multiple languages.

Existing methods to obtain a questionnaire in multiple languages

Multiple methods exist for obtaining a questionnaire in different languages. Each method has its own advantages and disadvantages. Traditionally, multiple language versions of a questionnaire have been achieved through the translation of an existing questionnaire. This process is referred to as a sequential model. Alternatives to this process are parallel and simultaneous development of a questionnaire in multiple language versions (Bullinger *et al.* 1993). The way in which researchers conduct these processes may vary. A review of the various methodologies of sequential, parallel and simultaneous instrument development is provided in the following section.

Sequential approach for multi-language versions

Previously in this chapter, the sequential process of adapting an original language questionnaire version (i.e., source) into one or more languages (i.e., target) was referred to as the linguistic process or translation. This has been the traditional method of adaptation. Over time, researchers have created many guidelines for this process. A review of relevant papers published between January 1966 and February 2003, identified in Medline and Embase, and a specific research in Mapi Research Institute database, revealed 18 key references for 12 translation guidelines (Table 2.1.3): among them three are unpublished. These guidelines can be grouped into two categories: those developed specifically for a questionnaire (FACT, SF-36, SIP, NHP and STAI) and those proposed for a broader range of questionnaires by various organizations (AAOS, Mapi Research Institute, Mathias and colleagues and MOT). The translation methodologies of the organizations that provided the translation guidelines currently applied are summarized in Table 2.1.4.

All guidelines fit the sequential model in that they began with an existing or source questionnaire, which is subsequently translated into target languages. These guidelines discuss various methods for addressing the subjectivity of PRO questionnaire translation. However, they provide relatively little information about the requirements, qualifications or characteristics of the people involved in the processes. All guidelines utilize a multi-step process that includes at least one forward translation, a backward translation, expert review, pre-testing with patients and investigation of the measurement properties of the translated versions. The guidelines differ in that they reflect theoretical differences between research groups, e.g., definitions of equivalence (Beaton *et al.* 2000; Stewart and Napoles-Springer 2000) and approaches for development (Bullinger *et al.* 1996) as well as the trade-offs made by each group, e.g., available resources (Mathias *et al.* 1994; Guyatt 1993).

Interestingly, translatability assessment, whose objective is to investigate relevance of concepts to be translated in other cultures and the feasibility of their translation, was mentioned in only one group's guidelines (MAPI Research Institute), although it limits the threat of bias and therefore constitutes an important step in the linguistic validation process. Performing a translatability assessment on the original version prior to questionnaire translation helps evaluate the relevance of the concepts in each of the target languages. Subsequently, any concepts carried by items that are identified as irrelevant for a target language can be considered for deletion or modification in the original version. Thus, when a questionnaire is considered for international research, it is recommended that translatability be assessed at the early development phase.

Certainly, instrument translation that utilizes a rigorous methodology and involves qualified teams is the appropriate method for obtaining other language versions of a previously developed instrument. However, when an instrument is not available or is under development, parallel and simultaneous development are valuable alternatives.

Table 2.1.3 Key references for translation guidelines

Scientific Advisory Committee of the Medical Outcomes Trust (2002). Assessing health status and quality of life instruments: attributes and review. *Quality of Life Research,* **11,** 193–205.

Skevington, S. M. (2002). Advancing cross-cultural research on quality of life: observations drawn from the WHOQOL development. *Quality of Life Research,* **11,** 135–144.

Conway, K., Mear, I., Giroudet, C., Acquadro, C. (2001). Mapi Research Institute's manual for the linguistic validation of HRQL questionnaires. Unpublished document.

Beaton, D. E., Bombardier, C., Guillemin, F., Ferraz, M. B. (2000). Guidelines for the process of cross-cultural adaptation of self-report measures. *Spine,* **25,** (24), 3186–3191.

Bullinger, M., Alonso, A., Apolone, G. *et al.* (1998). Translating health status questionnaires and evaluating their quality: the IQOLA approach. *J Clin Epidemiol,* **51,** (11), 913–923.

Herdman, M., Fox-Rushby, J., Badia, X. (1998). A model of equivalence in the cultural adaptation of HRQL instruments: the universalist approach. *Quality of Life Research,* **7,** 323–335.

Herdman, M., Fox-Rushby, J., Badia, X. (1997). Equivalence and the translation and adaptation of health-related quality of life questionnaires. *Quality of Life Research,* **6,** 237–247.

Bonomi, A. E., Cella, D. F., Hahn, E. A. *et al.* (1996). Multilingual translations of the Functional Assessment of Cancer Therapy (FACT) quality of life measurement system. *Quality of Life Research,* **5,** 309–320.

The Johns Hopkins University. Guidelines for translation of the Sickness Impact Profile. Unpublished Document. January 1996.

Ware, J. E., Keller, S. D., Gandek, B. *et al.* (1995). Evaluating translations of health status questionnaires: methods from the IQOLA project. *International Journal of Technology Assessment in Health Care,* **11,** (3), 525–551.

Mathias, S. D., Fifer, S. K., Patrick, D. L. (1994). Rapid translation of quality of life measures for international clinical trials: avoiding errors in the minimalist approach. *Quality of Life Research,* **3,** 403–412.

Sartorius, N., Kuyken, W. (1994). Translation of health status instruments. In J. Orley, W. Kuyken (eds) *Quality of Life Assessment: International perspectives,* pp. 3–18. Berlin, Heidelberg: Springer Verlag.

Guillemin, F., Bombardier, C., Beaton, D. (1993). Cross-cultural adaptation of health-related quality of life measures: literature review and proposed guidelines. *J Clin Epidemiol,* **46,** (12), 1417–1432.

European Group for Health Measurement and Quality of Life Assessment: Hunt, S. M., Alonso, J., Bucquet, D., Niero M., Wiklund, I., Mckenna, S. (1991). Cross-cultural adaptation of health measures. *Health Policy,* **19,** 33–44.

Hunt, S. M. (1986). Cross-cultural issues in the use of socio-medical indicators. *Health Policy,* **6,** 149–158.

Spielberger, C. D., Sharma, S. (1976). Cross-cultural measurement of anxiety. In C. D. Spielberger, R. Diaz-Guerrero (eds) *Cross-cultural Anxiety,* pp. 13–28. Washington: Hemisphere Pub.

Table 2.1.4 Overview of translation guidelines

Reference	Recruitment criteria	Forward translation	Back translation	Expert review	Content and face validity testing	Specificities
Medical Outcomes Trust Scientific Advisory Committee 2002	Not reported	At least two forward translations; synthesis of results.	At least one.	Yes, by lay and expert panels.		
World Health Organization Skevington et al. 2002	Team members described in detail with motivation for the requirements.	Two translators work together. Bilingual panel reviews translation and a monolingual panel 'tests' the instrument. Bilingual panel then modifies the translation.	Yes, one translation	Forward and back translations are administered to a bilingual group. Alternatively, a bilingual panel assesses equivalence.		
MAPI Research Institute Conway et al. 2001 Unpublished	Detailed requirements for each member of the team are specified in the paper. The entire process takes place in the target culture.	Two translators residing in the target country work independently. Results are synthesized in collaboration with the instrument's developer.	One translator with no knowledge of the source version.	Yes, in consultation with the developer.	Two parallel phases: Clinician's review (users) Cognitive debriefing with a sample of five to ten respondents	The method emphasizes clear justification and documentation of each step. International harmonization is also done when a PRO is linguistically validated in more than one language at the same time.

Reference	Translator qualifications	Forward translation	Back translation	Review committee	Pretest	Comments
American Association of Orthopedic Surgeons Beaton et al. 2000	Bilingual translators	Two translators work independently; synthesis conducted by the translators.	Two translators work independently with no knowledge of the underlying concepts.	Yes, methodologists, health professionals, language professionals and the translators.	Yes, n = 30–40 from the target setting, followed by interviews.	Method emphasizes clear justification and documentation of each step.
EuroQoL Group 2000 Unpublished	The guidelines specify that qualifications be reported.	Two native speakers in source (at least one with health-related experience) trained by the Project Manager and working independently. Synthesis conducted by two translators and the Project Manager.	Two back translators, native in English work independently on literal and 'polished' translation.	Yes, but it does not specify who makes the consensus version.	Eight subjects (preferably with low levels of education) including healthy individuals as well as patients respond to the PRO and are interviewed.	Detailed documentation is required.
EORTC Quality of Life Study Group Cull et al. 1998 Unpublished	Translators are native speakers, otherwise not specified.	Two (minimum) translators work independently. Reviewed by coordinator with the translators. Difficulties are resolved with the help of a new independent translator.	Two independent translators work independently.	Reviewed by coordinator with the translators. Difficulties are resolved with the help of a new independent translator.	Yes, n = 10–15 Individual interviews.	

Continued

Table 2.1.4 (*Continued*) Overview of translation guidelines

Reference	Recruitment criteria	Forward translation	Back translation	Expert review	Content and face validity testing	Specificities
IQOLA Bullinger *et al.* 1998	Not reported in these articles.	Minimum of two translators work independently and also rate difficulty. Synthesis of results first by original translators, then by two other translators who work independently	Yes, two translators evaluate the forward translation.	Yes, by US IQOLA team.	Yes, up to 50	Most rigorous method. Development time of a new version of the SF-36 is several years.
FACT Group Bonomi *et al.* 1996	Translators are native speakers of the target language, otherwise not reported.	Two translators: one living in US, one living in target country. Synthesis is developed by third translator	One by a fourth translator	Yes, reviewed by three to four bilingual health professionals from the target country.	Yes, 15–16 patients	
Johns Hopkins University – SIP 1996		Two translations who live in the target country (native tongue is the target language) and a focus group of two or more independent translators review each item and synthesize.	Yes, by at least one native in the source language.	A lay panel plus four to five experts review each item in the pooled forward translation, identify troublesome items and propose alternatives.	Yes, at least 50 'hedges' plus statistical testing to determine item and dimension weights in the target language. They also assess test-retest reliability and internal consistency.	The testing procedure is involved and time consuming.

European Group for Health Measurement and Quality of Life Assessment translation of the NHP Hunt et al. 1994	Panel members and other participants briefly described.	Translated by 8–12 from target population, consensus version produced. No synthesis of results is developed; however, 26 bilinguals respond to both original and consensus target version, differences compared.	Yes, for problem items only by teachers of English/target language.	Yes	Yes, subjects in the target culture responded to and discussed the PRO.	
Mathias et al. 1994	Certified translators, but not necessarily native speakers, all living in the source country.	One by a single translator.	Yes, by a different translator.	Yes, by the instrument developer.	Yes, three to five bilinguals living in the source country respond to both the original and target language versions. No focus group or debriefing step.	This method was used to simultaneously translate a PRO into 10 European languages and to modify the original. (International harmonization)
Spielberger et al. 1976	Psychologists, psychiatrist language experts. Academic grounding in psychometrics, test theory, extensive experience in the field in which translated scale will be used.	Number not specified. Synthesis of results referred to as preliminary translation step.	Yes.	Expert review.	On bilingual subjects.	Review of methods used to translate the STAI.

Parallel and simultaneous instrument development

Both parallel and simultaneous instrument development consider the relevance of concepts within constructs to each language from the beginning stage of questionnaire development. These two methods help ensure conceptual equivalence of concepts at each stage of questionnaire development, thereby producing a more robust measure. Such a measure will in theory be better adapted to different cultures and less sensitive to cultural specificities than questionnaires translated after the development process is complete (i.e., sequential).

These two processes begin with identification of relevant concepts in all final language versions. For the parallel process, items are generated in only one language (the source language) with subsequent translation into the target languages. In the simultaneous process, native speakers of each language from each country create items simultaneously. During the item generation process, both cultural differences and discrepancies in the language versions are resolved. In practical terms, no single source language is used in the simultaneous item generation process.

To be suitable for data pooling across languages, simultaneous questionnaire development should follow a standardized process. Simultaneous instrument development begins with the elicitation of important concepts in each culture based on patient interviews or focus groups. Results of interviews or focus groups are analyzed in each language to elicit a list of concepts. This list of relevant concepts in each language is utilized, along with verbatim quotes from patients, to develop items simultaneously in each language. Moreover, the overall preliminary structure and format of the instrument should be determined prior to developing items to ensure consistency across languages. This includes the conceptual model, the order of the domains in the questionnaire, response format and recall period. This defined structure (i.e., model) is then used to input generated items for each language version of the instrument. The simultaneous item generation process involves native representatives from each culture.

As with the development of all PRO questionnaires, each language version undergoes cognitive debriefing in each culture. The term 'debriefing' is commonly used because patients are asked to give their feedback on the questionnaire newly developed. This step is essential for determining conceptual equivalence. By interviewing patients in each country to assess their comprehension and to obtain their own explanations of the meanings of individual items, researchers can determine whether patients in different cultures understand the questions in the same way. Additionally, if proper and thorough cognitive debriefing methods are employed in the simultaneous development process, backward translation may not be necessary.

Examples of parallel development include the development of the European Organization for Research and Treatment of Cancer Quality of Life Questionnaire (EORTC QLQ-C30) (Cull *et al.* 1995), the European Quality of Life Questionnaire

(EQ-5D) (Brooks 1996). Although each of these questionnaires was developed following a parallel method, each varied in its process of development. For example, the EQ-5D was developed following discussions by multinational researchers from five countries. Questions were generated in one language and then forward and backward translated into multiple languages.

The World Health Organization Quality of Life Assessment (WHOQOL-100) (WHOQOL 1994; Power *et al.* 1999) is considered to be an example of a complex simultaneous development. The WHOQOL-100 development followed a methodology that included the development of a conceptual model and contribution of items from 15 centres around the world. From an initial pool of 1800 items, 236 were retained for the pilot testing. Repeated forward and backward translations were used to check the appropriateness of the items generated.

An other example of simultaneous instrument development is found in the work of Tanzer, Gittler and Ellis, who simultaneously developed an instrument in German and English to measure spatial ability (Tanzer *et al.* 1995).

When many languages are included, the burden and the complexity of implementing a simultaneous approach can be reduced by using a mix approach. The simultaneous approach is used for core languages, supplemented by a parallel approach or a translatability assessment for additional languages.

The three processes – sequential translation, parallel development and simultaneous development – use qualitative methods and evidence to target cross-cultural equivalence prior to the administration of the instrument in a population. After adapting a questionnaire into different languages, empirical evaluation of completed instruments is necessary for evaluating the equivalence of multiple language versions of a single instrument.

Existing methods to assess cross-cultural/metric equivalence

Multiple methods are employed to assess the construct validity and the metric properties of questionnaires. Their application for evaluating the cross-cultural equivalence of questionnaires deserves a stand-alone article. Although some of these methods are described fully in other chapters of this book, psychometric testing is a mandatory component of the assessment of cross-cultural equivalence. Thus, the most frequently used methods are discussed in this chapter. Currently, no guidelines address the testing of cross-cultural equivalence of PRO questionnaires for clinical research.

The most commonly used methods for assessing questionnaire structure and construct validity are exploratory factor analysis (primarily principal component analysis) and multi-trait scaling analysis. Although both analyses are based on correlations and are useful for assessing the construct validity of each version separately, they have several drawbacks when used to compare different language versions: (1) the qualitative nature of the results and the fact that they do not provide a global indice through which to judge the consistency/equivalence of the different language versions indicate that conclusions about equivalence are somewhat arbitrary; (2) the results are sample dependent and may be unstable; (3) the methods are insensitive to linear shift (a systematic shift with perfect correlation will not be detected with these correlation-based methods). Furthermore, when a questionnaire demonstrates similar factor loadings in various language groups, it does not imply that the scores of the instrument exhibit scalar or metric equivalence, as factor analysis is not appropriate for evaluating measurement units across cultures (Vijver and Leung 1997). However, results of a factorial analysis may enable the identification of differences in constructs and items deviant from expected loading, indicating that an inconsistent concept within the construct is being measured due to either poor translation or a specific cultural issue.

Structural equation modelling, including confirmatory factor analysis (Reise *et al.* 1993; Cary 1989) is more appropriate to evaluate the equivalence of constructs across different translations. Fit indices provide useful decision criteria regarding the validity of the overall structure across countries and for deviant items within constructs. These techniques have only been used in a few cases to evaluate a questionnaire cross-culturally (Keller *et al.* 1998; Marquis *et al.* 2001).

The use of more modern psychometric methods, such as Item Response Theory (IRT) (Thissen 1991; Lord and Norvick 1968; Rasch 1980; Raczek *et al.* 1998), provides a unique basis for evaluating cross-cultural equivalence through in-depth analysis of item performance, assessing their fit in the model and determining the overall quality of the model for evaluating the construct. IRT is a powerful tool used to assess the metric equivalence of scales.

Conclusion

Requirements for cross-cultural clinical research are not exactly the same as those for cross-cultural psychology. For cross-cultural clinical research, the ultimate goal is to pool data across languages in order to evaluate the effect of a treatment on an outcome measured by the same questionnaire. To achieve this objective, for each language, the concepts assessed by each item should be as identical as possible, the aggregation of items should result in the same constructs, and the metric of scales should be similar.

When a questionnaire has already been developed and used in one culture, the sequential approach based on a thorough translation is essential for controlling potential bias at the level of the items. A thorough translation process includes a forward–backward method implemented by a qualified team, followed by pilot testing with patients. However, this sequential approach relies on the assumption that the constructs of a questionnaire, and their content, are relevant and equivalent across cultures.

For questionnaires in development, the parallel approach and the simultaneous approach provide more insight regarding the relevance and suitability of constructs and their content across cultures (Table 2.1.5).

Table 2.1.5 Optimal approaches for handling cultural issues

Type of questionnaire	Optimal approach	Methods
For an existing questionnaire	Sequential approach	Thorough translation to obtain identical concepts in languages Content and construct imposed from the original culture into other cultures
For a questionnaire in development in one language, based on patient information collected in the same language	Translatability assessment followed by a sequential approach	Major cultural issues in concepts addressed before translation Amendment of the questionnaire based on translatability of concepts Thorough translation to obtain identical concepts in languages (facilitated by the translatability assessment) Content and construct imposed from the original culture into other cultures
For a questionnaire in development in one language, based on patient information collected in several languages	Parallel approach	Major cultural issues in concepts addressed before item generation Development of the questionnaire based on common, culturally relevant concepts Thorough translation to obtain identical concepts in languages (facilitated by the decision based on multicultural information) Common relevant content and construct across cultures
For a questionnaire developed simultaneously in several languages, based on patient information collected in different languages	Simultaneous approach	Major cultural issues in concepts and constructs addressed before item generation Development of the questionnaire based on common, culturally relevant concepts and on patient wording in different languages Thorough cognitive debriefing in different languages to ensure identical concepts in languages (facilitated by the decision based on multicultural information) Common relevant content and construct across cultures

Finally whatever the approach used, the linguistic stage should be followed by a psychometric evaluation that includes a test of the equivalence of the construct and the equivalence of the metric in order to produce a cross-culturally valid questionnaire for clinical research.

References

Apolone, G., De Carli, G., Brunetti, M., and Garattini, S. (2001). An evaluation of the EMEA recommendations on the use of quality of life measures in drug approval. *PharmacoEconomics*, **19**, (2), 187–195.

Beaton, D. E., Bombardier, C., Guillemin, F., and Ferraz, M. B. (2000). Guidelines for the process of cross-cultural adaptation of self-report measures. *Spine*, **25**, (24), 3186–3191.

Berry, J. W., Poortinga, Y. H., and Segall, M. H. *et al.* (1992). *Cross Cultural Psychology: Research and applications*. Cambridge, UK: Cambridge University Press.

Brooks, R. (1996). EuroQol: the current state of play. *Health Policy*, **37**, (1), 53–72.

Bullinger, M., Anderson, R., and Cella, D. *et al.* (2001). Developing and evaluating cross-cultural instruments from minimum requirements to optimal models. *Quality of Life Research*, **2**, 451–459.

Bullinger, M., Power, M. J., Aaronson, N. K., Cella, D. F., and Anderson, R. T. (1996). Creating and evaluating cross-cultural instruments. In B. Spilker (ed.) *Quality of Life and Pharmacoeconomics in Clinical Trials*, pp. 659–668, 2nd edn. Philadelphia: Lippincott-Raven Publishers.

Burke, L. (2000). Acceptable evidence for pharmaceutical advertising and labeling. DIA Workshop on Pharmacoeconomics and Quality of Life Labeling and Marketing Claims. New Orleans, LA October 3.

Burke, L. (2003). Progress in measuring PROs. Drug Information Association Conference. Baltimore, MD, 17 March 2003.

Cary, N. C. (1989). *SAS/STAT User's Guide*, Version 6, 4th edn.

CDC Chronic Disease Prevention (2002). *The Burden of Chronic Diseases and their Risk Factors: National and State Perspectives*. http://www.cdc.gov/nccdphp/burdenbook2002. Accessed November 2003.

CDC (1994). Prevalence of disability and associated health conditions – United States, 1991–1992. *MMWR* **43**, (40), 730–739.

Fieldstein, P. J. (1993). *Health Care Economics*, 4th edn. Albany, NY: Delmare Publishers Inc.

Gold, M. R., Siegel, J. E., and Russell, L. B. *et al.* (1996). *Cost-effectiveness in Health and Medicine*. New York: Oxford University Press.

Guyatt, G. H., Feeny, D. H., and Patrick, D. L. (1993). Measuring health-related quality of life. *Ann Intern Med*, **118**, 622–629.

Guyatt, G. H. (1993). The philosophy of health-related quality of life translation. *Quality of Life Research*, **2**, 461–465.

Herdman, M., Fox-Rushby, J., and Badia X. (1998). A model of equivalence in the cultural adaptation of HRQL instruments: the universalist approach. *Quality of Life Research*, **7**, 323–335.

Hui, C. H., Triandis, H. C. (1985). Measurement in cross-cultural psychology: a review and comparison of strategies. *Journal of Cross-Cultural Psychology*, **16**, (2), 131–152.

Keller, S. D., Ware, J. E. Jr., and Bentler, P. M. *et al.* (1998). Use of structural equation modeling to test the construct validity of the SF-36 health survey in ten countries: results from the IQOLA Project. *J Clin Epidemiol*, **51**, (11), 1179–1188.

Lord, F. M. and Norvick, M. R. (1968). *Statistical Theories of Mental Test Scores*. Reading: Addison-Wesley.

Marquis, P., Comte, S., and Lehert, P. (2001). International validation of the CLAU-S quality-of-life questionnaire for use in patients with intermittent claudication. *PharmacoEconomics*, **19**, (6), 667–677.

Mathias, S. D., Fifer, S. K., and Patrick, D. L. (1994). Rapid translation of quality of life measures for international clinical trials: avoiding errors in the minimalist approach. *Quality of Life Research*, **3**, 403–412.

Power, M., Bullinger, M., and Harper, A. (1999). The World Health Organization WHOQOL-100: tests of the universality of quality of life in 15 different cultural groups worldwide. *Health Psychology*, **8**, (5), 495–505.

Raczek, A. E., Ware, J. E., and Bjorner, J. B. *et al.* (1998). Comparison of Rasch and summated rating scales constructed from SF-36 physical functioning items in seven countries: results from the IQOLA Project. *J Clin Epidemiol*, **51**, (11), 1203–1214.

Rasch, G. (1980). *Probabilistic Models for some Intelligence and Attainment Tests*. Chicago, IL: University of Chicago Press.

Reise, S. P., Widaman, K. F., and Pugh, R. H. (1993). Confirmatory factor analysis and item response theory: two approaches for exploring measurement invariance. *Psychological Bulletin*, **114**, 552–566.

Schieber, G. J., Poullier, J. P., and Greenwald, L. M. (1993). Health spending, delivery and outcomes in OECD countries. *Health Affairs*, **12**, (12), 120–129.

Schipper, J., Clinch, J. J., and Olweny, C. L.M. (1996). *Quality of Life Studies: Definitions and conceptual issues. Quality of Life in Pharmacoeconomics in Clinical Trials*, 2nd edn. Philadelphia: Lippincott-Raven Publishers.

Sprangers, M. A., Cull, A., and Groenvold, M. *et al.* (1998). The European Organization for Research and Treatment of cancer approach to developing questionnaire modules: an update and overview. *EORTC Quality of Life Study Group. Quality of Life Research*, **7**, (4), 291–300.

Stewart, A. L. and Napoles-Springer, A. (2000). Health-related quality of life assessments in diverse population groups in the United States. *Medical Care*, **38**, (9), Suppl 2, 102–124.

Tanzer, N. K., Gittler, G., and Ellis, D. D. (1995). Cross-cultural validation of item complexity in a LLTM-calibrated spatial ability test. *European Journal of Psychological Assessment*, **11**, 170–183.

Thissen, D. (1991). *MULTILOG: Multiple, categorical item analysis and test scoring using item response theory*, version 6. Chicago, IL: Scientific Software.

Van de Vijver, F. J. R. and Leung, K. (1997). Methods and data analysis of comparative research. In J. W. Berry, Y. H. Poortinga, J. Pandey (eds) *Handbook of Cross-cultural Psychology*, pp. 257–300, 2nd edn, vol. 1. Chicago: Allyn and Bacon.

Vijver, F. J. R. and Leung, K. (1997). Methods and design. In F. J. R. Van de Vijver and K. Leung (eds) *Methods and data analysis for cross-cultural research*, pp. 27–58. 1st edn, vol. 1. California: Sage Publications.

WHOQOL Group. (1994). The development of the world health organization quality of life instrument (the WHOQOL). In J. Orley, W. Kuyken (eds) *Quality of Life Assessment: International perspectives*, pp. 41–57. Heidelberg, Germany: Springer Verlag.

2.2

Computerized adaptive testing and item banking

Jakob B. Bjorner, Mark Kosinski and
John E. Ware Jr

Introduction

Improving the validity and precision of our measurement tools and making them
more practical are constant challenges for the quality of life field. Computerized adaptive testing (CAT) holds great promise in helping us meet these challenges (see e.g.
Wainer *et al.* 2000). The basic idea of CAT is to have a computer to select the items that
seem most appropriate for a particular respondent (given our knowledge so far) and to
score the responses in way that allows us to compare the results with results from other
respondents answering a different set of items. This results in a quicker and more accurate assessment. To function, the CAT needs a set of rules for selecting the most appropriate items and scoring them on a common ruler, and a bank of items that can be
chosen for the test. Item banks contain information on the wording of each item, the
concept it measures, and its measurement characteristics according to a measurement
model. Most CAT-based assessments utilize a set of statistical models building on item
response theory (IRT, see also Chapters 1.5 and 2.3) to select items and to score the
responses. The combination of CAT and IRT provides several advantages compared to
current practice:

1. By selecting the most appropriate items for each person, assessment precision is
   optimized for a given test length and irrelevant items can be avoided.

2. Assessment precision can be adapted to needs of the specific application. For example, for a diagnostic purpose precision should be high for scores close to diagnostic
   cut-points, or test precision could be set high over all the score range for purposes
   of follow-up of individuals.

3. Assessments can be compared even if different items have been used or different
   precision levels have been specified.

4. Item banks can be expanded gradually by seeding and evaluating new items,
   without sacrificing backwards comparability.

5. By including items from traditional questionnaires in the item bank, it is possible to cross-calibrate widely used questionnaires.

6. The response process can be monitored in real time to ensure assessment quality and aberrant response patterns are explored.

7. At the end of the assessment, the respondent (or a health professional) can be given a score immediately, along with the guidelines on how to interpret the score.

Although some of these advantages can be achieved with other methodologies, the use of CAT and the careful analysis of items that is required for IRT modeling significantly improve assessment quality.

This chapter will be organized in the following way: We start by demonstrating the logic of CAT. We then describe how to build the item banks that underlie a working CAT and discuss practical aspects of CAT. Since discussions of CAT have almost exclusively taken place within educational testing, we briefly outline the differences between that field and applications in research on quality of life. Finally, we discuss some advanced topics and the future challenges for CAT in quality of life research. Throughout the chapter we rely heavily on examples from the CAT-based Headache Impact Test (HIT) (Ware *et al.* 2000, 2003; Bjorner *et al.* 2003a, 2003b). Readers may check out the HIT and the CAT-based assessments of generic health outcomes via the internet at *https://www.amihealthy.com*.

An example of CAT based on IRT methodology

The logic of a typical CAT is shown in Figure 2.2.1 (see also Wainer *et al.* 2000). The test begins with an initial estimate of the respondent's score (Step 1). This could be based on the response to an initial global question that is asked of all respondents, or on previous information about the respondent. A global question should be informative for the average person and have appropriate content for a first item. The initial score is used to select the most informative item, which is administered at Step 2. The answer is used at Step 3 to re-estimate the score. At Step 4, a respondent-specific confidence interval (CI) is computed for the score estimate. At Step 5, the computer determines whether any stopping rules have been fulfilled. If the stopping rule is test-precision the computer evaluates whether the CI is within specified limits. Once the standard is met, the computer either begins assessing the next concept or ends the battery. Otherwise, Step 2 is repeated for the next most informative item.

Figure 2.2.2 shows examples of the IRT models that are used to evaluate item information and estimate the persons IRT score (often represented by the Greek letter θ – *theta* – see Chapters 1.5 and 2.3). The figure illustrates the IRT models for three items concerning headache impact (the three upper plots) and the corresponding item information functions (lower plot). For these examples, we used the Generalized Partial Credit IRT model (GPCM) (Muraki 1997). Each curved line in the upper plots represents the models' prediction of the probability of choosing each of the item

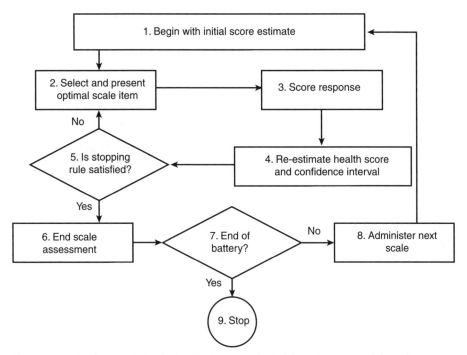

Fig. 2.2.1 Logic of computerized adaptive testing, adapted from Wainer *et al.* (2000).

response categories for various degrees of headache impact. The curves are called item characteristic curves (ICC) or trace lines (see Chapter 1.5). The horizontal axis is the headache impact IRT score, 'normed' so that the average headache sufferer in the USA has a score of 50; a positive score means more than average headache impact. The plots show that a respondent with a score of 50 has a 52 per cent probability of answering *A little of the time* to the question on the impact of headache on family interactions (Item 1), a 30 per cent probability of answering *None of the* time, a 16 per cent probability of answering *Some of the time* and low probabilities of choosing other categories. In contrast, to the question on needing help in routine tasks (Item 2) a respondent with a score of 50 has a much higher probability of choosing *None of the time/A little of the time* (which have been combined in this analysis) than any other response. The GPCM is characterized by two types of item parameters: thresholds and slopes. The item threshold parameters are the values on the horizontal axis where the item characteristic curves for two adjacent categories intersect, and the slope parameter (only one for each item) is a function of the slope of the curves (see Chapter 1.5). In Figure 2.2.2, item 3 has higher slope than item 2, which has higher slope than item 1.

The information functions, which express the contribution of each item to the overall test precision for various levels of headache impact, can be calculated from the IRT model (see Chapter 2.3).

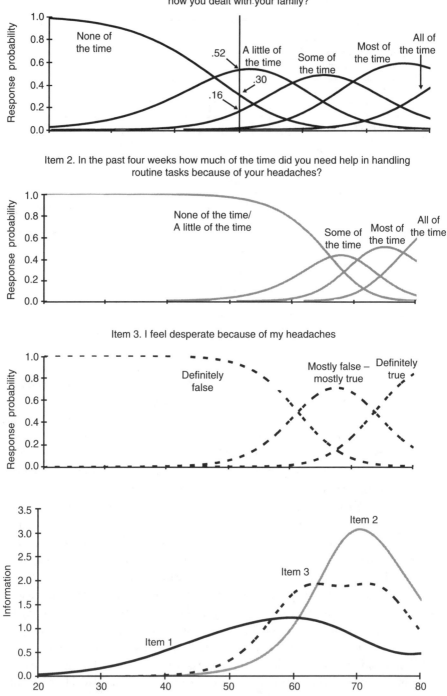

Fig. 2.2.2 Item characteristic curves and information functions.

Figure 2.2.3 shows an example of how the ICC and information functions are used in carrying out the tasks outlined in Figure 2.2.1. The upper part of Figure 2.2.3 shows the likelihood of various levels of headache impact for a person that has not yet answered any questions (the prior distribution). For headache impact, the prior distribution can be approximated by a normal distribution (Bjorner *et al.* 2003a). The mean (expected) IRT score is 50, but a wide range of values is possible (95 per cent prediction interval 30 to 70). Around a score of 50, item 1 has the highest information function (Figure 2.2.2), so this item is picked as the first item. Suppose the respondent replies *Some of the time* (plot below). The curve for this response choice (black line) is multiplied with the prior distribution, which produces the 'posterior distribution'. The expected value (mean) of this distribution is 57, and the prediction interval is 43 to 70, which is considerably narrower than for the prior distribution. However, this is still a wide confidence interval, and so Step 2 can be repeated by selecting the next most informative item. For scores around 57, item 3 has higher information function than item 2 and is thus the optimal second item. If one of the middle response categories is chosen, the response curve for these is multiplied with the previous likelihood – resulting in a new posterior distribution (score estimate 62, prediction interval 51 to 71). Finally, the answer to item 2 (*Some of the time*) results in an estimated score of 64 with a prediction interval of 55 to 71. No matter which or how many items are answered, the IRT score is on the same scale, and we achieve higher precision by asking more questions.

Development of an item bank for CAT

To achieve a CAT of high quality, we need an item bank (or 'item pool') containing a sufficient number of items fitting an IRT model. The methods outlined in Chapters 1.5 and 2.3 are also used when developing an item bank for a CAT. We briefly review the steps in item bank development.

Construct definition and item development

Meaningful assessments require clearly defined constructs. Careful specification of the subdomains of the constructs and the domains that are not part of the constructs ensures that the item bank covers all relevant aspects of the constructs. Often this involves specifying hypotheses to be tested in later stages, e.g. whether some domains can be seen as part of a common construct (dimension) or whether they should be treated as two separate constructs (dimensions). For example, for the HIT test a content analysis of previous questionnaires revealed six subdomains: headache pain, (impact of headache on:) role functioning, social functioning, energy, cognitive functioning, and mental health, indicating potential multidimensionality.

Good items are crucial for a well-functioning CAT. In principle, the criteria for good items do not differ between a CAT and a traditional questionnaire. In many standard

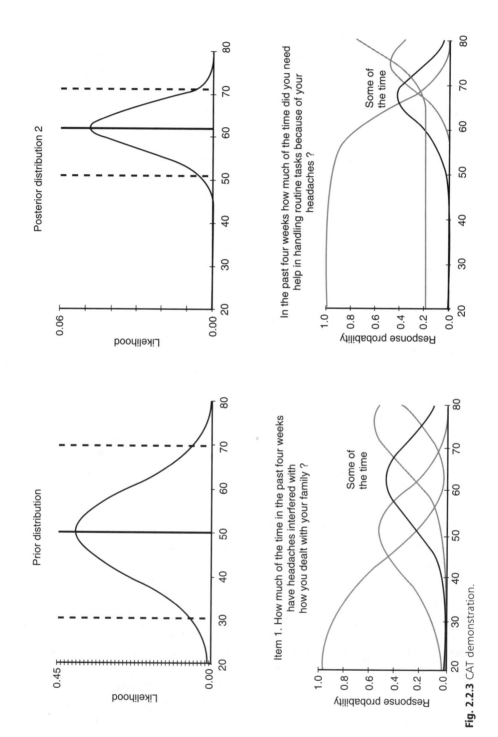

Fig. 2.2.3 CAT demonstration.

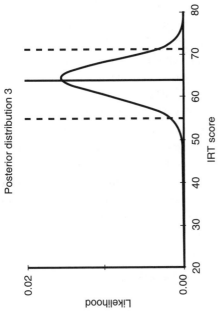

Posterior distribution 1

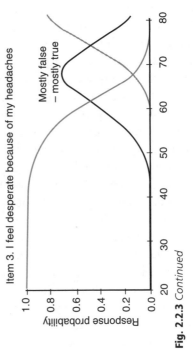

Posterior distribution 3

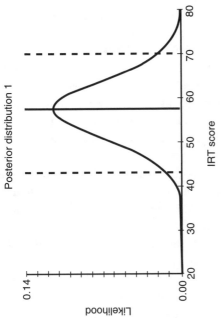

Item 3. I feel desperate because of my headaches

Mostly false – mostly true

Fig. 2.2.3 *Continued*

questionnaires, items are often presented in a grid to save space. However, in a CAT items are normally presented one at a time, so there is rarely a need to adapt the items to a grid format. If high measurement precision throughout the range of IRT scores is required, steps have to be taken to develop items that are relevant for the extremes of the scale. Such items often have poor item–total correlations or other psychometric properties, and therefore they tend to be lacking in traditional questionnaires. The measurement of minor disease impact is a challenge because items aimed at minor impact generally have lower slopes than items directed at major disease impact.

We recommend including items from existing questionnaires in the item bank, since this allows cross-calibrating of scores (so that the results of a CAT can be expressed in the metric of traditional questionnaires – see below). For the HIT, items were developed in several steps: the initial item pool was based on items from existing headache and migraine questionnaires; after gathering data and evaluating the IRT models for these items, we developed an additional pool of items – using the IRT results and input from clinicians.

Collecting data for item calibration and testing

To achieve precise estimates of item parameters and to check the model, we need a sufficient sample size with a sufficient spread over the range of quality of life to allow for estimation of all model parameters. Sample size requirements depend on the match between the item thresholds and the IRT score levels in the sample. However, even when the match is good, the sample has to be fairly large, so we can ignore errors in the estimates of item parameters. For the dichotomous two-parameter IRT model, simulation studies have found sample sizes of 500–1,000 to be sufficient (Tsutakawa and Soltys 1988; Tsutakawa and Johnson 1990). It is likely that similar sample sizes are required for the polytomous items. For very hard and for very easy polytomous items, some response categories are rarely used – presumably because few respondents score at the extremes covered by these item categories. In such circumstances, it might be helpful to oversample respondents in the ranges for which we want to establish good measurement precision.

Ideally, the data collection method for item calibration should be the same as the data collection method in the final CAT (most often a computer interface, although interviews, phone interviews, and automated phone interviews may also work well with a CAT). People tend to give more positive responses (better QoL) in personal telephone interviews than in self-administered postal surveys (McHorney et al. 1994) in particular for mental health questions (Bjorner et al. 2003c). We therefore expect differences (although not major) between IRT parameters for data gathered by interviews and by postal/computerized surveys – mainly for mental health and mainly for the threshold parameters. Major differences between computerized and paper and pencil surveys seem unlikely.

Fitting an IRT model and testing model assumptions

The statistical analyses of the item pool serves several purposes: to test model assumptions, to identify items and item response choices that do not function well, to select the best IRT model and to get item parameters.

We recommend that the following six steps are carried out in item bank development:

1. Basic descriptive analyses (proportion of missing, frequency distribution, skewedness etc.)

2. Test dimensionality and local independence

3. Initial analyses of item characteristic curves by non-parametric methods to detect potential problems for standard parametric IRT modeling

4. Fit an item-response model and test model fit

5. Test of differential item functioning (DIF) – see Holland and Wainer (1993) and Chapter 3.4

6. Test whether unfortunate choices of items could introduce bias/multidimensionality (random multidimensionality).

Steps 1–5 are described in other parts of this book (Chapters 1.5, 2.3, 3.4) and will not be discussed in detail here. However, we will briefly mention some of the lessons learnt in analyzing the HIT item pool.

Standard CAT requires that items measure only one dimension, and that this dimension explains all covariation between items – the assumption of *local independence* (see Chapter 1.5). Further, multidimensionality is also an important source of DIF (see Chapter 3.4). Although a fully unidimensional item bank is probably not achievable for most theoretically meaningful constructs, exploration of dimensionality is one of the most important parts of item analysis. The bank needs to be sufficiently unidimensional to make a single score meaningful and to ensure that item parameter estimates (and in turn person IRT scores) are not unduly influenced by problems of multidimensionality and local dependence between items. Many different methods exists for testing dimensionality and local dependence (Muthen and Muthen 2001; Holland and Rosenbaum 1986; Bock *et al.* 1988; Christensen *et al.* 2002; Stout *et al.* 1996; Muraki and Carlson 1995) (see Chapter 1.5). We rely strongly on exploratory and confirmatory factor analytic methods for categorical data (Muthen and Muthen 2001).

There are no definitive rules for deciding when multidimensionality or local dependence is of sufficient magnitude to prose problems. However, it is easy and important to test the robustness of the model. In case of potential multidimensionality, we recommend fitting an IRT model for each subdimension to see whether the item parameters and the IRT scores differ notably from the ones achieved if unidimensionality was assumed. In case of local dependence between a pair of items, we recommend examining whether item parameter–estimates change when one item of the pair is excluded. In the analysis of the HIT item pool, we applied both approaches and found no major problems.

Based on factor analytic results and tests of robustness, we may choose to exclude items with poor loadings from the pool, or split the item pool into two or more pools. However, milder cases of multidimensionality may be handled in a CAT by specifying item selection rules to ensure that every test includes items from all subdimensions, ensuring content balance. Cases of local dependency between pairs of items – which inflates slope parameters and leads to overestimation of precision – can be handled by estimating item parameters for each item separately and specifying item selection rules to ensure that only one of the items in the pair is selected during any CAT.

A problem unique to CAT is 'random multidimensionality'. Since the items used in any particular CAT are a subset of the items in the pool it is possible that the item selection procedure may introduce bias/multidimensionality by focusing on a narrow subdomain of the item bank. This might occur even if analyses of the total item pool do not indicate multidimensionality. Such problems might necessitate more sophisticated item selection procedures (to achieve content balance). In developing the HIT item pool we examined this problem using several methods: additional factor analyses of the subset of items that were frequently used in CAT simulations (see below), and examination of bias from different worst case scenarios of subsets of items. For the HIT item pool, we found no such problems.

Before fitting a parametric model, it is useful to examine non-parametric IRT models that allow visual inspection of the empirical item characteristic curves (Ramsay 1995). This allows further identification of poor items and response choices. Items can be excluded or a more general IRT model used (such as the nominal categories model instead of the GPCM), or response choices that do not discriminate can be collapsed. Items with low slopes have flat information functions and will therefore rarely or never be picked in a CAT (Ware *et al.* 2003). In this way, CAT is automatically protected against poor items. However, it is important to check whether some content areas are always omitted; if so, the CAT is assessing a narrower concept than intended.

Setting the metric

After the CAT has been developed, the researcher has to decide how the metric (IRT score) should be defined. In Rasch type models, the metric is often defined by the items: 0 is set as the mean of all item thresholds. In other IRT models, the metric is often defined by the population: the population mean is routinely set to 0, and the standard deviation to 1. However, calibration from one metric to the other is possible, as are other definitions of the metric. For generic health status measures it may be convenient to standardize the metric to a general population (e.g. US population), setting the mean to 50 and the standard deviation to 10. For disease-specific concepts, a mean defined by the general population may have little meaning. A more appropriate metric could be based on a well-defined population of people with the given disease. Note that the population that defines the metric need not answer all the questions – only enough questions to set the metric precisely.

CAT design and pretesting by simulations

To use the item bank in a CAT, item selection rules and stopping rules must be defined. Simulated CAT runs are very effective in evaluating the impact of various rules on test length, precision, and validity. One approach is to run simulations of a CAT on the data already collected (so-called 'real simulations') (Sands *et al.* 1997). These simulations can implement the steps shown in Figure 2.2.1. The total set of responses used to develop the item pool are used as input, but during the simulation the computer only reads the responses that correspond to the questions that would have been asked during a real CAT. Another possibility is to simulate item responses based on the IRT model, and use these simulated responses as input to the CAT; this is particularly useful when the item bank has been developed by linking items across several studies, so that no respondent has actually answered all items.

Figure 2.2.4 shows results of a 'real' simulation using the first item bank developed for the HIT. The line represents the standard error of measurement (SEM) for assessments using the total item bank (48 items), the dots represents SEM for CAT assessments using only the maximum information item selection rule and a stopping logic based on number of items administered (five items for all persons). The five-item CAT has a SEM that is below four points over most of the range, but higher for low impact.

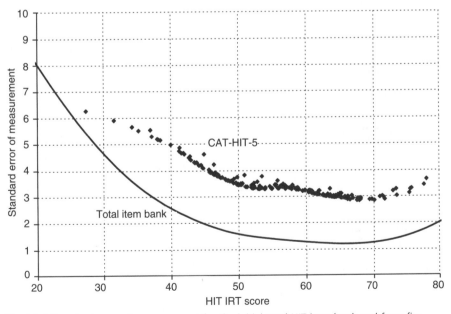

Fig. 2.2.4 Standard error of measurement for the initial total HIT item bank and for a five item CAT.

Additional analyses showed high concordance between the total score and the CAT score and lack of systematic deviations (bias). In worst-case CAT scenarios (where the least informative item was systematically chosen) the CAT score was much less precise but still without bias (results not shown).

Within the limits set by the total information in the item pool, the precision of a given CAT can be set to meet the need of a given situation. For the CAT–HIT, we decided that high precision was not necessary for minor headache impact. Therefore stopping rules were based on precision, but with requirements for precision varying over the range: <40 (SEM <7.5), 40–49 (SEM <4), 50–58 (SEM <3), 59–75 (SEM <2.75) and 75 + (SEM <4.8). While the mean number of items for a CAT with these specifications was still five, we achieve higher precision for people with severe headache impact, and people with minor impact were not burdened with many questions (see Ware *et al.* 2003). Table 2.2.1 summarizes the patterns of item usage given these stopping rules: 20 items

Table 2.2.1 Characteristics of the 20 items selected in simulations of CAT-HIT

Abbreviated Content	Domain	No. of Times Admin[1]	No. of Choices
How often is pain severe	Pain	1011	5
Restricted daily activities	Role	848	3
Feel too tired	Vit	541	5
Reduced activities, chores	Role	409	5
Fell frustrated	Emot	397	3
Restrict recreational activities	Role	397	3
Difficult achieve life goals	Role	265	3
I feel handicapped	Role	261	3
Reduced, non-work activities	Role	211	5
Limit ability to concentrate	Cog	166	5
Less likely to socialize	Soc	141	3
I am afraid to go outside	Emot	115	3
Unable social activities	Soc	76	4
Avoid social activities	Soc	63	5
Need help routine tasks	Role	48	4
Feel irritable	Emot	42	3
Difficult to focus attention	Cog	23	3
Work ability reduced	Role	18	5
Cancel work/daily activities	Role	18	4
Stress on relationships	Soc	1	3

were used in the 1011 simulations, but some were rarely used. The 20 items included all the conceptual subdomains outlined for the HIT. Thus, the CAT procedure did not lead to exclusion of specific subdomains.

CAT in practice

Establishing a working CAT requires a great deal of work beyond the psychometric analyses described above. Although a few software packages allow users to develop his/her own CAT, e.g. FastTest Pro (Weiss 2001), to date these packages have not included models for polytomous data.[1] Thus, until now the researcher has been forced to write CAT software for quality of life research. Among the issues that need to be considered in software development are:

1. Integrating maximum likelihood item selection with other item selection principles, e.g. defining rules to achieve content balance: see van der Linden (2000)

2. Visual appearance of items for different systems, screen setting etc.

3. Data security

4. Back-up in case of system failure

5. Should the respondent have the possibility of changing previous answers?

6. Check of data quality

7. Saving data from a CAT

8. Providing feedback to respondents, clinicians and other persons

9. Integration with existing patient information systems.

   Detailed discussion of these issues is beyond the present chapter, but we address some aspects of data quality evaluation and presentation of results.

Evaluating data quality

Using Figure 2.2.2 to evaluate the response pattern from our CAT example reveals that these responses (Item 1 – *Some of the time*, Item 2 – *Some of the time*, and Item 3 – *Mostly true*) are very likely for a person with a score estimate of 64 (the probabilities are 0.47, 0.35, and 0.63). However, let us consider another set of responses: Item 1 – *All of the time*, Item 2 – *Definitely false*, Item 3 – *Some of the time*. This combination of responses also leads to an estimated score of 64 (and a 95 per cent prediction interval of 55 to 71) but Figure 2.2.2 shows that these responses are much less likely (probabilities 0.02, 0.35, and 0.32). Another way to illustrate this is to compare the likelihoods of each response combination (0.106 vs. 0.002). Such comparisons of likelihoods form

---

[1] However, the next version of FastTEST (Version 2) is scheduled to include models for polytomous items.

the basis for IRT-based data quality indicators (Drasgow *et al.* 1985; van Krimpen-Stoop and Meijer 2002). Such indicators can serve as a warning signal to indicate potential misreading of items or a too simplistic IRT model (in this hypothetical example, headache impact might not be unidimensional after all).

Presentation of results

Although the IRT score is fine from a theoretical point of view, it is advisable to do as much work as possible to make the score easy to interpret for the respondent, the clinician, and the fellow researcher. Tools to do this are benchmarks and cross-calibration tables. One advantage of an IRT model is that it enables benchmarks from the content of the questionnaires: Figure 2.2.2 will, for example, quickly tell you that a typical person with a score of 50 will very rarely have need for help with routine tasks because of headaches.

Cross-calibration tables use the IRT score to predict scores on other (traditional) questionnaires on the same topic. Such tables establish comparability with results and interpretation guidelines already established from previous research using these questionnaires. If IRT parameters have been established for the items in a traditionally sum-scored scale, the expected sum score (for each level of the IRT score) can be estimated: (1) Calculate the expected item score (for each IRT score level) by calculating the product of the response choice probability and the response choice weight (e.g. *none of the time* = 1, *a little of the time* = 2 …) and sum over all response choices, (2) Sum the expected item scores (see e.g. Bjorner *et al.* 2003b). Figure 2.2.5 shows examples of expected score values on some traditional headache scales for each level of the HIT score.

CAT in educational testing and in quality of life research

CAT was mainly developed in the setting of educational testing, and most CAT research and all major books are based on this framework. Applications of CAT in QoL research differ from those in educational testing in three major areas: generation of items, choice of IRT models, and problems of item exposure.

Generation of items

To achieve precision over the full range of a scale, the total item bank needs a large number of items with sufficient diversity. In an educational test, generation of new items is done routinely and the pool of potential items can be seen as unlimited for many topics. In contrast, the number of ways questions can be asked about quality of life may be limited. Item banks based on pooling items from existing questionnaires may provide good measurement precision in some ranges, but insufficient precision at the extremes, in particular for people with relatively good quality of life. Thus, it is a challenge to develop new items targeted at specific ranges of quality of life. In our view, the potential for developing such items has not been fully explored yet.

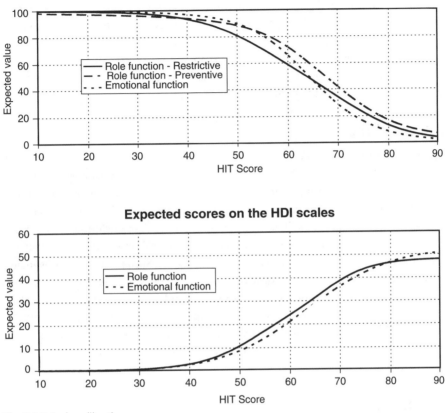

Fig. 2.2.5 Scale calibration.

IRT model

Educational tests most frequently use multiple-choice items that are scored right/ wrong and analyzed by dichotomous IRT models. Such items are only informative over a narrow range of the scale and uninformative at other levels, which can create problems if the CAT is started at an inappropriate level (van der Linden and Pashley 2000). In contrast, quality of life research mostly uses items that are scored on a rank scale (e.g. 1–5) and analyzed by polytomous IRT models (like the graded response model or the generalized partial credit model). Such items provide more information over a much broader range of scores. Therefore, the same level of precision can be attained with fewer items and the choice of prior distribution is less crucial. Furthermore, because of the many informative response choices for each item, a CAT will have power to detect response inconsistencies, even when items are targeted to the score level of the respondent (van Krimpen-Stoop and Meijer 2002).

Item exposure

In educational testing, the assessment needs to take place in a controlled environment and item content needs to be kept secret to avoid cheating. Countering these problems necessitates special test sites, large item pools, and complex procedures for item exposure control. In quality of life research, items are not kept secret and item exposure is thus much less of a problem. Thus, CAT in quality of life research can be simpler and much more cost-efficient than in educational testing.

Advanced topics

We have dealt with a bank of items that measure one unidimensional construct. In quality of life assessment, the researcher will often want to measure several related constructs and might want to gain measurement precision by utilizing information on the association between the different dimensions. Further, it might sometimes be more realistic to assume that some items are measuring more than one dimension. Both of these tasks can be accomplished by multidimensional CAT which allows simultaneous measurement of multiple dimensions (Segall 1996, 2000). Such models can be estimated by factor analytic methods for categorical data (e.g. Muthen and Muthen 2001) and the parameters for these models can be converted to IRT parameters (e.g. Gardner *et al.* 2002). Multidimensional CAT is an exciting area for future development, but can also be very computer-intensive. Currently only a small number of dimensions can be handled within reasonable computational time. Also, the interpretation of scores is more complex.

Conclusion

In this chapter we have tried to illustrate how CAT works and how CAT can be used to achieve more precise, relevant, and useful measurement. We conclude with another relevant question: what are the disadvantages of CAT? One potential disadvantage is mode of delivery: the traditional paper and pencil questionnaires that have been a robust and cost-efficient data collection method do not work with CAT, although some intermediate forms exist (Larkin and Weiss 1975). However, computerized administration of questionnaires will probably become much more frequent in the future, making the transition to CAT easier.

Since IRT is fairly explicit about model assumptions, criticism has been raised that the assumptions are too strong and not likely to be met with real data. In our opinion, the same assumptions are made implicitly in traditional measurement as are made explicitly in IRT. However, it is possible that CAT is less robust to violations of the measurement assumptions. Thus, careful checking of model assumptions is crucial for a successful implementation of CAT. Once model violations are identified, their impact can be evaluated and often corrected by selecting an appropriate adaptation of the CAT methodology. Thus, the real disadvantage of CAT is the cost for establishing large item banks of high quality.

Such increased costs seem justified when considering the measurement gains: reduction in response burden, increase in measurement precision, creation of a common metric, availability of real time quality control, and immediate feedback. CAT applications in the health field have been seen to have the potential to revolutionize how symptoms and treatment outcomes are assessed (NIH 2003). It is up to the researchers in quality of life assessment to carry that revolution forward.

Acknowledgements

We would like to thank Morten Aa. Petersen, Christopher Dewey, and Peter Fayers for helpful comments on a previous version of this chapter.

References

Bjorner, J. B., Kosinski, M., and Ware, J. E., Jr. (2003a). Calibration of an item pool for assessing the burden of headaches: an application of item response theory to the headache impact test (HIT). *Quality of Life Research*, **12**, 913–933.

Bjorner, J. B., Kosinski, M., and Ware, J. E., Jr. (2003b). Using item response theory to calibrate the Headache Impact Test (HIT) to the metric of traditional headache scales. *Quality of Life Research*, **12**, 981–1002.

Bjorner, J. B., Ware, J. E., Jr., and Kosinski, M. (2003c). The potential synergy between cognitive models and modern psychometric models. *Quality of Life Research*, **12**, 261–274.

Bock, R. D., Gibbons, R., and Muraki, E. (1988). Full-information item factor analysis. *Appl Psychol Measur*, **12**, 261–280.

Christensen, K. B., Bjorner, J. B., Kreiner, S., and Petersen, J. H. (2002). Tests for unidimensionality in polytomous Rasch models. *Psychometrika*, **67**, 563–574.

Drasgow, F., Levine, M. V., and Williams, E. A. (1985). Appropriateness measurement with polychotomous item response models and standardized indices. *British Journal of Mathematical and Statistical Psychology*, **38**, 67–86.

Gardner, W., Kelleher, K. J., and Pajer, K. A. (2002). Multidimensional adaptive testing for mental health problems in primary care. *Medical Care*, **40**, 812–823.

Holland, P. W. and Rosenbaum, P. R. (1986). Conditional association and unidimensionality in monotone latent variable models. *Ann Statist*, **14**, 1523–1543.

Holland, P. W. and Wainer, H. (1993). *Differential Item Functioning*. Hillsdale, NJ: Lawrence Erlbaum Associates, Inc.

Larkin, R. and Weiss, D. (1975). *An Empirical Comparison of Two-stage and Pyramidal Adaptive Testing* (Rep. No. 75–1). Minneapolis: University of Minnesota, Department of Psychology, Psychometric method program.

McHorney, C. A., Kosinski, M., and Ware, J. E., Jr. (1994). Comparisons of the costs and quality of norms for the SF-36 health survey collected by mail versus telephone interview: results from a national survey. *Medical Care*, **32**, 551–567.

Muraki, E. (1997). A generalized partial credit model. In W. J. van der Linden and R. K. Hambleton (eds) *Handbook of Modern Item Response Theory*, pp. 153–164. Berlin: Springer.

Muraki, E. and Carlson, J. E. (1995). Full-information factor analysis for polytomous item responses. *Appl Psychol Measur*, **19**, 73–90.

Muthen, B. O. and Muthen, L. (2001). *Mplus User's Guide*, Version 2, computer software. Los Angeles: Muthén and Muthén.

NIH (2003). *Re-Engineering the Clinical Research Enterprise*. Bethesda, MD: NIH.

Ramsay, J. O. (1995). *TestGraf – A Program for the Graphical Analysis of Multiple Choice Test and Questionnaire Data*, computer software. Montreal: McGill University.

Sands, W. A., Waters, B. K., and McBride, J. R. (1997). *Computerized Adaptive Testing: From Inquiry to Operation*. Washington, DC: American Psychological Association.

Segall, D. O. (1996). Multidimensional adaptive testing. *Psychometrika*, **61**, 331–354.

Segall, D. O. (2000). Principles of multidimensional adaptive testing. In W. J. van der Linden and C. A. W. Glas (eds) *Computerized Adaptive Testing, Theory and Practice*, pp. 53–74. Dordrecht: Kluwer Adacemic Publishers.

Stout, W., Habing, B., Douglas, J., Kim, H. R., Roussos, L., and Zhang, J. (1996). Conditional covariance-based nonparametric multidimensionality assessment. *Applied Psychological Measurement*, **20**, 331–354.

Tsutakawa, R. K. and Soltys, M. J. (1988). Approximation for Bayesian ability estimation. *Journal of Educational Statistics*, **13**, 117–130.

Tsutakawa, R. K. and Johnson, J. C. (1990). The effect of uncertainty of item parameter estimation on ability estimates. *Psychometrika*, **55**, 371–390.

van der Linden, W. J. (2000). Constrained adaptive testing with shadow tests. In W. J. van der Linden and C. A. W. Glas (eds) *Computerized Adaptive Testing, Theory and Practice*, pp. 27–52. Dordrecht: Kluwer Adacemic Publishers.

van der Linden, W. J. and Pashley, P. J. (2000). Item selection and ability estimation in adaptive testing. In W. J. van der Linden and C. A. W. Glas (eds) *Computerized Adaptive Testing, Theory and Practice*, pp. 1–25. Dordrecht: Kluwer Adacemic Publishers.

van Krimpen-Stoop, E. M. L. A. and Meijer, R. R. (2002). Detection of person misfit in computerized adaptive tests with polytomous items. *Applied Psychological Measurement*, **26**, 164–180.

Wainer, H., Dorans, N. J., Eignor, D., Flaugher, R., Green, B. F., and Mislevy, R. J. *et al.* (2000). *Computerized Adaptive Testing: A primer*, 2nd edn. Mahwah, NJ: Lawrence Erlbaum Associates.

Ware, J. E., Jr., Bjorner, J. B., and Kosinski, M. (2000). Practical implications of item response theory and computerized adaptive testing: a brief summary of ongoing studies of widely used headache impact scales. *Medical Care*, **38**, II73–II82.

Ware, J. E., Jr., Kosinski, M., Bjorner, J. B., Bayliss, M. S., Batenhorst, A., and Dahlof, C. G. *et al.* (2003). Applications of computerized adaptive testing (CAT) to the assessment of headache impact. *Quality of Life Research*, **12**, 935–952.

Weiss, D. J. (2001). *FastTEST Pro*, Version 1.6, computer software. St. Paul: Assessment Systems Corporation.

Developing a questionnaire using item response theory: a case study of fatigue

David Cella, Jin-Shei Lai, Kim Davis, Kelly Dineen, Stacie Hudgens and Richard Gershon

Introduction

Fatigue is a common problem in most chronic medical conditions. For example prevalence estimates for significant fatigue have been documented in cancer (Cella *et al.* 1993, 1997, 2001; Vogelzang *et al.* 1997; Winningham *et al.* 1994; Irvine *et al.* 1994; Blesch *et al.* 1991), multiple sclerosis (Schur 1989; Liang *et al.* 1984), Parkinson's disease (Friedman and Friedman 2001, 1993; Karlsen *et al.* 1999; Krupp and Pollina 1996) and HIV (Breitbart 1998; Cunningham 1998). Because fatigue is a symptom associated with so many conditions, its evaluation is included in many HRQoL instruments, both generic and condition-specific. There are also many stand-alone self-report measures of fatigue. Given the number of available self-report fatigue measures, why develop another? Despite the diversity of available approaches to measuring fatigue (or perhaps because of it), there is no common measurement for this common symptom. As a result, today's consumer of HRQoL instruments must select a fatigue measurement that is tied to the context of the larger questionnaire and patient sample on which it was evaluated. Because it is so common and important, it would be desirable if a standard metric for fatigue could be applied across multiple conditions and fatigue questionnaires. This would improve communication regarding the meaning of study results and the magnitude of a treatment benefit. If its validity across diseases was independent of the sample upon which it was originally evaluated, and its questions could be shown to be representative of various levels of an underlying fatigue continuum, it would then be possible to compare people across different studies, even if they answered different subsets of the fatigue questions, because the fatigue score would be expressed on the common underlying metric. A common measurement for fatigue would therefore be possible, even if different questions from the overall pool of questions ('item bank') are administered to different respondents.

In this chapter, we describe one method for developing a measure of fatigue using item response theory (IRT). We emphasize that this method does not describe a 'new instrument', meant to compete with other instruments and eventually be yet another in the compendium. Rather, we describe the application of a measurement model to create an item bank to measure fatigue, with the ultimate goal of positioning items from any other instrument along one continuum of fatigue defined by this bank.

For the past 15 years, we have been developing and refining various HRQoL questionnaires, including measurement of fatigue and its perceived impact on functioning. Within the scope of IRT, a definable and distinctive component of any collection of questions is the 'item bank'. An item bank is a collection of questions (and their rating scales) that individually and collectively contribute information on the position of any tested person along the continuum defined by the items in the bank (Cella and Chang 2000). A useful item bank is 'loaded' with more questions than are needed in any one assessment; these questions can have come from multiple sources (questionnaires). Furthermore, once in the bank, subsets of the items can be extracted to create multiple variations of 'short forms' for clinical research or practice. The goal of an item bank is to help assess patients precisely by including questions that cover the entire underlying continuum, or 'latent trait', which in the present example is fatigue. An item bank consists of a sufficient number of items that are positioned on the defined continuum based on their psychometric properties. Knowledge of the psychometric properties of the items can inform the creation of various short forms, with content based upon clinical relevance of the questions, or the matching of the position of the item with the average position of the patients along the continuum. For example, chronic fatigue sufferers could be asked questions that target severe fatigue, whereas general ambulatory outpatients could be asked questions about tiredness at the end of the day.

An item bank can also enable adaptive testing which asks a select number of questions sequenced according to the amount of information they provide (Hays *et al.* 2000). Typically, due to the many computations required in real time, a computer is used for adaptive testing, and this is then referred to as computerized adaptive testing (CAT). CAT is a measurement methodology that combines innovative measurement models (i.e., IRT) with technology in an adaptive manner, the goal of which is to provide precise estimates of a patient's level of HRQoL/symptom. Of particular importance, CAT allows for real-time assessments and interpretation over time. We now offer a brief overview of IRT and then describe a series of steps to develop a fatigue item bank as a component of a larger HRQoL measurement system. It is one of several possible approaches, offered as an example of an IRT application to HRQoL assessment.

Item Response Theory (IRT)

A fundamental feature of IRT is that item location is related to the estimated amount of a patient's latent trait. A core concept of IRT is the item characteristic curve (ICC) which illustrates the relationship between a patient's level of the trait being measured (e.g., fatigue), and the probability of a patient making a specific response on the items being administered. This curve displays two item properties: item difficulty (or location) and item discrimination (or slope). Item difficulty refers to the location of the item on the measurement continuum, the same continuum that is used to describe the respondent's level on the measured trait. (Thus, items can be targeted to people by selecting those whose probability of endorsement is near 50 per cent for a given person or group of people). Item discrimination describes how well an item can differentiate between patients below and above the location of the item on the continuum (Baker 2001; Thissen and Orlando 2001). The steeper the slope of the curve, the better the item discrimination. However, this property only reflects the discrimination of the item in its middle (steepest) section, and the slope changes along the continuum for each item. Using probability models, IRT mathematically describes the relationship between a respondent's underlying level of the trait being measured and the location ('difficulty') of the item administered on the same continuum. A useful set of items will cover the full range of the continuum. By using fatigue as an example, some items are likely to be endorsed even by a person with little fatigue (e.g., 'I get tired at the end of a long day') and others are unlikely to be endorsed unless a person has a great deal of fatigue (e.g., 'walking from one room to another is exhausting'). IRT models allow one to 'calibrate' items in an instrument by their locations on the latent trait. This in turn allows one to be selective about which items are administered. Very fatigued people can be administered items that are targeted to differentiate people with significant fatigue. Similarly, people with limited fatigue can be administered items that distinguish mere absence of fatigue from a high degree of energy.

Numerous models fall into the IRT family. IRT was first proposed for use with rating scales more than 25 years ago (Andrich 1978; Bock 1972). In rating scale HRQoL applications, the 1-parameter logistic (1-PL) model and the 2-PL model are most commonly used. 1-PL is based upon the assumption that the probability of a patient endorsing a particular response category in an item is based solely upon his/her fatigue level relative to the location of that item on the fatigue continuum. Discrimination in the model is fixed at a constant. The 2-PL model additionally considers how well that item discriminates among persons with different levels of fatigue (i.e., discrimination). While the merits of these models are subject to ongoing debate, all unidimensional IRT models specify that only one trait is being estimated by the items in the scale and all calibrate items onto this trait. The 1-PL model is a simpler but more restrictive model that requires a smaller sample size of about 200 patients to achieve stable item calibrations (Hambleton 1989; Linacre 1994). In contrast, the 2-PL model requires at least 500 patients to produce stable estimates (Hambleton 1989). Selecting the appropriate model depends on factors such as sample size and the degree of item fit.

Steps to develop an item bank

Figure 2.3.1 outlines a series of steps used to develop a useful item bank. The four general steps include: (1) determining the latent trait being measured and the target population, (2) creating an item pool, (3) examining dimensionality of items, and

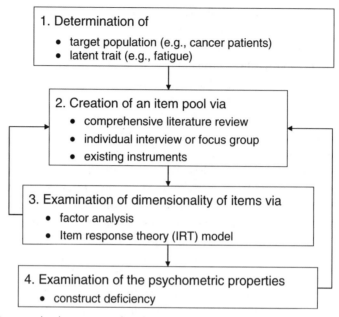

Fig. 2.3.1 Steps to develop a comprehensive measurement system/item bank.

(4) examining the psychometric properties of the items. Some steps may be repeated in an iterative process in order to refine the item bank.

Determining the latent trait and the target population

The context for measurement is important. Before embarking on creating the bank, we first determine what we want to measure (the latent trait, construct, or continuum), who we want to measure (i.e., the target population), and how we intend to measure the construct within that target population. When the target population is diverse, or is from a diagnostic group to be compared to a different group, researchers tend to use generic HRQoL instruments to achieve comparability. However, by their design generic questionnaires tend to be less responsive than targeted scales in detecting important differences or changes in a particular trait (Hays 2004; Vickery 2004). An item bank of questions tapping a targeted HRQoL component such as fatigue can solve this dilemma by making targeted concepts measurable generically. Using IRT, this can be achieved by positioning a sufficient number of items across the continuum to enable the user to select from a bank of items measuring targeted constructs (e.g., fatigue). The selected items can be ones targeted appropriately to the relevant disease. In this way, the user can realize precision equal to or better than that of a targeted questionnaire, with generalizability that rivals that of generic instruments.

In a preliminary attempt to evaluate a generic instrument's potential for perform-ance in an item bank used across diverse patient groups, we examined the psychomet-ric properties of 10 physical functioning (PF-10) items from the generic MOS SF-36 questionnaire (Bode *et al.* 2003a). We evaluated item performance among patients with diagnoses of cancer, multiple sclerosis, HIV, and stroke. By item performance (i.e., fit to the measurement model) dimensionality of the items, location along the measure-ment continuum, and difference in item location based on diagnosis, we found that half (five) of those 10 items could be used in a common core bank which, for our pur-poses, formed the basis for a larger physical functioning item bank intended for people with chronic medical conditions. Results indicated that the item calibrations for these five core items could be fixed at the level determined from the combined sample and used to link the data across diagnostic groups, while items that exhibited differential item functioning (DIF) could be treated as separate items for each group and allowed to have different locations in the bank. Similarly, because our goal is to derive a fatigue item bank to be applied across different patient groups, we planned to evaluate whether items for which there are data across diagnostic groups indeed perform similarly across those groups.

Creating an item pool

An item pool can be created by writing new items, using items from existing instru-ments, or both. New items can be generated via individual interview (e.g., cognitive interview) of patients and clinicians, or by conducting patient/clinician focus groups. There is a great time-saving advantage to using existing instruments when possible, so long as there are suitable data available to confirm the appropriateness of the items for the bank. Beginning with well-studied and evaluated questions enables rapid defini-tion of the underlying latent trait, and appraisal of any bank deficiencies, such as floor and ceiling effects. Whether the initial items in the bank are existing or newly written, careful content review is essential during the early stage of building a bank. Comprehensive literature reviews and consultations with experts facilitate compilation of previously tested items. They also help to clearly define the construct(s) being measured to enable the writing of new items to appropriately cover the measurement continuum and eliminate gaps in coverage.

Recently, we have developed several preliminary item banks, starting with items from existing instruments. Most of the over 500 items in the Functional Assessment of Chronic Illness Therapy (FACIT) measurement system (Cella 1997) were written based on input from patients and clinical (content) experts. These and other items, often generously provided by their developers, comprise a pool of questions available for selection based on analysis of available data. Item selection starts with a review of existing items to determine conceptual fit with the latent trait and applicability to the target population. This is done in consultation with patients and clinical experts, and informed by comprehensive literature review. Analysis of the resulting item pool varies based on the availability of data. If data are available for some items, an initial item bank can be created by linking different datasets. Bode *et al.* (2003b) detailed methods to create an initial item bank by using existing datasets.

However, when previously-collected data are not available, one must field test items to evaluate their level of contribution to the item bank. We have implemented this approach in the development of several item banks such as physical function (Bode *et al.* 2003b), cancer pain (Bode *et al.* 2003a; Lai *et al.* submitted), bowel function in prostate cancer (Lai *et al.* 2003a), cancer-related fatigue (Lai *et al.* 2003b, in press), and emotional distress. All banks demonstrate good fit to a unidimensional measurement model, a stable hierarchy of item locations, and reasonable coverage of the measurement continuum, as determined by both IRT and classical test theory methods.

Examining the dimensionality of items

Once items have been compiled and sufficient data have been collected, there are many analytic methods designed to test the underlying dimensionality of the items. Within the classical test theory framework, factor analytic methods have been used to describe similarities in responses to items that form different factors or constructs. Exploratory (i.e., to determine the number of factors defined by a set of items) and confirmatory (i.e., to confirm a hypothesized factor structure in which factors are fixed a priori) analyses with rotations that maximize simple structure of item loadings on factors have typically been used (Baker 1989). The measurement model portion of structural equation modeling has also been used to evaluate hypothesized underlying factors (Lunz and Bergstrom 1994; Bunderson *et al.* 1989). These classical methods use the inter-correlations among the raw responses to the items to form the factors; unfortunately, these correlations are sample-specific and may be compromised by the ordinal (as opposed to interval) nature of the data. Recently, IRT methods have been used to examine patterns of responses to items which are not as prone to sample dependence and the ordinal nature of item responses (Cella *et al.* 1996; Fisher 1997; Reise *et al.* 1993).

Examining the psychometric properties of items

Typically, when a scale is constructed from a set of items, it is intended that those items cover the complete spectrum of the construct being measured, at least when it is applied to the target population. Often in practice this does not occur, with the most common problem being inadequate coverage at the floor (very unhealthy people) or ceiling (very healthy people) of a trait. Insufficient coverage of a segment of the continuum is known as construct deficiency, whereas redundant coverage (more questions than needed at a given location) is referred to as construct saturation. Since redundant items provide the test developer the luxury of choosing various items to meet user preferences and patient characteristics, construct saturation is not a concern in an item bank, as it is understood that only a few of the redundant questions will be asked of any one patient. However, action is needed where construct deficiency exists. It can be overcome by positioning items on the trait being measured from the least severe to the most severe. IRT can be used to examine if this action is successful. For example, the most severe item in a fatigue item hierarchy would only be endorsed by people with the greatest amount of fatigue (e.g., 'Fatigue prevents me from getting out of bed'). Construct deficiencies can be classified into either statistical construct deficiency or clinical construct deficiency.

Statistical construct deficiency refers to the acceptable amount of distance across the measurement continuum which is not covered by a maximally-discriminating item or, to some degree, a maximally-discriminating step between two adjacent response categories within an item. We have set the maximum allowable uncovered distance of 0.30–0.50 log transformed units (logits).

Clinical construct deficiency, evidence of poor content validity, is suggested if an important aspect of the symptom or functional area is not queried by the items in the bank. Assurance of clinical coverage can only be obtained through engagement of patients and clinical experts during the process of building and evaluating the item bank. In addition to expert input, literature review helps inform the appropriateness of item content to the population of interest. In response to both statistical and clinical deficiency, the item bank team uses an item-writing approach that estimates the targeted gaps by examining existing items in the vicinity and discussion with clinical experts. This effort is followed by re-testing new items concurrent with existing items in the target population.

Item banking is an ongoing, iterative process. Modification (e.g., adding new items or revising existing items) to the initial item pool is necessary when (1) the bank shows unacceptable evidence of multidimensionality (see Figure 2.3.1 arrow from box 3 to box 2); or (2) when construct deficiency is found (see Figure 2.3.1, arrow from box 4 to box 2). For the remainder of this chapter, we illustrate the development of a fatigue item bank, targeted to cancer patients but with potential applicability to other patient populations and the general population.

An illustration: Development of a cancer-related fatigue bank

Prevalence reports of cancer-related fatigue (CRF) range from 60 to 90 per cent (Cella *et al.* 2001; Cella 1997; Vogelzang *et al.* 1997; Winningham *et al.* 1994; Irvine *et al.* 1994; Blesch *et al.* 1991) making fatigue one of, if not the most, common symptom associated with cancer and its treatment. Fatigue has been demonstrated to have a major negative impact on other aspects of HRQoL (Cella 1997; Cella *et al.* 1993; Ferrell *et al.* 1996; Irvine *et al.* 1994; Yellen *et al.* 1997) for patients both on and off treatment. While the past few years have witnessed increased attention to the need for improved assessment of fatigue (NCCN 2003), there is still a significant amount of uncertainty regarding the optimal tools for assessment and frequency with which to assess fatigue. As fatigue emerged as a prominent problem in cancer, several measures were developed to assess it such as the Multidimensional Fatigue Inventory (Smets *et al.* 1995), Fatigue Assessment Instrument (Schwartz, Jandorf, and Krupp 1993), Brief Fatigue Inventory (Mendoza *et al.* 1999), Profile of Mood States subscales (POMS, McNair, Lorr, and Droppelman 1971), the Piper Fatigue Scale (Piper *et al.* 1989), and the Fatigue Symptom Inventory (Hann *et al.* 1998). These scales result in over 200 items that are currently in use to assess fatigue. The existence of all of these instruments provides the potential to create a comprehensive item bank for cancer-related fatigue. Many of these questions are similar in content and scaling, and they are highly correlated with one another (Mendoza *et al.* 1999; Yellen *et al.* 1997). Some of these instruments are treated as unidimensional (e.g., FACIT-F), while others claim to be multidimensional (e.g. the Piper Fatigue Scale). The creation of an item bank allows one to draw from all available measures such that the most accurate estimate of CRF is obtained. Ultimately, the goal for the fatigue item bank was to develop, define and quantify cancer-related fatigue in order to maximize the precision and clinical relevance of each question.

Initial fatigue item bank

We began the banking process by developing an initial fatigue item bank consisting of common items that can assess fatigue in both anemic cancer patients and the general US population (Lai *et al.* 2003b). Two data sets were analyzed in this study: 1,022 anemic cancer patients, randomly selected from a pool of 2,369 anemic cancer patients, (Cella *et al.* 2002; Demetri 1998) and a random-digit dial sample of 1,010 from the general US population, unscreened for medical conditions (Lai *et al.* 2003). All subjects answered the 13-item FACIT-Fatigue scale (Yellen *et al.* 1997). A polytomous extension of the Rasch dichotomous model was utilized in the analysis (Andrich 1978). Items were retained in the core bank if two criteria were met. First, items needed to fit the assumption of one parameter logistic (Rasch) model, in which the ICC slope of all items in the scale should be equal. This assumption was tested by using the mean square (MnSq) fit statistic. Items with MnSq less than or equal to 1.4 (that is, with no more than 40 per cent unexplained variance) were considered to meet the above assumption and therefore, were considered for retention in the bank. The second criterion was that there could be no significant differential item function (DIF) across samples.

 Results showed that four items had MnSq values greater than 1.4 when anemic cancer patients and the general US population were analyzed separately. Three items demonstrated DIF across these two samples. It is noteworthy that these three items were among the four items that did not fit the Rasch model in both cancer patients and the general population. Together, the evidence for item misfit and DIF supported the exclusion of these four items from the core item bank; among these four items, two were measuring the low end of the fatigue continuum for both samples. Thus, based on the combined criteria of acceptable item fit statistics in both samples and non-significant DIF results, we decided to keep nine items plus the screening item ('I have a lack of energy') to comprise the initial fatigue item bank. These 10 items were then positioned on a fatigue continuum along with the score distributions for each sample (shown in Figure 2.3.2). Reported fatigue (transformed into a 0–100 possible score range) was clearly more severe among the cancer patient sample than the general population: general population mean = 72.6 (SD = 18.4), median = 70.8 (SD = 18.4); cancer patients mean = 41.8 (SD = 19.0), median = 43.8 (SD = 19.0); t(2030) = 37.2, $P < 0.001$. The positioning of item locations on the same figure as the sample distributions allows one to visually determine the extent of floor and ceiling effects by sample. The majority of cancer patients (83 per cent) and the general population (67 per cent) report a level of fatigue that falls within the range of available item-category locations. However, among cancer patients, 16 per cent demonstrated a floor effect, defined as having an estimated score below the lowest item-category average measure (i.e., 23.4). On the other end of the continuum, however, fewer than 2 per cent demonstrated a ceiling effect, defined as having an estimated score higher than the highest item-category average measure (80.8). In contrast, less than 1 per cent of the general population showed a floor effect and yet, one-third of the sample (33 per cent) showed a ceiling effect. This illustrates the importance of considering the target population for bank application. The bank showed deficiencies at the floor for cancer patients and at the ceiling for the general population.

An operational fatigue item bank

Based upon these results, new items were written to expand the bank from 10 (nine core items and one screening item) to 92 items in an attempt at addressing the ceiling and floor effects in the initial fatigue core item bank. A new sample of 301 cancer patients from the metropolitan Chicago area was tested. The psychometric properties of the items were examined using the infit MnSq and DIF criteria described above. Twenty items did not meet these criteria and were deleted from the pool. The final 72 items satisfied Rasch measurement requirements and demonstrated high Cronbach's alpha (0.99) and moderate to high item-total correlations (range = 0.51 – 0.85). These 72 questions are presented in Appendix 1. This testing confirmed the hierarchy (i.e., order of the items on the continuum) of the original 10 items and positioned the other 62 along the same hierarchy, now adequately representing the full range of fatigue experienced by people with cancer. We view the item overlap (i.e., multiple items sharing the same location on the continuum) as a strength of the item bank, so long as people are not exposed to too many items from one location or to items with overlapping (redundant) content in a given administration from the bank. This size bank (72 items) provides an ample supply of related questions from which to choose when developing short-forms or adaptive tests.

The comparison of 'self-reported fatigue' and 'item-response category measures' showed that average self-reported fatigue was well-covered by the item-response categories.

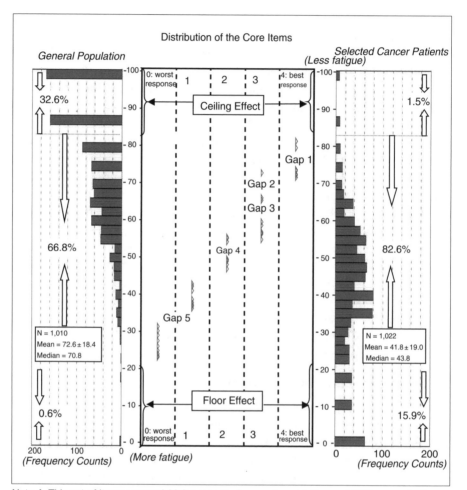

Distribution of the Core Items

General Population

Selected Cancer Patients (Less fatigue)

Note A This set of items covered 66.8 per cent of general population and 82.6 per cent of cancer patients. Among cancer patients, 15.9 per cent of subjects demonstrated a floor effect, 1.5 per cent demonstrated a ceiling effect. On the contrary, only 0.6 per cent of general population demonstrated a floor effect and 32.6 per cent demonstrated a ceiling effect.

Note B 'Gap' means no item (along with response category) available to measure fatigue on subjects who locate on the corresponding area of the fatigue continuum in a sensitive manner. Gap 1 is between 73.3 and 79.0, gap 2 between 65.8 and 71.4, gap 3 between 59.4 and 65.3, gap 4 between 49.7 and 54.1, and gap 5 between 31.7 and 36.6.

Note C For negatively worded item, (best response) 4 = *not at all*, 3 = *a little bit*, 2 = *somewhat*, 1 = *quite a bit*, and (worst response) 0 = *very much*. For positively worded item, (best response) 4 = *very much*, 3 = *quite a bit*, 2 = *somewhat*, 1 = *a little bit*, and (worst response) 0 = *not at all*.

Fig. 2.3.2 Comparison between range of item locations (9 core items) and fatigue level on selected cancer patients and general population. Each represents the location of an item-category combination. From Lai *et al.* 2000, reprinted with permission from Springer.

We did not find floor effects and found only minimal ceiling effects (7/301 = 2.3 per cent). Only one significant gap was found on the higher end (less fatigue/better quality of life) of the fatigue continuum. Based on these results, we concluded that our item writing successfully addressed the construct deficiency in the initial core fatigue item bank.

Moving into CAT: Test and item information function

CAT selection of item administration sequence is driven by a computational algorithm that evaluates the information functions of the items individually (item information function) and collectively (test information function). Individual item and test information functions for the 72 fatigue items included in the bank were therefore computed to examine how precisely this item bank estimated levels of fatigue experienced by this sample of patients. An information function estimates the maximum accuracy with which a subject's fatigue level can be estimated over the total fatigue continuum (Timminga and Adema 1995; Baker 2001). The mathematical formula for calculating information function can be found in Timminga and Adema (1995) and Wright and Masters (1982). The amount of information provided by an item/test is related to the precision with which fatigue is estimated at a specific location. Information is affected by the (1) number of test items, (2) quality of test items, and (3) match between item location and subject fatigue level (Baker 2001). Information functions do not depend on the distribution of examinees over the latent construct. The ideal information function theoretically would be a horizontal line and all subjects would be estimated with the same precision along the continuum defined by the test.

Then, item selection for people whose measurement lies at a given location can be oversampled from the target location. Unfortunately, such an information function is almost impossible to achieve in reality. More commonly, the typical shape is a bell-shaped curve in which fatigue at middle-range levels is measured more precisely than at the extremes. This is of considerable importance to both the test developer and the test consumer, since it means that the precision with which a subject's fatigue is estimated depends upon where the subject is located on the fatigue continuum. For clinical purposes, our concern was focused more on the items at the lower end of the continuum (i.e., moderate to severe fatigue). Figure 2.3.3 depicts the precision level of this item bank for the sample along the fatigue continuum. The x-axis of both upper and lower graphs is the fatigue continuum (in equal interval logit units) with more fatigue on the left end and less fatigue on the right end. The upper histogram is patient distribution and the graph at the lower portion of the figure is the error function (standard error, SE) derived by using this formula. By aligning the graphs along the same continuum it allows investigators to identify areas for bank improvement. Using an arbitrary, a priori threshold for adequate precision set at SE < 0.5, we found 95 per cent of samples were precisely measured by using this bank. All patients with SE greater than 0.5 were those who did not report severe fatigue. We, therefore,

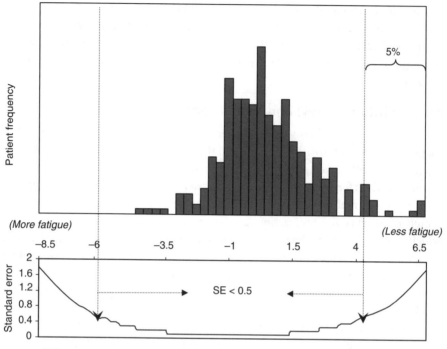

Fig. 2.3.3 Demonstration of the measurement precision of the fatigue item bank to the current sample.

concluded that this bank can precisely estimate cancer-related fatigue for patients who need clinical attention (Lai *et al.* in review).

Short-forms

Once one has a well-calibrated fatigue item bank, it is possible to draw short-form assessments that are highly precise (Kosinski *et al.* 2003). Because all items drawn from the bank are previously calibrated onto one common continuum and reported on a common metric, a short-form can serve as a means for group comparisons in settings such as multicenter clinical trials. Consequently, investigators can compare fatigue among diverse groups of patients, even if they answered different questions. Multiple short-forms can be developed from an item bank, with content and item location based upon the assessment goal and the characteristics of the patient population. This can provide flexibility of administering whichever is more convenient and more practical to the clinics. Short-forms constructed from the bank allow for brief, yet tailored, static tests targeted at the population of concern, thereby maximizing precision with a small number of questions. And yet, it remains possible to express results on a common metric shared by other investigators who may well have used other questions in the bank.

The item parameter, or calibrations, allow for this practice in settings where CAT is not feasible or desired. Following the development of an operational and psychometrically sound fatigue item bank, we have created a six-item short-form that could be used in clinical trials and other situations where group data are the unit of analysis. This particular short-form was intended to provide the same precise fatigue measure as the full fatigue item bank along the continuum. These six items (see Appendix 1 for full fatigue item bank and the fatigue short-form) together demonstrated good psychometric properties: all met pre-set measurement criteria, and the range of fatigue covered was similar to that covered by the complete bank of 72 items.

Conclusion

Because fatigue is a subjective phenomenon and lacks a clear objective criterion for verification, its measurement has challenges for both clinicians and researchers. While self-report is standard, the approach presented here provides a structure for a well-defined self-reported fatigue assessment driven by a testable measurement model. Precise measurement of fatigue has potential applications in many clinical settings, including screening, defining targeted subpopulations in need of services, and measuring change in level of fatigue over time. IRT-based measurement offers the opportunity to advance clinical applications of health status measurement by contributing to the definition of the latent trait being measured, and organizing the items – and response categories within those items – along a continuum of severity. With enough response categories across enough questions, a complete item bank for fatigue can be constructed and implemented clinically. Assessment flexibility, including multiple short-forms and CAT is then enabled while retaining a common metric. This chapter highlighted the issues to consider when developing a measure using IRT, and illustrated steps we took to achieve this goal in the development of a fatigue item bank. We began the banking process by developing a core item bank across a sample of anemic cancer patients and a general US population sample. This approach allowed us to compare cancer patients to a general US population sample. It can further permit investigators to compare fatigue scores across different patient populations using the same fatigue continuum.

In conclusion, when measuring HRQoL and related symptoms associated with medical conditions, the use of IRT has some distinct features that enable one to nicely complement what has been achieved using classical test theory. These features include the opportunity for deep, comprehensive coverage of each construct; flexibility in choice of questions used; flexibility in degree of precision obtained; availability of multiple short forms; interval measurement contributing to improved statistical power; and capability for individual assessment using computerized adaptive testing. The IRT applications described here can be applied to other related HRQoL measurement efforts across different conditions.

References

Andrich, D. (1978). A rating formulation for ordered response categories. *Psychometrika*, **43**, 561–573.

Baker, F. B. (1989). Computer technology in test construction and processing. In R. L. Linn (ed.) *Educational Measurement*, 3rd edn, pp. 409–428. New York, NY: Macmillan.

Baker, F. B. (2001). *The Basics of Item Response Theory. ERIC Clearinghouse on Assessment and Evaluation.* College Park, MD: University of Maryland.

Blesch, K. S., Paice, J. A., Wickham, R., Harte, N., Schnoor, D. K., Purl, S., *et al.* (1991). Correlates of fatigue in people with breast or lung cancer. *Oncology Nursing Forum*, **18**(1), 81–87.

Bock, R. D. (1972). Estimating item parameters and latent ability when responses are scored in two or more nominal categories. *Psychometrika*, **37**, 29–51.

Bode, R. K., Cella, D., Lai, J.-S., and Heinemann, A. W. (2003a). Developing an initial physical function item bank from existing sources. *Journal of Applied Measurement*, **4** (2), 124–136.

Bode, R. K., Lai, J.-S., Cella, D., and Heinemann, A. W. (2003b). Issues in the development of an item bank. *Archives of Physical Medicine and Rehabilitation*, **84** (4 Suppl 2), S52–S60.

Breitbart, W. (1998). Fatigue in ambulatory AIDS patients. *Journal of Pain and Symptom Management*, **15**, 159–167.

Bunderson, C. V., Inouye, D. K., and Olsen, J. B. (1989). The four generations of computerized educational measurement. In R. L. Linn (ed.) *Educational Measurement*, 3rd edn, pp. 367–408. New York, NY: Macmillan.

Cella, D. (1997a). *Manual of the Functional Assessment of Chronic Illness Therapy (FACIT) Measurement System.* Evanston, IL: Center on Outcomes, Research and Education (CORE), Evanston Northwestern Healthcare and Northwestern Universit.

Cella, D. (1997b). The Functional Assessment of Cancer Therapy-Anemia (FACT-An) scale: A new tool for the assessment of outcomes in cancer anemia and fatigue. *Seminars in Hematology*, **34** (3, Suppl 2), 13–19.

Cella, D. and Chang, C-H. (2000). A discussion of item response theory and its applications in health status assessment. *Medical Care*, **38**(Suppl. II): II66–II72.

Cella, D., Davis, K., Breitbart, W., and Curt, G. (2001). Cancer-Related Fatigue: Prevalence of proposed diagnostic criteria in a United States sample of cancer survivors. *Journal of Clinical Oncology*, **19**(14), 3385–3391.

Cella, D. F., Lloyd, S. R., and Wright, B. D. (1996). Cross-cultural instrument equating: Current research and future directions. In B. Spilker (ed.) *Quality of Life and Pharmacoeconomics in Clinical Trials*, 2nd edn, pp. 707–715. New York: Lippincott-Raven.

Cunningham, W. (1998). Constitutional symptoms and health-related quality of life in patients with symptomatic HIV disease. *American Journal of Medicine*, **104**, 129–136.

Demetri, G. D., Kris, M., Wade, J., Degos, L., and Cella, D. (1998). Quality-of-life benefit in chemotherapy patients treated with epoetin alfa is independent of disease response or tumor type: results from a prospective community oncology study. Procrit Study Group. *Journal of Clinical Oncology*, **16**(10), 3412–3425.

Ferrell, B., Grant, M., Dean, G. *et al.* (1996). "Bone tired:" The experience of fatigue and its impact on quality of life. *Oncology Nursing Forum*, **23**, 1539–1547.

Fisher, W. P. Jr. (1997). Physical disability construct convergence across instruments: Towards a universal metric. *Journal of Outcome Measurement*, **1**, 87–113.

Friedman, J. H. and Friedman, H. (2001). Fatigue in Parkinson's disease: a nine-year follow-up study. *Movement Disorders*, **16**, 1120–1122.

Friedman, J. H. and Friedman, H. (1993). Fatigue in Parkinson's disease. *Neurology*, **43**, 2016–2018.

Hambleton, R. K. (1989). Principles and selected applications of item response theory. In R. L. Linn (ed) *Educational measurement*, 3rd edn , pp. 147–200. NY: American Council on Education.

Hann, D. M., Jacobsen, P. B., Azzarello, L. M., Martin, S. C., Curran, S. L., Fields, K. K. *et al.* (1998). Measurement of fatigue in cancer patients: development and validation of the Fatigue Symptom Inventory. *Quality of Life Research*, **7**, 301–310.

Hays, R. D. (2005). Generic versus disease-targeted instruments. In P. Fayers and R. D. Hays (eds) *Assessing Quality of Life in Clinical Trials*. Oxford: Oxford University Press.

Hays, R. D. and Revicki, D. A. (in press) Reliability and Validity (including Responsiveness). In P. Fayers and R. D. Hays (eds) *Assessing Quality of Life in Clinical Trials*. Oxford: Oxford University Press.

Hays, R. D., Morales, L. S., and Reise, S. P. (2000). Item response theory and health outcomes measurement in the 21st century. *Medical Care*, **38**, II28–II42.

Irvine, D., Vincent, L., Graydon, J. E., Bubela, N., and Thompson, L. (1994). The prevalence and correlates of fatigue in patients receiving treatment with chemotherapy and radiotherapy. A comparison with the fatigue experienced by healthy individuals. *Cancer Nursing*, **17**(5), 367–378.

Karlsen, K., Larsen, J., and Tandberg, E. *et al.* (1999). Fatigue in patients with Parkinson's disease. *Movement Disorders*, **14**, 237–241.

Kosinski, M., Bayliss, M. S., Bjorner, J. B., Ware, J. E., Garber, W. H., Batenhorst, A., *et al.* (2003). A six-item short-form survey for measuring headache impact: The HIT-6™. *Quality of Life Research*, **12**(8), 963–974.

Krupp, L. and Pollina, D. (1996). Mechanisms and management of fatigue in progressive neurological disorders. *Current Opinion in Neurology*, **9**(6), 456–501.

Lai, J.-S., Eton, D. T., and Cella, D. (2003a). Measuring bowel function in prostate cancer patients. *Annals of Behavioral Medicine*, **23** (Supplement), S066.

Lai, J-S., Cella, D., Chang, C-H., Bode, R., and Heinemann, A.W. (2003b). Item Banking to improve, shorten and computerize self-reported fatigue: An illustration of steps to create a core item bank from the FACIT-Fatigue Scale. *Quality of Life Research*, **12**, 485–501.

Lai, J.-S., Cella, D., Dineen, K., Bode, R., Von Roenn, J., Gershon, R., and Shevrin, D. (2005) Item banking to improve measurement of cancer-related fatigue. *Journal of Clinical Epidemiology*, **58**, 190–197.

Lai, J-S., Dineen, K., Reeve, B. B., Von Roenn, J., Shevrin, D., McGuire, M., *et al.* (in review). *An Item Response Theory based pain item bank can enhance measurement precision*.

Liang, M., Rogers, M., and Larson, M. *et al.* (1984). The psychosocial impact of systemic lupus erythematosus and rheumatoid arthritis. *Arthritis and Rheumatism*, **27**, 13–19.

Linacre, J. M. (1994). Sample size and item calibration stability. *Rasch Measurement Transactions*, **7**, 328.

Lunz, M. E. and Bergstrom, B. (1994). Computer adaptive testing: A national pilot study. In M. Wilson (ed), *Objective Measurement: Theory into Practice, Volume* **2**, pp. 103–114. Norwood NJ: Ablex Publishing.

McNair, D. M., Lorr, M., and Droppelman, L. F. (1971). Manual for the Profile of Mood States. San Diego: Educational and Industrial Testing Service.

Mendoza, T. R., Wang, X. S., Cleeland, C. S., Morrissey, M., Johnson, B. A., Wendt, J. K., and Huber, S. L. (1999). The rapid assessment of fatigue severity in cancer patients: Use of the Brief Fatigue Inventory. *Cancer*, **85**, 1186–1196.

Nail, L. M. and Winningham, M. L. (1995). Fatigue and weakness in cancer patients: The symptoms experience. *Seminars in Oncology Nursing*, **11**(4), 272–278.

National Comprehensive Cancer Network (2003). *NCCN Clinical Practice Guidelines in Oncology: Cancer-related Fatigue.* Available: www.nccn.org.

Piper, B. F., Lindsey, A. M., Dodd, M. J., *et al.* (1989). The development of an instrument to measure the subjective dimensions of fatigue. In S. G. Funk, E. M. Tornquist, M. T. Champagne, L. Archer Copp, and R. A. Wiese (eds). *Key aspects of comfort management of pain and nausea.* Philadelphia: Springer.

Piper, B. F., Dibble, S. L., Dodd, M. J., Weiss, M. C., Slaughter, R. E., and Paul, S. M. (1998). The revised Piper Fatigue Scale: Psychometric evaluation in women with breast cancer. *Oncol Nurs Forum,* **25**, 711-717.

Reise, S. P., Widaman, R. F., and Pugh, K. H. (1993). Confirmatory factor analysis and item response theory: two approaches for exploring measurement invariance. *Psychological Bulletin,* **114**, 552–566.

Schur, P. (1989). Clinical features of SLE. In W. N. Kelly, E. D. Harris, Jr, S. Ruddy, and C. B. Sledge (eds) *Textbook of Rheumatology.* Philadelphia, PA: W. B. Saunders.

Schwartz, J. E., Jandorf, L., and Krupp, L.B. (1993). The measurement of fatigue: A new instrument. *J Psychosom Res.* **37**(7), 753–762.

Smets, E. M. A., Garssen, B., Bonke, B., and DeHaes, J. C. J. M. (1995). The Multidimensional Fatigue Inventory (MFI) psychometric qualities of an instrument to assess fatigue. *Journal of Psychometric Research,* **39**, 315–325.

Thissen, D. and Orlando, M. (2001). Item Response Theory for items scored in two categories. In D. Thissen and H. Wainer (eds). *Test scoring* (pp. 74-140). Mahwah, NJ: Lawrence Erlbaum Associates.

Timminga, E. and Adema, J. J. (1995). Test construction from item banks. In G. H. Fischer and I. W. Molenaar (eds). *Rasch MODELS: Foundations, recent developments, and applications,* pp. 111–130. New York: Springer-Verlag Inc.

Vickery, B. (forthcoming). Developing disease-targeted health-related quality of life measures for neurologic conditions. In P. Fayers and R. Hays (eds) *Assessing Quality of Life.* Oxford: Oxford University Press.

Vogelzang, N. J., Breitbart, W., Cella, D., Curt, G. A., Groopman, J. E., Horning, S. J., *et al.* (1997). Patient, caregiver, and oncologist perceptions of cancer-related fatigue: Results of a tripart assessment survey. The Fatigue Coalition. *Seminars in Hematology,* **34**(3 Suppl 2), 4–12.

Winningham, M., Nail, L., Burke, M., *et al.* (1994). Fatigue and the cancer experience: The state of the knowledge. *Oncology Nursing Forum,* **21**, 23–36.

Wright, B. D. and Masters, G. N. (1982). *Rating Scale Analysis: Rasch Measurement.* Chicago, IL: MESA Press.

Yellen, S. B., Cella, D. F., Webster, K., Blendowski, C., and Kaplan, E. (1997). Measuring fatigue and other anemia-related symptoms with the Functional Assessment of Cancer Therapy (FACT) measurement system. *Journal of Pain and Symptom Management,* **13**, 63–74.

Appendix 1: 72-item Fatigue Bank*

1. **I have had enough energy to exercise strenuously.**
2. I have had enough energy to play sports.
3. I have had enough energy to lift heavy objects.
4. I have been too tired to lift heavy objects.
5. I feel fatigued.
6. I feel tired.
7. I have had enough energy to exercise moderately.
8. I have energy.
9. I have a lack of energy.
10. **I have been too tired to exercise moderately.**
11. I have felt energetic.
12. I have had enough energy to exercise lightly.
13. **I have had enough energy to get through the day without resting.**
14. I have felt worn out.
15. Fatigue interferes with my ability to work.
16. I have been too tired to clean the house.
17. Fatigue interferes with my ability to do household chores.
18. I have been too tired to exercise lightly.
19. I am able to do my usual activities.
20. Fatigue interferes with my social activities.
21. I have trouble starting things because I am tired.
22. I have had enough energy to clean the house.
23. I have trouble finishing things because I am tired.
24. I have been too tired to do errands.
25. I have been so tired that I need to rest during the day.
26. Fatigue interferes with my mood.
27. Fatigue interferes with my family life.
28. I have been too tired to do my normal household chores.
29. I need to sleep during the day.
30. I have been too tired to go out with my friends.
31. I have had enough energy to do errands.
32. I have been too tired to take a short walk.
33. I am frustrated by being too tired to the things I want to do.
34. I have had enough energy to climb more than one flight of stairs.
35. I have been too tired to enjoy the things I do for fun.
36. Fatigue makes me depressed.
37. Fatigue interferes with my ability to concentrate.
38. I have been too tired to prepare a meal.
39. I have had enough energy to go out with my friends.
40. I am too tired to climb more than one flight of stairs.

41. I feel listless ('washed out').
42. I have had enough energy to do my normal household chores.
43. I have had enough energy to enjoy the things I do for fun.
44. I have been too tired to concentrate.
45. I have been too tired to go out with my family.
46. I have had enough energy to carry groceries.
47. I have to limit my social activity because I am tired.
48. I have been too tired to enjoy life.
49. I have been too tired to leave the house.
50. I need help doing my usual activities.
51. I have been too tired to carry groceries.
52. I have had enough energy to go out with my family.
53. I feel weak all over.
54. I have had enough energy to feel happy.
55. I have had enough energy to enjoy life.
56. I have been too tired to feel happy.
57. I have been too tired to write a letter.
58. I have had enough energy to write a letter.
59. I have been too tired to read.
60. **I have been too tired to think clearly.**
61. I have had enough energy to concentrate.
62. I have been too tired to climb one flight of stairs.
63. I have had enough energy to climb one flight of stairs.
64. I have had enough energy to leave the house.
65. I have had enough energy to read.
66. Fatigue interferes with my ability to eat meals.
67. I have been too tired to watch television.
68. I am too tired to eat.
69. I have been too tired to eat.
70. **I have been too tired to take a bath or shower.**
71. I have had enough energy to take a bath or shower.
72. **I have had enough energy to eat.**

---

* Questions in bold text comprise the sample short form described in the text. Response options to all questions are:

None of the time
A little of the time
Some of the time
Most of the time
All of the time

Context effects and proxy assessments

Elaine McColl and Peter Fayers

Introduction

Responses to subjective questions – such as those concerning quality of life – are open to external influences, and a patient may answer the same question very differently according to the context. Thus, for example, previous questions might influence answers by focusing attention on specific issues, or by affecting the patient's mood or attitude; perhaps the setting (home/hospital) or mode of administration (e.g. self-completed paper-based questionnaire, computer touch-screen, or interview) might have an impact. This chapter reviews the literature regarding the impact of such effects on HRQoL assessment. This is a rapidly changing field, and we make no pretence of having carried out a formal systematic review – but we believe that the conclusions faithfully represent current knowledge on this subject. We also draw extensively on the work carried out in survey research since the 1970s, and in particular recommend as further reading the books by Schuman and Presser (1981), Sudman and colleagues (1996) and Tourangeau and co-workers (2000) for comprehensive reviews of research into the cognitive processes involved in responding to survey questions.

The model of the cognitive processes proposed by Tourangeau and colleagues (2000) provides a theoretical basis for context effects. It identifies four stages in producing an answer: comprehension; retrieval; judgment; response. It suggests that, in the limited time available to respond to a questionnaire, respondents do not carry out an in-depth trawl of all relevant beliefs and experiences, but instead are likely to retrieve only a small sample of memories and feelings. This is especially true if they seek to minimize the amount of cognitive effort they put in ('satisfice'). Furthermore, this mental sample is likely to be biased in favour of those beliefs and experiences that are currently most accessible. Both the physical setting in which the questionnaire is completed, and the mind set induced by other questions, can affect accessibility, thus producing context effects.

Question and instrument ordering effects

In evaluations of health technologies, it is generally agreed that a combination of generic and condition-specific measures of HRQoL is required. Condition-specific and generic measures are also often used in combination to establish the validity of newly developed instruments, or the applicability of existing measures in new populations. Yet there is little consensus about which should be administered first, or whether questions on quality of life should precede or follow those on other topics (e.g. patient characteristics, use of health services). In validation studies, some experts recommend administering the instruments in a randomized order, while others favour placing the instrument to be validated first, especially if it is designed as a stand-alone instrument. Developers' instructions for many instruments state that their questionnaire should be put first – which presents an insoluble challenge for studies where multiple instruments are used. By implication, these recommendations suggest that instrument order matters, and that responses to a particular instrument (or to questions within an instrument) may be influenced by the preceding questions. Empirical evidence for these recommendations is seldom cited.

Four specific types of question order effects have been proposed – saliency, redundancy, consistency and fatigue. There is also the possibility of rapport and learning effects, and it has been suggested that question order can lead to both consistency and contrast effects (Schuman and Presser 1981). This is supported by Tourangeau and colleagues' model (1988; 2000), which implies that previous questions can: affect the interpretation of subjective items, influence the specific beliefs and experiences which are accessed or retrieved, influence the dimensions, standards or norms applied in making the required judgment, and affect how an answer is reported. Such context effects can operate both in favour of greater apparent consistency and greater contrast. Collectively, these concepts underpin the common wisdom that general questions should precede those about more specific issues. This view is reflected, for example, in the recommendations about the administration of the generic SF-36 before other questionnaires (Ware *et al.* 1993), and the cancer-specific EORTC QLQ-C30 before site-specific modules (Sprangers *et al.* 1998).

A major factor in questionnaire response rates is whether the subject matter is relevant, appropriate and interesting (salient) to the target population. In general surveys it has been shown that respondents' attention will be captured if the opening items address their interests and concerns, and they are then likely to answer every question because of a 'completion tendency' (Roberson and Sundstrom 1990). There is little evidence, however, that this effect translates to quality of life assessments. McColl and colleagues (2003) found no significant differences in questionnaire response rates when condition-specific instruments for asthma or angina (which could be seen as being more salient) were placed before or after generic quality of life instruments. It seems likely that, in the context of a clinical trial or other HRQoL research study, respondents consider all questions on their well-being, both general and disease-specific, to be relevant and important. Compliance with questionnaire completion protocol can also be enhanced by explaining the purpose of the study and the importance of completing the questionnaire.

Fatigue effects are manifested when respondents tire as they work through the questionnaire. In extreme cases, they may abandon the questionnaire part way through. More usually, fatigue leads to greater accidental or deliberate omission of later items, or to more stereotypical responses such as endorsing the same response category for all items; stereotypical responses and increasing frequency of omissions for later items are both commonly observed on HRQoL questionnaires in clinical trials. The risk of fatigue is one reason for administering first whichever quality of life instrument taps the primary outcome in a trial. On the other hand, learning effects occur when respondents become more familiar with the cognitive tasks of responding as they proceed through the questionnaire. For example, they may become more proficient in using response scales, leading to a lower rate of item non-response to later questions. In their study, McColl and colleagues (2003) used item non-response rates to test for fatigue and learning effects. The angina questionnaire was 13 pages long and contained 73 items while the asthma questionnaire was 17 pages long and contained 94 items; in both, demographic questions followed the quality of life items. Item non-response rates were very low throughout, and there was no significant ordering effect with respect to the pattern of missing data.

Rapport effects relate to the positioning of items of a sensitive or personal nature. It is generally held that these items are best placed later in a questionnaire, once a feeling of trust has been established with the respondent. This may result both in lower rates of item non-response and in more 'truthful' (valid) responses. However, findings from experiments in general surveys with the placement of personal questions are equivocal and there is no empirical evidence from quality of life research on the topic of rapport. Despite this, it is strongly recommended to place sensitive or embarrassing questions at the end of a HRQoL questionnaire, because some patients may become offended or distressed and then cease completing the questionnaire. For example, it is relevant to ask prostate and gynaecological cancer patients about sexual activity and problems, but it has frequently been observed that in many cultures, and especially in older patients, this may lead to serious compliance issues. Patients may be more willing to answer if they are told *why* these questions are being asked, while compliance with questionnaire completion may be improved if responding to these items is made optional.

Context effects, including redundancy and consistency effects, are generally a function of the relative placement of items. Questions appearing earlier in the questionnaire may provide a frame of reference for the interpretation and answering of later questions. One means by which consistency effects may be evoked is the 'norm of reciprocity', whereby responses are consciously or subconsciously brought into line with each other, perhaps to present a more consistent image to an interviewer or researcher.

Consistency effects may also result from 'priming' – preceding questions bring certain issues to the forefront of the respondent's mind, and thereby make certain beliefs and experiences more accessible in answering later items. This notion of priming is implicit in the placement at the end of the instrument of the global health rating item in the EORTC QLQ-C30; it is assumed that preceding questions on role functioning, social and emotional well-being will indicate to the respondents that these issues, not just physical well-being, should be taken into account in assessing overall quality of life.

There is limited empirical evidence to support the existence of a priming effect. David and colleagues (1999) experimented with the placement, as the first or last item, of a global question on evaluation of health (normally the first item) within a self-completed SF-36 questionnaire. When this question appeared first, there was a tendency for patients to report better health; however, this trend was only statistically significant when those subjects with 'middle' responses (very good – good – fair) were considered. David and colleagues suggested that, 'once reminded of their poor health by respond-ing to the entire SF-36', respondents might downgrade their overall self-assessment when the global item appeared last. Briancon and colleagues (2001) randomized the order of the SF-36 and a visual analogue scale (VAS) to assess general health. They demonstrated an interaction between gender and instrument position with respect to VAS ratings, but scores on the eight sub-scales of the SF-36 were not affected by the relative placement of the two instruments.

Conversely, contrast effects arise when the order in which questions are presented leads to greater differences between responses. If a general question follows more spe-cific questions, respondents may mentally redefine the general item to subtract what now seems redundant information. In HRQoL assessments, subtraction could make responses to generic instruments different when those instruments are administered after condition-specific measures ('my general health, *excluding* the issues I have just reported on'). However, empirical evidence from a number of studies (Barry *et al.* 1996; Wu *et al.* 1997; Leidy *et al.* 2000; McColl *et al.* 2003) does not support the notion of 'subtraction' effects, or indeed of any impact of instrument ordering on scores on either the generic or condition-specific instruments. In more than 70 comparisons across these four studies, only two differences reached statistical significance at the 5 per cent level, and the observed differences were all in the negligible to small range (effect sizes less than 0.5).

Nor does empirical research provide strong support for the concept of consistency effects in quality of life assessments, with the exception of the priming effect described above. Three studies (Leidy *et al.* 2000; Letley and Garratt 2000; McColl *et al.* 2003) have investigated the effect of instrument ordering on the internal consistency of responses. Their findings are equivocal; for the most part, observed values of Cronbach's α were not significantly different between the two versions. Of the statisti-cally significant differences, some favoured placing the condition-specific instrument first, others the generic first. However, even these differences were sufficiently small as to be unlikely to alter conclusions about instrument reliability.

Mode of administration

Mode of questionnaire administration is one of the first decisions to be made when collecting quality of life data. Essentially the choice is between interviewer-administration (either face-to-face or by telephone) or self-completion by the respondent (either by post or, for example, in a clinic). Both face-to-face and telephone interviews can be computer-assisted. There is also growing interest in computerized administration of self-completion questionnaires, either using conventional keyboard entry or touch-screen methods. Survey researchers are generally agreed that each mode of question-naire administration has its advantages and disadvantages in respect of the quantity and quality of data collected (Table 2.4.1).

Response rates

Interviewer administration relieves the respondent of the burden of recording the responses, and the interviewer can probe and prompt for further details. Thus it may be possible to use longer questionnaires, and collect more detailed and complex data. It has also been suggested that overall response rates will be higher because of reduced respondent burden, and that, with face-to-face administration, refusal bias is reduced by the social interaction with the interviewer. However, evidence from quality of life studies is equivocal and in many cases runs counter to received wisdom. For example, Aneshensel and colleagues (1982) randomized individuals to face-to-face or telephone interviews and found a slightly higher, though not statistically significant, rate of response in the telephone interview group (82 per cent versus 80 per cent). McHorney and colleagues (1994) found that significantly more of those randomized to postal self-completion of the SF-36 responded (79 per cent) than for telephone interview (69 per cent), but after excluding those who completed the survey by a mode other than that originally assigned, the difference was not statistically significant.

High response rates reduce the risk of non-response bias (although they are not in themselves a guarantee of an unbiased sample). McHorney and colleagues (1994) found evidence of non-response bias for both modes of administration, with non-respondents having less education, lower income and being less likely to be in employ-ment; however, only for age was the nature of the non-response bias different between the two modes of administration.

Low response rates and non-response bias are particularly relevant in surveys, where participant recruitment and data collection are part of the same process; postal surveys of HRQoL frequently report compliance rates of about two-thirds. In clinical trials, participants will generally have agreed to participate prior to collection of quality of life data, and there is evidence that compliance rates of over 95 per cent are attainable if the objectives are explained to patients and they are given encouragement (Sadura *et al.* 1992). Thus in clinical trials the effect of mode of administration on overall response rates may not be so marked.

Table 2.4.1 Advantages and disadvantages of different modes of questionnaire administration (adapted from De Vaus (1991) after Dillman (1978)).

	Face-to-face interviews	Telephone interviews	Postal questionnaires
Response rates			
General population samples	Usually best	Usually lower than face-to-face	Poor to good
Special population samples	Usually good	Satisfactory to best	Satisfactory to good
Representative samples			
Avoidance of refusal bias	Depends on good interviewer technique	Depends on good interviewer technique	Poor
Control over who completes the questionnaire	Good	Moderate	Poor to good
Gaining access to a named selected person	Good	Good for those with telephones	Poor to good
Locating the named selected person	Good	Good	Good
Ability to handle:			
Long questionnaires	Good	Moderate	Satisfactory to poor
Complex questions	Good	Moderate	Moderate to poor
Boring questions	Good	Moderate	Poor
Item non-response	Good	Good	Moderate
Filter questions	Good	Good	Moderate to poor
Question sequence control	Good	Good	Poor
Open-ended questions	Good	Good	Poor
Quality of answers			
Minimize social desirability responses	Poor	Moderate	Satisfactory
Ability to avoid distortion due to:			
Interviewer characteristics	Poor	Moderate	Good
Interviewer's opinions	Moderate	Moderate	Good
Influence of other people	Moderate	Good	Poor
Allows opportunities to consult	Moderate	Poor	Good
Implementing the survey			
Ease of finding suitable staff	Poor	Moderate	Good
Speed	Poor	Good	Poor
Cost	Poor	Moderate	Good

Mode of administration may also affect item non-response patterns. Item non-response rates could be lower with interviewer-administration, because the burden of recording responses falls on the interviewer and risk of respondent fatigue effects is lessened. However, item non-response to sensitive questions may be greater in the presence of an interviewer, because of the embarrassment factor. Computer-assisted administration can also reduce item non-response rates, because the system can be programmed to prompt for a response or even to prevent progression to the next item until a response is entered (when appropriate, response options for 'not applicable' or even 'don't want to say' may be permitted). There is growing evidence from HRQoL studies to support the acceptability of computer-based questionnaires and their impact in minimizing item non-response rates – as reported in Chapter 4.5.

Validity and reliability

Mode of administration may affect the validity and reliability of responses, but the relative merits of different modes is unclear. In theory, interviewers can clarify and explain questions, ensure that they are answered in the correct sequence, and implement complex filter and skip instructions. However, these advantages are less relevant when highly structured instruments, such as most quality of life measures, are employed. There is also the risk that interviewers, or even people assisting with a self-completion questionnaire, may introduce both random and systematic errors, and for this reason many instruments intended for use in clinical trials carry the recommendation that, whenever possible, competent patients should complete the questionnaire on their own in private, and without assistance. Random errors, for example due to interviewer inaccuracy in recording answers, are possibly of minor importance. Systematic effects, or bias, are more serious. Systematic effects include those due to the interviewer alone, such as differential probing for a substantive response or acceptance of 'don't know' answers, and those that are due to the interviewer–respondent interaction, in particular social desirability bias, whereby respondents may systematically try 'to please the doctor' or other staff by reporting a higher than actual quality of life, or may under-report in an effort to gain further health care. Although these latter biases may occur irrespective of the mode of administration, they are likely to be more pronounced in interviews.

Effects of the order in which response categories are presented ('response order' effects) have also been postulated to differ with mode of administration. 'Primacy' effects (the tendency to select the first apparently appropriate response category) may occur more frequently in self-completion (including postal) questionnaires, and where cue cards are presented to respondents by interviewers, while 'recency' effects (the tendency to select response options towards the end of the offered list) are more likely under interviewer administration (including telephone interviews) where the respondent simply listens to a list of responses read out by the interviewer. The rationale for these proposed effects is the difference in stimulus – visual versus auditory – coupled with the tendency to satisfice (Krosnick 2000).

Several studies have compared scores on quality of life instruments across different modes of administration, with varying findings. McHorney and colleagues (1994) found that their postal survey yielded less favourable health ratings than the telephone survey, and suggested that the former mode offers greater anonymity for reporting sensitive and personal information. In Aneshensel and colleagues' survey (1982), a significantly greater number of face-to-face interview respondents reported restricted activity days (due to disability) compared with telephone respondents. By contrast, Wu and colleagues (1997) found no significant differences in scores on the EuroQol or MOS-HIV between face-to-face and telephone interviews, with the exception of the MOS-HIV social functioning scale, where significantly lower scores were found for telephone interview (60.0 versus 72.1, a moderate effect size of 0.6 with respect to the reference value of face-to-face interview). Litaker (2003) compared conducted pair-wise comparisons of paper-and-pencil, computer touch-screen and web-based administration of the Rhinoconjunctivitis Quality of Life Questionnaire (RQLQ) and the Work Productivity and Activity Impairment (WPAI) instrument. Although no mode effects were observed for the RQLQ, respondents completing the web-based version of the WPAI reported higher scores on average than those completing the pencil-and-paper and touch-screen versions, with the latter difference reaching statistical significance. Ryan and colleagues (2002) found minimal differences in SF-36 scale scores between electronic and paper versions of the instrument; the largest difference was −2.8 points for the social function scale, equivalent to a negligible effect size of 0.11, using the traditional paper-based version as the reference. A problem in interpretation of all of these findings, however, is the absence of an objective 'gold standard' by which to judge which mode yields the more valid responses.

Feasibility and acceptability

Many investigators are reporting that respondents prefer computer-aided questionnaires, with either keyboard or touch-screen data entry, over paper-based versions – see Chapter 4.5. There can also be substantial time and cost savings in terms of data entry and verification. Telephone interviewing, on the other hand, is likely to be one of the more expensive options, although less costly than travelling to interview patients at home.

Place of administration

Some researchers (e.g. Osoba 1992) caution against postal administration or allowing respondents to take questionnaires home to complete. Their rationale is that greater variability of surroundings and time of completion may affect responses. More importantly, it is impossible to know whether respondents have indeed completed the questionnaire themselves or the extent to which they have been influenced by the opinions of others. It is easier to control and standardize the setting in a hospital environment.

However, hospital settings may prime respondents to focus on negative aspects of their health and well-being, and therefore to report poorer quality of life than they would in the normal home environment. Social comparisons might also be made with other patients, which could result in biased responses. An experiment in which respondents completed a general health status measure twice in a group setting led to their reporting better health status on average when a wheelchair-bound individual was introduced to the group, presumably because of downward social comparisons (M Couper, personal communication, 2003).

Completion of a health status or quality of life questionnaire when confined to or attending hospital may introduce confounding factors. Ziebland (1994) suggests that hospitalization might of itself lead to greater anxiety and depression, and role performance may be reduced, not only by the illness or injury leading to hospitalization, but also because of the hospital routine (e.g. being confined to bed or one room for the convenience of hospital staff rather than out of medical need). Empirical evidence of the effect of setting on quality of life reports is scant, partly because of the difficulty in designing and implementing comparative studies. Bardsley and colleagues (1992) found no effect of hospitalization on scores on the Nottingham Health Profile and Muntner and co-workers (2000) reported similar psychometric properties for the Asthma Quality of Life Questionnaire during acute hospitalization and subsequently at an outpatient visit (the setting for which it was originally designed). By contrast, Jenkinson and colleagues (1993) found that 36 per cent of rheumatoid arthritis patients who were originally recruited as inpatients had significantly poorer scores on the mobility scale of the Functional Limitations Profile (FLP), despite very similar scores on other domains and on clinical tests. They concluded that the apparently marked restriction of physical function was largely an artefact of the combination of a reference period of 'today' with statements such as 'I stay in one room' and 'I only get about in one building' in the FLP mobility scale. Ziebland (1994) cautions about the interpretation of comparisons of pre-discharge and post-discharge data in situations where such effects might occur.

Proxy effects

Quality of life is essentially subjective and it is the individual who experiences that life who is best placed to report on it. However, there are circumstances in which assessments of health status, functioning and quality of life are desirable, but where the individual concerned is not capable of self-reporting because of old age, communication difficulties or cognitive impairment. In such circumstances patient responses will either be missing or of dubious validity. Proxy respondents – either health professionals or relatives – provide a valuable alternative. Failure to use proxy respondents could result in over-estimates of health status and quality of life, or biased estimates of the impact of an intervention, since it is likely to be the frailest and most ill individuals who are unable to provide self-reports. Proxy assessments may also be required for very young children.

There have been a large number of studies across a range of conditions comparing proxy assessments with patients' self-assessments, but many have used small sample sizes. The results have been usefully summarized by several authors. Sprangers and Aaronson (1992) initially reviewed 49 studies that compared proxies and patients with chronic disease, and in 2002 focused on a further 23 more recent studies (Sneeuw *et al.* 2002). McPherson and Addington-Hall (2003) reviewed 30 studies of patients at the end of life; only six studies, in cancer, overlapped between the reviews of these two groups of investigators. Lampic and Sjödén (2000) reviewed 22 studies of cancer patients' psychological concerns and needs; again there was a small overlap (seven studies). A further contribution to this debate is the meta-analysis by Janse and colleagues (2004), focusing on quality of life as assessed simultaneously by physicians versus patients (including both children and adults) using the same validated generic or condition-specific quality of life questionnaire. Of 1,316 articles initially identified by their research strategy, only 12 met the inclusion criteria in full, in the sense of providing strictly comparable assessments; only six (all relating to paediatric populations) were appropriate for inclusion in a meta-analysis.

When considering the adequacy of proxy ratings, it is important to distinguish between group-level assessments – as in clinical trials – and individual-patient assessments. For group assessments and comparisons, we are primarily concerned with the impact on the means (or other group summaries, such as medians), as this amounts to bias; we are also concerned to avoid extra 'noise' or imprecision due to proxy assessment, as increased variability will affect the standard deviation and reduce the power to detect differences. When monitoring individual patients, we are rather more concerned with the level of agreement between proxies and patients – as, for example, reflected statistically by the intra-class correlation, or more simply by the percentage of cases in which there is perfect agreement or close agreement. Thus it is possible to have 'high or good agreement' from the perspective of group comparisons, but inadequate agreement for useful individual-patient assessments.

Findings from studies across a range of conditions show that agreement between individual patient and clinicians' (or other health care providers') ratings, both of symptoms and of quality of life impairment, is generally only weak to moderate. Although discrepancies in both directions have been reported, the most common finding is that, relative to patient ratings, clinicians tend to rate the patients as having slightly lower levels of functioning and health, and slightly more symptomatology. They also tend to overestimate the levels of anxiety, depression and distress. On the other hand, minor symptoms and the more common symptoms tend to be under-reported – perhaps because if a symptom is characteristic of all patients with a particular illness, then minor cases of that symptom are regarded as not worthy of noting unless they cause particular distress. Thus it has been observed that the level of disagreement is usually greater in respect of patients with less severe symptoms or impairment. Agreement about the presence of symptoms is usually better than agreement about symptom intensity, and as might be expected agreement is strong for concrete and visible symptoms but weak for dimensions such as anxiety and depression. Overall, most reviewers suggest that agreement between patients and clinicians – or other health care providers – is poor for individual patients, but is reasonably good for group comparisons, and that the bias in group means is likely to be small in terms of effect sizes (median overall effect sizes ranged from 0.03 to –0.28, where effect size equals mean difference divided by standard deviation).

There are a number of possible explanations for this lack of concordance. Clinical training emphasizes symptom frequency and severity for diagnosis and treatment, so it is not surprising that clinicians may focus primarily on these more easily observable and measurable aspects, while patients also consider symptom-related disability, and the impact on quality of life. Patients and clinicians may also use different frames of reference in their assessments, with patients considering their own past experiences of symptoms or an ideal state of health, while health care professionals may implicitly compare a given patient to other patients whom they have treated. A patient may regard their pain as being very severe, whereas to clinicians that pain may appear trivial compared to the extreme suffering observed in many other patients. However, it has also been suggested that patients' ratings may frequently be biased for a variety of reasons, and cannot necessarily be accepted as a gold standard. Thus patients may report low levels of symptoms and psychosocial concerns to avoid presenting themselves as a burden to family or others, to please the health care staff, or may over-report because they fear their treatment may be reduced. A few studies have used multiple raters (physician, nurse, significant other) and have noted that patients frequently differ from all the observers. Two possible explanations are that the observers were equally unaware of the patients' health experience, or that the validity of the patients' scores is called into question. A more likely explanation may be that patients adapt to their illness, learn to cope, and in various ways 'response shift' (see Chapter 4.4); thus only the patients themselves can say how their illness impacts on their inner sense of quality of life, observers merely see the physical signs.

Similar mismatches are found in comparisons of the ratings of patients and 'significant others', including spouses, other relatives and informal caregivers. In general, concordance between patients and significant others appear to be better than that between patients and health professionals, with intraclass correlations between 0.60 and 0.70 for physical domains of quality of life, and of the order of 0.50 for psychosocial domains. The closer the significant other, the closer the agreement.

Overall, substantial discrepancies between proxies and patients are only reported in a minority of cases, and judgements of proxies appear to be reasonably accurate, especially for the more physical symptoms and observable aspects of quality of life. For clinical trials, it will usually be preferable to use proxy ratings than to have missing data, but best of all is to obtain the patients' self-rating. However, there is still a need for large studies which further investigate the adequacy of proxy ratings, factors affecting the discrepancies, and methods of improving proxy reports.

One group of patients inadequately represented in existing reviews are the cognitively impaired, for example those with Alzheimer's disease, or those in palliative care and with delirium. Although there have been a number of studies investigating proxies in these important groups of patients, proxy-patient comparisons inevitably have to focus on the milder end of the spectrum where the patients are able to provide a coherent self-assessment (and where, by definition, proxy assessments are less essential). It is not clear how well one can extrapolate from these findings to more severe cases, and indeed there is philosophical debate about the meaning of quality of life in severely ill patients, with some investigators holding the view that absence of symptoms and suffering must be the most important objective for the demented. It remains unclear as to the adequacy of proxy ratings, and at what level of cognitive impairment they should be used.

Children, especially young ones, may also need to be assessed by proxies and present special problems. Eiser and Morse (2001) reviewed 14 such studies. Many of the issues are covered in Chapter 5.3. As with studies of the cognitively impaired, direct comparisons of proxies and self assessments have to rely on studies in children with adequate comprehension skills – the older ones. And again there are questions about downward extrapolation – can we be sure that results for older children will apply to those too young to answer for themselves? In older children, it has been reported that, as for adults, there is greater agreement with proxies about physical symptoms and observable functioning. There is no clear conclusion as to whether parents perceive the illness to have greater impact than their child. Agreement is better between parents and chronically ill children compared to parents and healthy children. It is therefore suggested that ratings be obtained from both parents and children.

Conclusions and recommendations

Question and instrument ordering

Empirical evidence for ordering effects within or across HRQoL questionnaires remains weak and inconsistent across studies. Thus there appears to be no intrinsic merit in placing generic instruments before condition-specific or vice versa, although there is some indication of priming or framing effects which may or may not support placing global 'overall quality of life' questions at the end of a questionnaire.

It seems prudent to reduce the effects of fatigue by keeping questionnaires brief and relevant. The most important and informative items may be best placed at the beginning, and sensitive, personal or potentially embarrassing items towards the end. But the principal reason for the frequent statements (a) 'use our instrument first' and (b) 'do not alter the order of items on our questionnaire, and place any new items at the end' remains the unsubstantiated fear that, unless proven otherwise, bias could conceivably result. In the absence of evidence to the contrary, it does seem prudent to maintain a standardized order of questionnaires within a clinical trial. Also, to facilitate comparisons across studies, if possible try to adhere to the same order as used by others.

Mode of administration

Neither expert opinion nor empirical evidence indicates the superiority of any one mode of administration in all respects or in all settings. The choice of mode of administration therefore needs to be made on a study-by-study basis, taking into account: the mode for which the instrument of choice was designed and validated (adapting an instrument for a new mode of administration is not be undertaken lightly, and will generally require further testing); the study population (for example, do sensory or motor impairments preclude some modes?); the method and timing of participant identification, recruitment and follow-up (for example, if there they are not being followed up in clinic, telephone, postal or web-based delivery may be more appropriate); and the resources available for data collection (face-to-face interviews being much more resource intensive than any other approach). Trade-offs between the quantity and/or quality of data that can be collected and the financial and opportunity costs of collecting those data may be required. As with ordering effects, evidence suggests that mode of administration effects on quality of life scores are likely to be small. Nonetheless, caution is needed in employing mixed modes within a single study; if multiple methods of data collection are used, testing for mode effects should be carried out before pooling data across methods.

Place of administration

In trials where patients are identified and recruited in hospital or clinic settings, it is usually appropriate and administratively convenient to collect quality of life data in that setting. In some studies, such as trials of certain surgical interventions, the most appropriate timing of initial HRQoL assessments will be on a hospital ward during inpatient stay, although completion of subsequent follow-up questionnaires may be in the outpatient clinic or the patient's own home. In such situations, care should be taken that the setting for completion is not a confounding factor, as in the study by Jenkinson and colleagues (1993). Moreover, because the setting may influence the response, for any given follow-up, all respondents should complete the questionnaire in the same place; if this is not feasible, tests for setting effects should be carried out before pooling data.

Use of proxies

The majority of studies have shown differences between self-reports and proxy ratings of symptoms and quality of life, though the observed effect sizes are generally small. Proxies tend to rate the patients as having slightly lower levels of functioning and health, and slightly more symptomatology, though this general pattern may vary with the nature of the proxy and of the disease. In collecting quality of life data, the ideal informant is the individual experiencing the life. However, when respondents are incapable of responding themselves, the use of a well-chosen proxy (the balance of evidence favours close relatives) is better than having missing data.

Moreover, in a well-designed double-blind randomized controlled trial, the mismatch between patient and proxy ratings should be similar across the different arms of the trial, and estimates of the effects of one treatment relative to another should be unaffected. However, estimates of absolute treatment effect could be biased. For example, if clinicians rate symptoms as less severe at baseline (potentially a floor effect), and patient and clinician ratings converge over time, any comparisons of changes in symptom severity that are based on clinicians' ratings are likely to underestimate the impact of treatment (McColl 2003). Problems could also arise when there is an imbalance in the use of proxy versus self-reports across the different arms of the trial, with the source of the report constituting a confounding factor. Where a mix of proxy and self-reports are used, care should be taken in pooling data; where matched proxy- and self-ratings are available for some individuals, the pattern of concordance between the paired ratings could be used to adjust all proxy scores.

References

Aneshensel, C. S., Frerichs, R. R., Clark, V. A., and Yokopenic, P. A. (1982). Telephone versus in-person surveys of community health status. *American Journal of Public Health*, **72**, 1017–1021.

Bardsley, M. J., Venables, C. W., Watson, J., Goodfellow, J., and Wright, P. D. (1992). Evidence for the validity of a health status measure in assessing short-term outcomes in cholecystectomy. *Quality in Health Care*, **1**, 10–14.

Barry, M. J., Walker-Corkery, E., Chang, Y., Tyll, L. T., Cherkin, D. C., and Fowler, F. J. (1996). Measurement of overall and disease-specific health status: does the order of questionnaires make a difference? *Journal of Health Services Research and Policy*, **1**, 20–27.

Briancon, S., Empereur, F., Guillemin, F., and Hercberg, S. (2001). Effect of VAS orientation and ordering of general perception of health vas within a quality of life questionnaire. *Quality of Life Research*, **8**, 650.

David, K. M., Ganiats, T. G., and Miller, C. (1999). Placement matters: stability of SF-36 EVFGP responses with varying placement of the question in the instrument. *Quality of Life Research*, **8**, 623.

de Vans, D. A. (1991). *Surveys in social research* (3rd edn). London: UCL Press.

Dillman, D. A. (1978). *Mail and telephone surveys: the total design method*. New York: John Wiley and Sons, Inc.

Eiser, C. and Mores, R. (2001). Can parents rate their child's health-related quality of life? Results of a systematic review. *Quality of Life Research*, **10**, 347–357.

Janse, A. J., Gemke, R. J. B. J., Uiterwal, C. S. P. M., van der Tweek, I., Kimpen, J. L. L., and Sinnema, G. (2004). Quality of life: patients and doctors don't always agree: a meta-analysis. *Journal of Clinical Epidemiology*, **57**, 653–661.

Jenkinson, C., Ziebland, S., Fitzpatrick, R., Mowat, G., and Mowat, A. (1993). Hospitalisation and its influence upon results from health status questionnaires. *International Journal of Health Sciences*, **4**, 13–19.

Krosnick, J. A. (2000). The threat of satisficing in surveys: the shortcuts respondents take in answering questions. *Survey Methods Centre Newsletter*, **20**, 4–8.

Lampic, C. and Sjödén, P-O. (2000). Patient and staff perceptions of cancer patients' psychological concerns and needs. *Acta Oncologica*, **39**, 9–22.

Leidy, N. K., Legro, M., Schmier, J., Zyczynski, T., McHorney, C., and Coyne, K. (2000). Does order of administration affect subject response on generic and condition-specific measures of health related quality of life? *Quality of Life Research*, **9**, 337.

Letley, L. and Garratt, A. (2000). Questionnaire length and internal reliability: a randomised study [poster presentation]. Society for Social Medicine 43rd Annual Scientific Meeting, Norwich, September 2000.

Litaker, D. (2003). New technology in quality of life research: are all computer-assisted approaches created equal? *Quality of Life Research*, **12**, 387–393.

McColl, E. (2004). Best practice in symptom assessment: a review. *Gut*, **53** (Suppl. iv), 49–54.

McColl, E., Eccles, M. P., Rousseau, N., Steen, I. N., Parkin, D. W., and Grimshaw, J. M. (2003). From the generic to the condition-specific? Instrument order effects in quality of life assessment. *Medical Care*, **41**, 777–790.

McHorney, C. A., Kosinski, M., and Ware, J. E. Jr. (1994). Comparisons of the costs and quality of norms for the SF-36 health survey collected by mail versus telephone interview: results from a national survey. *Medical Care*, **32**, 551–567.

McPherson, C. J. and Addington-Hall, J. M. (2003). Judging the quality of care at the end of life: can proxies provide reliable information? *Social Science and Medicine*, **56**, 95–109.

Muntner, P., Sudre, P., and Perneger, T. V. (2000). Comparison of the psychometric properties of the Asthma Quality of life Questionnaire (AQLQ) among 115 asthmatic adults assessed during acute hospitalization and as outpatients. *Quality of Life Research*, **9**, 987–995.

Osoba, D. (1992). The quality of life committee of the clinical trials group of the National Cancer Institute of Canada: organization and functions. *Quality of Life Research*, **1**, 211–218.

Roberson, M. T. and Sundstrom, E. (1990). Questionnaire design, return rates, and response favorableness in an employee attitude questionnaire. *Journal of Applied Psychology*, **75**, 354–357.

Ryan, J. M., Corry, J. R., Attewell, R., and Smithson, M. J. (2002). A comparison of an electronic version of the SF-36 General Health Questionnaire to the standard paper version. *Quality of Life Research*, **11**, 19–26.

Sadura, A., Pater, J., Osoba, D., Levine, M., Palmer, M., and Bennett, K. (1992). Quality of life assessment: patient compliance with questionnaire completion. *Journal of the National Cancer Institute*, **84**, 1023–1026.

Schuman, H. and Presser, S. (1981). *Questions and Answers in Attitude Surveys: Experiments on question from wording and content.* New York: Academic Press.

Sneeuw, K. C., Sprangers, M. A., and Aaronson, N. K. (2002). The role of health care providers and significant others in evaluating the quality of life of patients with chronic disease. *Journal of Clinical Epidemiology*, **55**, 1130–1143.

Sprangers, M. A. G. and Aaronson, N. K. (1992). The role of health care providers and significant others in evaluating the quality of life of patients with chronic disease: a review. *Journal of Clinical Epidemiology*, **39**, 743–760.

Sprangers, M. A. G., Cull, A., Bjordal, K., Groenvold, M., Aaronson, N. K., and Blazeby, J. (1998). The European Organisation for Research and Treatment of Cancer approach to developing questionnaire modules: an update and overview. *Quality of Life Research*, **7**, 291–300.

Sudman, S., Bradburn, N. M., and Schwarz, N. (1996). *Thinking about answers. The application of cognitive processes to survey methodology.* 1st edn. San Francisco: Jossey-Bass Inc.

Tourangeau, R. and Rasinski, K. A. (1988). Cognitive processes underlying context effects in attitude measurement. *Psychological Bulletin*, **103**, 299–314.

Tourangeau, R., Rips, L. J., and Rasinski, K. (2000). *The Psychology of Survey Response*. Cambridge: Cambridge University Press.

Ware, J. E. Jr, Snow, K. K., Kosinski, M., and Gandek, B. (1993). *SF-36 Health Survey Manual and Interpretation Guide*. Boston: New England Medical Centre.

Wu, A. W., Jacobson, D. L., Berzon, R. A., Revicki, D. A., van der Horst, C., Fichtenbaum, C. J., Saag, M. S., Lynn, L., Hardy, D., and Feinberg, J. (1997). The effect of mode of administration on Medical Outcomes Study health ratings and EuroQol scores in AIDS. *Quality of Life Research*, **6**, 3–10.

Ziebland, S. (1994). Measuring changes in health status. In C. Jenkinson (ed.) *Measuring Health and Medical Outcomes*, pp. 42–53. London: UCL Press.

Section 3

Analysis

Analysing longitudinal studies of QoL

Diane Fairclough

Introduction

Longitudinal data occur in most QoL investigations because we are interested in how a disease or an intervention affects an individual's functioning and well-being over time. These studies of health-related QoL consider measurement from one of two perspectives. In the first, the end points are expressed in the metric of the QoL scales, whereas in the second group the end point is expressed in the metric of time. The latter group includes outcomes such as Quality Adjusted Life Years (QALYs) that are discussed elsewhere in this book (Chapter 6.2). In studies where the end points are expressed in the metric of the QoL scales, QoL assessment is generally incorporated into the study by administering questionnaires at multiple time points before, during, and sometimes after an intervention, with the goal of characterizing the patient's health-related QoL in a longitudinal fashion.

Several issues influence the choice of the appropriate methods of analysis: timing of assessments, multiple end points and comparisons, and missing data. The presence of multiple end points presents two potential problems: that of controlling Type I errors for multiple comparisons and finding strategies for presenting QoL results in a way that is clinically meaningful and easily interpretable (Korn and O'Fallon 1990). Missing data is a concern because of the potential for biased estimates of QoL when the reasons for missing data are related to factors that affect the patient's QoL. The timing of assessments and the multiple end points arising from longitudinal studies are central to the discussion of alternative methods of analysis presented in this chapter. Missing data is addressed in the following two chapters (3.2, 3.3).

Models for longitudinal data

The design and timing of HRQoL assessments depends on the disease, its treatment and the scientific question. In some studies, the timing of assessments depends on events, phases of treatment or disease states. Other studies have periodic evaluations based on the time elapsed since the beginning of treatment or the onset of the disease. These event-driven and time-driven designs have corresponding analytic models: repeated measures models and growth curve models. In a repeated measures model, *time* is conceptualized as an ordered categorical variable. Each assessment must be assigned to one category. In a growth curve model, *time* is conceptualized as a continuous variable.

In some trials, either analytic design is appropriate. In other cases, there will be clear reasons for preferring one or the other of these approaches.

Event- or condition-driven designs

When the objective of the study is to compare HRQoL in subjects experiencing the same condition, assessments are planned to occur at the time of clinically relevant events or to correspond to specific phases of the intervention. These designs are more common when the intervention or therapy is of limited duration. For example, one might consider a simple design with a pre- and post-intervention assessment when comparing the QoL after two surgical procedures. Another design might include one assessment to measure QoL prior to, during and after therapy. Many variations are possible. For example, there may be reasons to believe that differences in HRQoL may exist during only the early or later periods of therapy. In this case, the design would include a minimum of two assessments during therapy. Studies with a limited number of phases of interest in the scientific investigation, where QoL is expected to be constant during those phases, are amenable to an event-driven design.

An example of an event-driven design is a breast cancer trial of adjuvant therapy designed to compare a 16-week dose-intensive regimen with a more traditional 24-week regiment (Fetting *et al.* 1998) Three assessments of QoL where planned: prior to, during and after therapy. The assessment prior to therapy was within 14 days of the start of chemotherapy. The assessment during therapy was approximately 12 weeks after the start of chemotherapy, allowing sufficient time for patients to be experiencing the cumulative effects of both regimens and not yet experience the psychological lift that occurs at the end of treatment. The assessment following therapy was to occur four months after the completion of therapy regardless of when that occurred. Thus, the timing of the off therapy assessment was likely to vary considerably among the patients.

When the scientific questions involve a more extended period of time or when the phases of the disease or its treatment are not distinct, the longitudinal designs are based on time. These designs are appropriate for chronic conditions where therapies are given over extended periods of time. For example, in studies of therapies for patients with advanced cancer, therapy is generally given until there is evidence that it is ineffective or occasioned unacceptable toxicity. Thus, the duration of therapy is indeterminate at the onset of the study. Obvious examples would include treatment of chronic conditions such as diabetes and arthritis. Timing in these designs is based on regularly spaced intervals (e.g., every three months), sometimes more frequent initially (e.g. every month for three months then every three months).

Repeated measures models

Repeated measures models are used in longitudinal studies with event-driven designs where there is a strong conceptual identity for each assessment. Repeated measures models may also be useful in some studies with a limited number (two to four) of assessments. If the timing of the longitudinal assessments occurs within predefined windows of time, then it is feasible to classify each of the assessments uniquely as one of the repeated measures.

Assignment of assessments to a planned assessment time (landmark) may become difficult in studies with more frequent assessments. These studies typically have variable follow-up intervals with increasing rates of dropout. The process of defining windows of time for each assessment becomes increasingly difficult. If the windows are wide, an individual may have more than one observation within the window. This will require the analyst to discard all but one of the observations occurring within that window. Not only will this reduce the statistical power of the study, but it may also lead to biased estimates, depending on how the observations are selected or discarded. For example, bias may occur if discarded assessments were delayed when individuals were experiencing toxicity. Using narrow intervals may lead to fewer subjects with data at each landmark. This creates instability of the estimation of both the means and the covariance. In summary, one of the restrictions associated with the choice of a repeated measures model for the analysis of the trial is the necessity of identifying each assessment with each landmark.

Multiple Univariate Analyses

The most commonly used method of analysis for repeated measures designs consists of univariate analyses at each time point using test procedures such as t-tests, ANOVA, or Wilcoxon rank sum test. While simple to implement, this approach has several disadvantages (de Klerk 1986; Pocock *et al.* 1987; Matthews *et al.* 1990; Fairclough 2002). First, the large number of comparisons often fails to answer the clinical question but rather presents a confusing picture. Specifically, the probability of concluding that there are significant differences in QoL when none exist (the Type I error) increases as the number of comparisons increase. Finally, the estimates obtained from these univariate analyses are biased if the missing data are not completely at random (See Chapter 3.3 for a more detailed discussion).

Multivariate analyses

A very useful approach for repeated measures is to use likelihood-based multivariate methods such as MANOVA when there is no missing data or models for incomplete repeated measures when there is ignorable missing data (Dempster *et al.* 1977; Jennrich and Schluchter 1986). (See Chapter 3.3 for a discussion of ignorable versus non-ignorable missing data.) In the adjuvant breast cancer study described previously, a repeated measures model for incomplete data (SAS Institute 1992) was used to estimate the means associated with the three phases within the two treatment groups (Table 3.1.1) as well as estimates of change between the three phases. The results clearly indicate no differences between the two groups prior to or following therapy, and a significantly lower score during therapy on the 16-week regimen.

Table 3.1.1 Repeated measures analysis of Breast Chemotherapy Questionnaire (BCQ) scores in the adjuvant breast cancer trial

Treatment	Pre-Therapy	On-Therapy	Post-Therapy	Change from Pre- to On-Therapy	Change from Pre- to Post-Therapy
24 week	7.57 (0.13)	6.82 (0.17)	8.01 (0.13)	−0.74 (0.14)	0.44 (0.13)
16 week	7.75 (0.14)	6.31 (0.18)	8.09 (0.14)	−1.44 (0.15)	0.34 (0.14)
Difference	−0.18 (0.19)	0.51 (0.24)*	−0.09 (0.19)	−0.69 (0.20)***	−0.10 (0.19)

* $P < 0.05$, *** $P < 0.001$.

Growth curve models and time-driven designs

The term *growth curve model* comes from early applications to describe changes in height and weight as a function of age. Typically, these measurements were taken at different ages for each child in a study. Curves were fit to the data to estimate the typical height or weight for a child as a function of age. The same concept is relevant when we want to describe changes in HRQoL as a function of time. The curves can be defined in many ways but are most often described by a polynomial function or a piecewise linear regression. The simplest example of a growth curve model is a straight line.

Growth curve models are useful in several settings. The first is when the timing of assessments differs widely among individuals. Growth curve models are also useful in studies with a large number of HRQoL assessments in which it is feasible to model changes over time with a smaller number of parameters than is required for a repeated measures model. Growth curve models are most useful for clinical trials with missing and mistimed observations, time-varying covariates and a large number of potential repeated measures. An example is a prospective longitudinal study of QoL in 68 terminal cancer patients in which patients were assessed every 3 to 6 weeks until death (Hwang *et al.* 1996; 2003) in which the research focus was the patterns of change in QoL over time prior to death. A second example is a proposed study having the primary research question, 'Is QoL better or worse because of disease changes or toxicity?' QoL change will be evaluated with time-varying covariates, including changes in disease status and the occurrence of treatment-related toxicity, in a growth curve model.

In most cases, growth-curve models include polynomial functions of the actual time of assessment relative to some reference point. While carefully selected models may provide a good fit to the data, the higher order terms (those other than intercept and slope) are difficult to interpret. An alternative parameterization of a growth curve model is a piece-wise linear regression where we assume that the change is approximately linear over limited periods of time. In these models, we can estimate and compare the average rate of change of the outcome during specific intervals of time. Figure 3.1.1 illustrates these alternative forms of growth curve models of the Trial

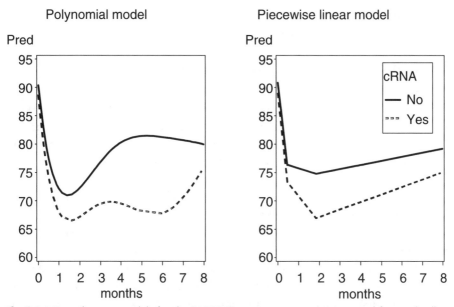

Fig. 3.1.1 Growth curve models for the FACT-TOI score among patients treated for renal cell carcinoma. Reproduced with permission from Fairclough, D. L. (2002), Chapter 3, *Design and Analysis of Quality of Life Studies in Clinical Trials*. Chapman & Hall/CRC, Boca Raton, USA).

Outcome Index of the Functional Assessment of Cancer Treatment (FACT-TOI) for a trial to evaluate cis-retinoic acid as part of a therapeutic regimen for renal cell carcinoma. The figure on the left is a cubic polynomial model. The figure on the right is a piecewise-linear model with nodes at the time of the first two on-therapy assessments.

Multiple end points

In most clinical trials, investigators assess HRQoL longitudinally over the period of treatment and, in some trials, subsequent to treatment. Each assessment involves multiple scales that measure general and disease-specific HRQoL domains. As a result, addressing the problem of multiple comparisons is one of the analytic challenges in these trials (Korn and O'Fallon 1990). Not only are there concerns about Type I errors, but also large numbers of statistical tests generally result in a confusing picture of HRQoL that is difficult to interpret (de Klerk 1986). There are three general approaches to reduce the impact of multiplicity:

1. *a priori* specification of a limited number of *confirmatory* tests

2. multiple comparison procedures including alpha adjustments (e.g., Bonferroni) and closed multiple testing

3. summary measures or statistics.

In practice, a combination of focused hypotheses, summary measures and multiple comparison procedures is necessary in most clinical trials.

Limiting the number of confirmatory tests

One strategy for handling the multiple testing is to specify a limited number of comparisons (generally no more than three) in the design of the trial (Gotay *et al.* 1992). While this is a valid approach, in practice investigators are reluctant to ignore the remaining data. Specifying primary and secondary comparisons is a related strategy, but if formal hypothesis testing is performed on all end points the issues of interpretation of the multiple comparisons remains.

Multiple comparison procedures

Multivariate tests, such as Hotelling's T and Likelihood Ratio tests, can be used to control the Type I error of the multiple comparisons. These statistics, however, test a hypothesis of no treatment differences against a general alternative. Specifically, they ask the general question, 'Are there differences in QoL at *any* point in time?' and are not sensitive to persistent differences over time. These tests may sometimes be hard to interpret when the results are counterintuitive (de Klerk 1986). For example, the test may be "statistically" significant when QoL is better in one treatment arm at one time point and the other treatment at another time point, and not significant when one treatment appears to have consistently better QoL over time (Fairclough and Gelber 1996). To illustrate, consider the two hypothetical examples displayed in Figure 3.1.2. In the example on the right, the measure of HRQoL is consistently better in one treatment during all four post-baseline assessments. In the example on the left, one treatment has a negative impact at the time of the second assessments that disappears by the third assessment and begins to reverse by the end of the observation period. Although the differences between the groups in both examples are of clinical interest, in most clinical trials one would wish to have test procedures that are more sensitive to (or have greater power to detect) the consistent differences.

An alternative method to address this problem is to utilize a multiple-comparisons procedure. The simplest and best known is the conservative Bonferroni procedure, in which only those tests with p-values that are less than α/K are declared to be statistically significant, where α is the overall Type I error and K is the number of tests (or comparisons) performed. The adjusted p-values are computed by multiplying the raw p-value by the number of tests (K).

$$p_k^{adj} = \min(Kp_k, 1), k = 1 \ldots K$$

An example of a less conservative approach is a sequentially rejective Bonferroni adjustment procedure (Hochberg 1988) in which the smallest p-value is compared to α/K, the next smallest to $\alpha/K-1$, and the largest to α.

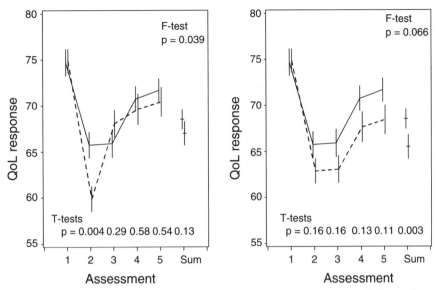

Fig. 3.1.2 Hypothetical studies with consistent differences in HRQoL over time (left) or a large difference at a single point in time (right). Summary measure is the mean of the post-baseline assessments. Means are joined by horizontal line. Vertical lines indicate 1 standard error. F-test indicates multivariate test of group differences at assessments 2, 3, 4 and 5. t-tests indicate test of group difference at that assessment or for the summary measure. Reproduced with permission from Fairclough, D. L. (2002), Chapter 10, *Design and Analysis of Quality of Life Studies in Clinical Trials*. Chapman & Hall/CRC, Boca Raton, USA).

The procedure is illustrated with a hypothetical example with five tests of hypotheses. Table 3.1.2 displays the ordered p-values. If we were using the traditional Bonferroni adjustment, the critical values for all tests would correspond to $\alpha/5$ and only one of the tests would be considered statistically significant at $\alpha = 0.05$. In contrast, using the Hochberg procedure, the critical values correspond to $\alpha/5$, $\alpha/4$, $\alpha/3$, $\alpha/2$, and $\alpha/1$ respectively and four of the tests would be rejected at $\alpha = 0.05$.

Table 3.1.2 P-value adjustments for a hypothetical example with five hypothesis tests

Ordered p-values	$P_{(1)}$	$P_{(2)}$	$P_{(3)}$	$P_{(4)}$	$P_{(5)}$
Unadjusted p-values	0.006	0.011	0.018	0.021	0.20
Hochberg adjusted p-values	0.030	0.042#	0.042*	0.042	0.20
Bonferroni adjusted p-values	0.030	0.055	0.090	0.105	1.00

$*P_{(3)}^{adj} = \min(3p_{(3)}, p_{(4)}^{adj}) = \min(0.054, 0.042)$

$^{\#}P_{(2)}^{adj} = \min(4p_{(2)}, p_{(3)}^{adj}) = \min(0.044, 0.042)$

This example also illustrates how the above procedure maintains the monotonicity of the adjusted p-values. If the raw p-values were simply multiplied by 5, 4, 3, 2, and 1 respectively, the adjusted p-values would be 0.030, 0.044, 0.052, 0.042, and 0.20. With the naive adjustment, smaller unadjusted p-values would have larger adjusted p-values and the hypothesis associated with $p_{(3)}$ would not be rejected when a hypothesis with a smaller unadjusted value was rejected. The exact procedure for computing the adjusted p-values is an adaptation outlined by Hochberg and proceeds as follows:

Rank the K p-values from largest $p_{(K)}$ to smallest $p_{(1)}$.
Largest p-value has no adjustment: $p_{(K)}^{adj} = p_{(K)}$
The remaining p-values are adjusted as follows:

$$p_{(K-1)}^{adj} = \min(2p_{(K-1)}, p_{(K)}^{adj}),$$
$$p_{(K-2)}^{adj} = \min(3p_{(K-2)}, p_{(K-1)}^{adj}), \ldots$$
$$p_{(1)}^{adj} = \min(Kp_{(1)}, p_{(2)}^{adj}).$$

Summary measures and statistics

Another approach is the use of summary measures (de Klerk 1986; Pocock *et al.* 1987; Cox *et al.* 1992) or global statistics (Tandon 1990). The use of summary measures (QoL indices) across the multiple domains measured by most QoL instruments is an unresolved issue among QoL researchers. Some groups of researchers prefer to report results by displaying the entire profile of the various domains. Others rely heavily on indices constructed from scales measuring various domains. There are three strategies that are commonly used to combine the scores on the various domains. In the first, scores from each of the domains are weighted by the number of items in each domain; in most cases the indices are computed by summing the responses to each of the individual items. Ideally, one would hope that the number of items in each domain reflected the relative importance of that domain. But in practice, the number of items in each domain generally is an artifact of the instrument development process. In the second strategy, all domains are given an equal weight. The scores for each domain are converted to a common scale, generally from 0–100, and then the domain scores are averaged. The third method, using factor analysis to determine the weights, is less common among QoL scales, but has been applied to the most widely used measure of health status, the SF-36, to create physical and mental component scores (PCS and MCS). The primary advantage of these indices is that they simplify the presentation of the results, reduce the number of comparisons, and potentially increase the power. The limitation is that changes that occur in different directions in two or more of the domains may not be evident in these indices. When an analyst uses a summary measure, it is advisable to examine the results for each of the components. Similarly, when interpreting the results it is important to understand how the summary measure was constructed (Simon *et al.* 1998).

The use of summary measures across time is generally less controversial. Examples include post-treatment mean, (de Klerk 1986; Matthews *et al.* 1990; Frison & Pocock 1992) mean change relative to baseline (Frison & Pocock 1992), last value minus baseline (Frison & Pocock 1992), average rate of change over time (or slope) (Matthews *et al.* 1990), maximum value (de Klerk 1986; Pocock *et al.* 1987; Matthews *et al.* 1990), area under the curve (Matthews *et al.* 1990; Cox *et al.* 1992) and time to reach a peak or a pre-specified value (Pocock *et al.* 1987; Matthews *et al.* 1990).

There are several reasons for the use of summary measures in the analysis of a longitudinal study of QoL (Fairclough 1996). The primary advantage of these summary measures is that they are often easier to interpret than the multivariate methods described previously. Not only is the number of comparisons reduced, but also measures such as the rate of change and the area under the curve are familiar concepts in clinical medicine. Summary measures and statistics also have greater power to detect small but consistent differences that may occur over extended periods of time or multiple domains of HRQoL. In contrast to the Bonferroni correction or a general multivariate test (Hotelling's T), summary statistics are more sensitive to the settings where there are consistent differences over time.

The primary weakness of summary measures or statistics is that differences in specific domains of HRQoL or transient differences at specific points in time may be obscured. Investigations that are confirmatory, designed to test the question of differences in overall HRQoL, may benefit from the use of summary measures. This is especially useful in studies where early toxicity in one treatment group may be balanced by later improvements in disease control. In contrast, studies that have a more exploratory objective of identifying the aspects of HRQoL impacted by the disease or a particular therapy may not benefit from the use of summary measures or statistics.

Choosing a summary measure or statistic

The choice of which summary measure or statistic should be selected as the end point in a clinical trial depends on the objective of the investigation, expected pattern of change across time, and patterns of missing data. Consider several possible patterns of change in QoL across time (Figure 3.1.3). One pattern might be a steady rate of change over time reflecting either a constant improvement in QoL over time (Figure 3.1.3A) or a constant decline over time. This pattern of change suggests that the rate of change or slope would be a good choice of a summary measure for this population. In contrast, other measures, such as the change from baseline to the last measure, might not be desirable if patients who fail earlier and thus drop out from the study earlier have smaller changes than those patients with longer follow-up.

An alternative profile might be a rapid change initially with a subsequent plateau after the maximum therapeutic benefit is realized (Figure 3.1.3D). Examples include two clinical trials of adjuvant therapy for breast cancer (Fetting *et al.* 1998; Levine *et al.* 1988).

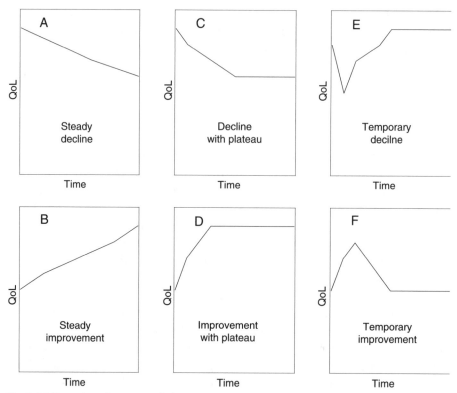

Fig. 3.1.3 Examples of patterns of change in QoL over time. Reproduced with permission from Fairclough, D. L. (1998), Chapter 13, *Quality of Life Assessment in Clinical Trials: Methods and Practice*, (1st edn), M. J. Staquet, R. D. Hays, and P. Fayers (eds). Oxford University Press, New York.

This profile illustrates the importance of identifying the clinically relevant question *a priori*. If the objective is to identify the therapy that produces the most rapid improvement in QoL, the time to reach a peak or pre-specified value would be a good choice. If, in contrast, the ultimate level of benefit is more important than the time to achieve the benefit, then a measure such as the post-treatment mean or mean change relative to baseline might be desirable.

A third pattern of change might occur with a therapy that has transient benefits or toxicity (Figure 3.1.3E and 3.1.3F). For example, individuals may experience transient benefits and then return to their baseline levels after the effect of the therapy has ceased. Alternatively, a toxic therapy for cancer may significantly reduce QoL during therapy, but ultimately result in a better QoL following therapy than the patient was experiencing at the time of diagnosis (Fetting *et al.* 1998; Levine *et al.* 1988). For these more complex patterns of change over time, a measure such as the area under the curve might be considered as a summary of both early and continued effects of the therapy.

Summary measures versus statistics

The terms *summary measures* and *summary statistics* are often interchanged. The following definitions are used in this chapter. A *summary measure* reduces the repeated observations on each individual to a single number. The procedure is first to summarize the data within an individual subject by calculating a single value (summary measure) for each individual and then to perform an analysis of the summary measures. For example, we can estimate the rate of change experienced by each individual using ordinary least squares (OLS), and then apply a two-sample t-test to compare the estimates in two treatment groups. In contrast, a *summary statistic* reduces the measurements on a group of individuals to a single value. Data are initially analyzed using multivariate techniques for longitudinal models, and summary statistics are constructed from the estimates of the parameters. For example, the mean rate of change (or slope) for each treatment group is estimated using a mixed-effects model and the differences in the slopes between the two treatment groups tested.

Constructing summary measures

The manner in which missing data are handled differs for summary measures and statistics. If there are no missing data, then the results from two approaches are virtually identical. When the period of observation varies widely among subjects or data collection stops for some reason related to the outcome, construction of summary measures is challenging. Analytic models for incomplete longitudinal data are chosen to produce unbiased estimates of the group means that are in turn used to construct the summary statistics. In contrast, rules must be constructed to handle missing assessments on an individual basis when constructing a summary measure. All of the following approaches make assumptions that may or may not be reasonable in specific settings, and it is advisable to examine the sensitivity of the conclusions to the various assumptions. Easy fixes without careful thought only hide the problem. Many of the procedures for constructing summary measures assume data are missing completely at random (MCAR) (Omar *et al.* 1999) and are inappropriate in studies of HRQoL.

For example, if intermediate observations are missing, one could interpolate between observations. This approach assumes that these intermediate missing values are random, and that the previous and following measures are taken under similar conditions. Interpolation is reasonable when the expected pattern of change over time is roughly linear (Figure 3.1.3A, B) or constant. Interpolation would not make sense in studies where temporary changes are expected (Figure 3.1.3 E, F). Interpolation also assumes that the missingness is not the result of some event, such as an episode of acute toxicity, which would cause the patient to miss the assessment and have poorer HRQoL.

Dropout and other causes of differences in the length of follow-up among individuals is another challenge. For a patient who dropped out, carrying the last value forward or extrapolating from the last two observations could be used to impute the last measurement. The most popular approach is to carry the value of the last observation forward. Unfortunately, this strategy is often implemented without careful thought. This may be a reasonable strategy if the expected pattern of change within individuals is either a steady improvement (Figure 3.1.3B), or improvement with a plateau (Figure 3.1.3D). But with other patterns of change (Figure 3.1.3A, C, E), this strategy would bias the results in favor of interventions with early dropout.

Assigning zero for persons who have died is a valid approach for HRQoL scores that are explicitly anchored at zero for the health state of death. These are generally scores measured using time trade-off (TTO), standard gamble (SG), or another preference technique. However, the majority of HRQoL instruments are developed to maximize discrimination among patients. In these instruments, a value of zero would correspond to the worst possible outcome on every question. Assigning zero also has some statistical implications. If the proportion of deaths is substantial, the observations may mimic a binomial distribution and the results approximate a Kaplan–Meier analysis of survival. When the number of deaths is small, the zero values will violate the multivariate normal distribution assumptions of the analysis methods.

Another method proposed for combining information across repeated measures uses ranks (O'Brien 1984). The measurements on all subjects are ranked at each time point and then the average of the ranks across the n time points is computed for each individual. If the reasons for missing data were known and one could make reasonable assumptions about the ranking of QoL in patients at each time point, one could possibly adapt this approach to a study with missing data. For example, it would not be unreasonable to assume that the QoL of patients who died or left the study due to excessive toxicity was worse than the QoL of those patients who remained on therapy. They would then be assigned the lowest possible rank for measurements scheduled after death or during the time of excessive toxicity.

Average rate of change (slopes)

When the changes over time are approximately linear, the average rate of change (or slope) may provide an excellent summary of the effect of an intervention. When there is virtually no dropout during the study or the dropout occurs only during the later part of the study, it is feasible to fit a simple regression model to the available data on each individual. This is often referred to as the ordinary least squares slope (OLS slope). Obviously, slopes for each individual can be estimated if all subjects have two or more observations. However, the estimates of the slope will have a large associated error when the available observations span a short period of time relative to the entire length of the study.

Area under the curve (AUC)

Another measure summarizing HRQoL over time is the area under the curve (AUC) of the HRQoL scores plotted against time (Matthews *et al.* 1990; Cox *et al.* 1992). The AUC for the *i*th individual can be estimated using a trapezoidal approximation from the observed scores (Figure 3.1.4). The area of each trapezoid is equal to the product of the height at the midpoint $(Y_{ij}+Y_{i(j-1)})/2$ and the width of the base (t_j-t_{j-1}). The total area under a curve for the ith subject with J assessments is calculated by adding areas of a series of trapezoids:

$$AUC_i = \sum_{j=2}^{J}(t_j - t_{j-1})(Y_{ij} + Y_{i(j-1)})/2.$$

With a little algebraic manipulation, this calculation can also be expressed as a weighted function of the HRQoL scores where the weights are determined by the spacing of the assessments over time:

$$AUC_i = (t_2 - t_1)/2 * Y_{i1} + \sum_{j=2}^{J-1}(t_{j+1} - t_{j-1})/2 * Y_{ij} + (t_J - t_{J-1})/2 * Y_{iJ}.$$

When the data are complete, this computation is straightforward. However, strategies for handling missing data need to be developed. For example, if intermediate observations are missing, one could interpolate between observations. If a patient dies during the study, the minimum QoL score could be assigned at that time point. For a patient who dropped out, the last measurement could be inferred either by

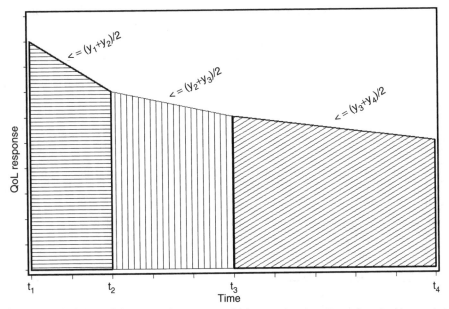

Fig. 3.1.4 Calculation of the AUC using a trapezoidal approximation. Reproduced with permission from Fairclough, D. L. (2002), Chapter 10, *Design and Analysis of Quality of Life Studies in Clinical Trials*. Chapman & Hall/CRC, Boca Raton, USA).

carrying the last value forward or extrapolating from the last two observations. Each of these approaches makes assumptions that may or may not be reasonable in specific settings, and it would be advisable to examine the sensitivity of the conclusions to the various assumptions.

The issue of selecting a strategy for computing the AUC also occurs when patients die during the study. One strategy is to extrapolate the curve to zero at the time of death; though this strategy may not be very sensible when the scale is not anchored by 0 being dead or as bad as being dead. Other proposed strategies include assigning values of the minimum HRQoL score for that individual or the minimum HRQoL score for all individuals (Hollen *et al.* 1997). One strategy will not work for all studies. Whichever strategy is chosen, it needs to be justified and the sensitivity of the results to the assumptions examined.

Fayers and Machin (2000) describe one alternative, the average AUC, which may be useful in some settings where the length of follow-up varies among subjects. This summary measure is calculated by dividing the total AUC by the total time of observation. The summary measure is AUC_i/T_i where T_i is the total time of observation for the *i*th individual. If the research question concerns the average HRQoL of patients during a limited period, such as the duration of a specific therapy, this may be a reasonable approach. However, if early termination due to toxicity or lack of efficacy results in similar or higher summary scores, then the results are biased. This is illustrated in Figure 3.1.5, where the average areas are the same for the two curves, but the scores decline more rapidly in the subject who terminated the study early. As always, the choice between these two approaches depends primarily on the research question.

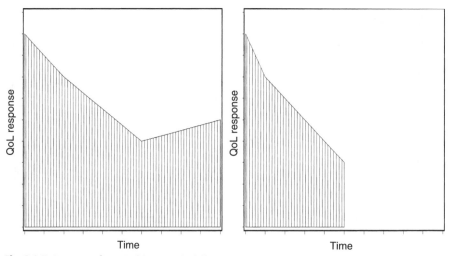

Fig. 3.1.5 Contrast of two subjects with different lengths of follow-up. Both subjects have the same AUC when adjusted by each individual's length of follow-up.

Univariate analysis of summary measures

After constructing the summary measures for each individual, statistical tests (e.g., two-sample t-test, Wilcoxon Rank Sum test) are used to compare treatment groups. In most cases these tests assume that the observations are independent and identically distributed. The assumption of homogeneity of variance of the summary measures is often violated when the duration of follow-up is vastly different among subjects. For example, slopes estimated for individuals who drop out of the study early will have greater variation than slopes for those who complete the study. One solution is to weight the slopes using their standard errors, giving greater weight to those individuals with the longest follow-up. Unfortunately, unless dropout is random, this approach may bias the analysis. The alternative procedure is to ignore the possible heterogeneity by giving equal weight to all subjects.

Constructing summary statistics

In contrast to summary measures, summary statistics are constructed by combining group measures over time. Examples of these group measures are the parameter estimates from growth curve models or means from repeated measures models. In practice, the use of summary statistics rather than summary measures is often preferable, because it may be much easier to develop a model-based method for handling missing data than to develop strategies for imputing each individual missing value required to compute the summary measures.

The general procedure for the construction of summary statistics is to obtain parameter estimates ($\hat{\beta}_{hj}$) for the hth treatment group and then reduce the set of estimates to a single summary statistic:

$$\hat{S}_h = \sum_{j=1}^{J} w_j \hat{\beta}_{hj}$$

In a repeated measures model, the parameter estimates are generally estimated means for each of the repeated assessments ($\hat{\mu}_{hj}$) adjusted for important covariates. A simple summary measure is the average of the post-baseline means. In a growth curve model, the parameter estimates are the intercepts, slopes, and higher order terms of the polynomial or piecewise regression model.

This approach of constructing summary measures can also be used to estimate the area under the curve (AUC) for the hth treatment group. When the data are analyzed using a repeated measures model, the AUC can be estimated by using a weighted function of the means (trapezoidal approximation):

$$\hat{S}_h = \sum_{j=2}^{J} (t_j - t_{j-1})(\hat{\mu}_{hj} + \hat{\mu}_{hj-1})/2$$

where $t_i \ldots t_j$ are the planned times of the repeated measures. Alternatively, if a polynomial model is used to estimate the change over time then the AUC can be estimated by integration

$$\hat{S}_h = \int_{t=0}^{T} \sum_{k=0}^{K} \hat{\beta}_{hk} t^k = \sum_{k=0}^{K} \frac{T^k}{k+1} \hat{\beta}_{hk}$$

Summary

The choice of the appropriate methods of analysis for longitudinal studies of health status and quality of life strongly depends on the research question and is influenced by the timing of assessments and the presence of missing data. Because QoL is a multidimensional concept, interpretation of results from multiple scales measured repeatedly over time is an additional challenge. In this chapter, strategies for determining the type of model (repeated measures versus growth curves) and minimizing the impact of multiple comparisons were discussed. While issues are important, perhaps the most challenging task is the clear definition of the research question upon which all choices among these strategies depends.

References

Cox, D. R., Fitzpatrick, R., Fletcher, A. E., Gore, S. M., Spiegelhalter, D. J., and Jones, D. R. (1992). Quality-of-life assessment: Can we keep it simple? *J R Statist Soc A*, **155**, 353–393.

de Klerk, N. H. (1986). Repeated warnings re repeated measures. *Aust N Z J Med*, **16**, 637–638.

Dempster, A. P., Laird, N. M., and Rubin, D. B. (1977). Maximum likelihood from incomplete data via the EM Algorithm. *Journal of the Royal Statistical Society (B)*, **39**, 1–38.

Fairclough, D. L. (1996). Quality of life in cancer clinical trials: Now that we have the data, what do we do? *J. Appl. Stat. Sci.*, **4**, 253–269.

Fairclough, D. L. (2002). Analytic methods for ignorable missing data. In D. L. Fairclough (ed.) *Design and Analysis of Quality of Life Studies in Clinical Trials*, pp. 93–114. Boca Raton: Chapman & Hall/CRC.

Fairclough, D. L. and Gelber, R. D. (1996). Quality of life: Statistical issues and analysis. In B. Spilker (ed.) *Quality of Life and Pharmacoeconomics in Clinical Trials*, 2nd edn, pp. 427–435. Philadelphia: Lippincott-Raven.

Fayers, P. M. and Machin, D. (2000). *Quality of Life: Assessment, Analysis and Interpretation*, Chapters 3–7. Chichester, England: John Wiley and Sons Ltd.

Fetting, J. H., Gray, R., Fairclough, D. L., Smith, T. J., Margolin, K. A., Citron, M. L., Grove-Conrad, M., Cella, D., Pandya, K., Robert, N., Henderson, I. C., Osborne, C. K., and Abeloff, M. D. (1998). Sixteen-week multidrug regimen versus cyclophosphamide, doxorubicin, and fluorouracil as adjuvant therapy for node-positive, receptor- negative breast cancer: an Intergroup study. *J Clin Oncol*, **16**, 2382–2391.

Frison, L. and Pocock, S. J. (1992). Repeated measures in clinical trials: analysis using mean summary statistics and its implications for design. *Stat Med*, **11**, 1685–16704.

Gotay, C. C., Korn, E. L., McCabe, M. S., Moore, T. D., and Cheson, B. D. (1992). Building quality of life assessment into cancer treatment studies. *Oncology (Huntingt)*, **6**, 25–28; discussion 30–32, 37.

Hochberg, Y. (1988). A sharper Bonferroni procedure for multiple tests of significance. *Biometrika*, 75, 800–802.

Hollen, P. J., Gralla, R. J., Cox, C., Eberly, S. W., and Kris, M. G. (1997). A dilemma in analysis: issues in the serial measurement of quality of life in patients with advanced lung cancer. *Lung Cancer*, 18, 119–136.

Hwang S. S., Chang V. T., Fairclough D. L., Cogswell J., and Kasimis, B. (2003). Longitudinal quality of life in advanced cancer patients: Pilot study results from a VA medical center. *Journal of Pain and Symptom Management*, 25, 225–235.

Hwang, S. S., Chang, V. T., Fairclough, D. F., Hoch, K., Latorre, M., and Corpion, C. (1996). Longitudinal measuremnt for quality of life and symptoms in terminal cancer patients. *Proceeding of the American Society for Clinical Oncology* (Abstract).

Jennrich, R. I. and Schluchter, M. D. (1986). Unbalanced repeated-measures models with structured covariance matrices. *Biometrics*, 42, 805–820.

Korn, E. L. and O'Fallon, J. (1990). For the Statistics Working Group: Quality of life assessment in cancer clinical trials: statistical considerations. *Report on the workshop on Quality of Life Research in Cancer Clinical Trials*. Division of Cancer Prevention and Control, National Cancer Institute.

Levine, M. N., Guyatt, G. H., Gent, M., De Pauw, S., Goodyear, M. D., Hryniuk, W. M., Arnold, A., Findlay, B., Skillings, J. R., and Bramwell, V. H. *et al*. (1988). Quality of life in stage II breast cancer: an instrument for clinical trials. *J Clin Oncol*, 6, 1798–1810.

Matthews, J. N., Altman, D. G., Campbell, M. J., and Royston, P. (1990). Analysis of serial measurements in medical research. *BMJ*, 300, 230–235.

O'Brien, P. C. (1984). Procedures for comparing samples with multiple end points. *Biometrics*, 40, 1079–1087.

Omar, R. Z., Wright, E. M., Turner, R. M., and Thompson, S. G. (1999). Analysing repeated measurements data: a practical comparison of methods. *Stat Med*, 18, 1587–1603.

Pocock, S. J., Geller, N. L., and Tsiatis, A. A. (1987). The analysis of multiple end points in clinical trials. *Biometrics*, 43, 487–498.

SAS Institute. (1992). The Mixed Procedure. Chapter 16. In: *SAS Technical Report T-229, SAS/STAT software, changes and enhancements*, pp. 289–366. Cary NC: SAS Institute Inc.

Simon, G. E., Revicki, D. A., Grothaus, L., and Vonkorff, M. (1998). SF-36 summary scores: are physical and mental health truly distinct? *Medical Care*, 36, 567–572.

Tandon, P. K. (1990). Applications of global statistics in analysing quality of life data. *Statistics in Medicine*, 9, 819–827.

3.2

Preventing missing data

Dennis A. Revicki and Diane L. Fairclough

Introduction

Health-related quality of life (HRQoL) and other patient reported outcomes are frequently incorporated into clinical trial protocols to evaluate the effects of treatments on patient functioning and well-being. The value of HRQoL data is in extending the understanding of safety and clinical efficacy end points, and in providing the patient's perspective in assessing the outcomes of health care interventions. Although there are some unique challenges to including HRQoL measures in randomized clinical trials, these end points should be treated no differently than clinical effectiveness end points. It is important to ensure that there is a rationale for including HRQoL outcomes in clinical studies and that there are clearly articulated research questions regarding the HRQoL end points.

The problem of missing HRQoL data is a significant source of selection bias in some clinical trials. Missing data are most often observed in cancer clinical trials (Bernhard *et al.* 1998), those involving long-term follow-up of patients with chronic diseases, and those involving patients with life threatening diseases or with poor survival prognosis. Missing HRQoL data is sometimes inevitable, given that for some clinical trials disease progression results in deterioration in health status or death. Clearly, the extent and nature of missing data depends on the patient population, duration and complexity of the clinical trial, data collection methods, and respondent burden issues (Fairclough, in press). This chapter focuses on sources and procedures for preventing or minimizing missing data in the HRQoL components of clinical trials.

Types of missing data in clinical trials

Two major types of missing HRQoL data can be identified: missing items within instruments (item non-response) and completely missing assessments (unit non-response) (Fayers *et al.* 1998). Reasons for failure to complete all the items within a HRQoL survey vary, but may be because of inattentiveness in completing the questionnaire, feeling too ill or distressed to make responses, sensitivity of the questions, or that questions are not understood or are considered not applicable (Fayers *et al.* 1998). In many studies, missing item rates are less than 1 per cent for any specific question, but these levels of missing data can accumulate across multi-item instruments.

Some items, especially about sexual dysfunction or other sensitive content, tend to be more likely to be missing. Why are missing item data a problem? The main effects include a loss of power, that is, insufficient data to make any conclusions from the clinical trial, and bias in the results of the data analyses. Assuming that a HRQoL instrument includes 30 items and missing data is distributed uniformly across respondents, a 1% missing item rate results in about 25% of subjects with at least one missing item response. If there is an association between the reason of incomplete response and the item content, these biases can be exacerbated. Although there are procedures available for imputing sub-scale scores in the presence of missing item data (see Fairclough, Chapter 3.3 in this volume; Fayers *et al.* 1998) and most instrument manuals contain guidelines for scoring when there are some missing items, minimizing missing item data is important.

Rates of missing HRQoL form data range from less than 1% to more than 50%, depending on the patient disease population and the complexity and duration of the clinical trial. The key consideration is that once the HRQoL form is missing, since it depends on patient responses at the time of assessment, it cannot be retrospectively reconstructed. Missing baseline (pre-treatment) assessments are particularly problematic since they obviate understanding the patient's HRQoL before treatment, and create problems for the statistical analysis of within and between treatment changes.

There are several patterns of missing HRQoL data, including intermittent missing forms and that attributable to dropout from the clinical trial. Missing form data may be due to administrative reasons (e.g., research coordinator forgot to give HRQoL questionnaire to subject during study visit) or patient-based reasons (e.g., deteriorating health status, mortality, study dropout). Missing HRQoL data are consistent with several missing value mechanisms, missing completely at random (MCAR), missing at random (MAR), or missing not at random (MNAR) (Rubin 1976; Little and Rubin 1987). In many cases, missing HRQoL and patient based outcome data in clinical trials is MAR or NMAR. Depending on the extent and nature of missing HRQoL form data, significant bias may be introduced into treatment comparisons and the statistical analyses. There are significant methodological challenges in the statistical analysis of HRQoL outcomes when missing data is MAR or MNAR (Fairclough 1998; Troxel *et al.* 1998; Fairclough 2002; Fayers and Machin 2000).

Sources of avoidable missing HRQoL data

Study methodological factors

Sources of avoidable missing HRQoL data are attributable to methodological factors, logistical and administrative factors, or patient-based reasons (Bernhard *et al.* 1998). Careful attention to the research design, instrument selection, data collection timing and frequency, motivation for the study, and decisions to include HRQoL measures should be part of the initial protocol and study design process. In the past, HRQoL outcomes were sometimes considered an afterthought and included after the research protocol was completed, resulting in the HRQoL data collection viewed as optional by study investigators. The frequency of assessments and duration of a study can result in more missing HRQoL data. A decrease in HRQoL follow-up form completion rates is often observed in long-term studies. Baseline assessments are necessary, but sometimes difficult to gather given the other competing logistical components involved in entering a subject in a clinical trial (i.e., diagnostic procedures, informed consent, randomization). In addition, subjects with no baseline HRQoL are much more likely to have missing follow-up assessments (Hahn *et al.* 1998).

The selection of psychometrically sound and relevant HRQoL measures for clinical trials is necessary. Long and complicated instruments increase respondent burden and result in increased missing item or form data. HRQoL measures need to be appropriate for the patient population under study. Unless the HRQoL component to the clinical trial is fully integrated into the research protocol, there is a greater possibility that the HRQoL part will not be well implemented, resulting in increased missing data. These methodological factors are all preventable through well-conceived HRQoL protocols (Gotay *et al.* 1992; Nayfield *et al.* 1992; Osoba 1992; Fayers *et al.* 1997; Fayers and Machin 2000; Hahn *et al.* 1998).

Study logistical and administrative factors

Missing item level data and HRQoL form data are most often due to problems with study personnel not understanding and/or implementing the HRQoL data collection protocol as specified, or due to ambiguity in the research protocol. In addition, sometimes research coordinators, based on their perceptions, do not administer the HRQoL questionnaires to the patients because they believe the patient is too ill to complete the questionnaires. A survey of 29 centers participating in one or more of three randomized trials for lung and head and neck cancer found that a high proportion of missing HRQoL data was potentially preventable (Hopwood *et al.* 1997). The three most frequently reported problems were unavailability of research staff to administer the questionnaires or to assist subjects, unavailability of questionnaires, and staff perceptions that the subject was too ill to complete the HRQoL assessments. Appropriate protocol development and planning by the investigators and providing adequate resources for participating clinical centers have the potential to address the first two problems, and education of study personnel is needed to address the third. Other reviews of reasons for missing HRQoL form data reach similar conclusions (Bernhard *et al.* 1998; Fayers *et al.* 1998; Curran *et al.* 1998).

The data collection and management procedures clearly depend on the patient population and research questions, the HRQoL instruments, number of centers and subjects enrolled in the study, and economic factors (Bernhard *et al.* 1998). Even if there is a well-developed and sound clinical trial design and protocol, logistical and administrative factors can interfere with implementation. Various modes of administration (e.g., self-completed in clinic, telephone or interactive voice recognition system interviewing, computer-administered, or mail surveys) can be used to collect the HRQoL data. There are advantages and disadvantages in terms of missing data associated with each method of instrument administration. Study staff need to be carefully trained and monitored, with anticipation of potential problems that may occur, and adequate center funding for personnel and data management.

One major source of missing HRQoL data occurs when the study site clinicians and research support staff involved with the clinical trial are not committed to the HRQoL part of the clinical trial. Without this motivation and commitment, the fidelity and implementation of the HRQoL will be compromised. Key factors related to compliance with HRQoL components of trials (defined as the percentage of completed HRQoL assessments) include institutional factors (i.e., size of centers, low accrual centers), chemotherapy compliance, commitment of the center physician investigator, or staff oversight (i.e., forgetting to administer the HRQoL questionnaires) (Bernhard *et al.* 1998; Olschewki 1998; Hahn *et al.* 1998). Most of these administrative sources of missing HRQoL data can be addressed with the implementation of standard quality control procedures.

Patient-related factors

Patient-related factors are also associated with HRQoL compliance rates. Previous research has indicated that older age (i.e., the very old), lower education, cancer metastases, baseline performance status and baseline HRQoL scores all are related to rates of missing HRQoL data (Bernhard *et al.* 1998; Hahn *et al.* 1998; Mosconi *et al.* 1998; Osoba and Zee 1998; Bernstein *et al.* 2002). For example, a recent study by Bernstein *et al.* (2002), in patients with chronic hepatitis C, demonstrated that decreases from baseline in fatigue, vitality, and physical functioning were associated with increased rates of study dropout. Many study patients are motivated to provide the HRQoL assessments, although some may need additional encouragement to complete the forms. The primary patient-related factors associated with missing HRQoL data relate to deteriorating health status and mortality, especially in clinical trials in advanced disease. While this source of missing HRQoL data is not really preventable, the use of proxy respondents and other procedures may provide some insight into the HRQoL of the patients. Finally, cultural factors may influence completion of the HRQoL instruments, especially related to sexual function and other sensitive domains, although this is not always a serious problem (Ganz *et al.* 1998).

Procedures for preventing missing HRQoL data

While analytic strategies exist for dealing with missing form data, they are less satisfactory than prevention. Some missing data, such as that due to death or disease progression, is not preventable. In general, however, the best strategy is primary prevention: missing data should be minimized at the design and implementation stages of the clinical trial protocol (Fairclough and Cella 1996; Young and Maher 1999). In most studies, a nurse or research coordinator is responsible for administering the HRQoL questionnaire to the patient. Various pressures and constraints facing study coordinators can result in missing data, including lack of time and perceived physician support, inadequately specified study protocols, lack of knowledge of the justification and rationale for collecting HRQoL data, lack of reminders, and lack of adequate sites for questionnaire completion (Young and Maher 1999). Thus, having clearly specified procedures in the protocol for collecting HRQoL is the first step in minimizing missing data. This information should include the data collection protocol if the treatment schedule is disrupted, procedures for when the patient requires assistance, and a system for prompting nurses/research personnel that a HRQoL assessment is due (Gotay et al. 1992; Cella 1995; Fairclough and Cella 1996). It is also important to consider alternative methods to obtain follow-up data when patients do not complete questionnaires. Patients, research assistants, and primary investigators should be educated about the importance of collecting these assessments on all patients willing to complete them. Reluctance to approach all patients on all occasions will lead to selection bias. The timing and duration of assessments should also be reasonable, and fit the research questions and disease indication. Practical considerations regarding frequency of assessments and duration of follow-up are important.

Study planning and protocol development

Preventing missing HRQoL data and compliance enhancement require careful research protocol planning, comprehensive education, training and monitoring of data collection personnel, and successful site level and centralized study data management (Hahn et al. 1998; Fayers and Machin 2000). Several study groups have developed guidelines for developing and implementing HRQoL protocols as part of randomized clinical trials (Nayfield et al. 1992; Gotay et al. 1992; Osoba 1992; Fayers et al. 1997; Hahn et al. 1998). There are a number of protocol-related procedures that can be implemented to prevent or minimize the amount of missing HRQoL data in clinical trials. Most of these procedures focus on ensuring that the protocol is clearly developed and described, specific clinical site personnel are identified, clinical center training is adequate and that study manuals are developed.

Early in the study protocol development phase, special consideration needs to be given to the rationale and importance of the HRQoL component to the study, its feasibility, and the study design and methods. In many clinical trial groups, a separate outcomes subcommittee or other group oversees and reviews study methods associated with HRQoL and other patient-reported outcomes. Once a study concept is approved, a rigorous and comprehensive protocol development phase follows, with special focus on instrument selection, timing of HRQoL assessments, and special provisions for handling problems in the HRQoL data collection procedures

(Hahn *et al.* 1998; Fayers and Machin 2000). The HRQoL part of the clinical trial protocol should avoid unnecessarily complicated methods and data collection schedules.

HRQoL instruments need to be selected that are relevant to the research questions and patient population, which possess adequate psychometric characteristics, and that are not overly burdensome to the patients. It is important to ensure that the readability of the survey items matches the target group's literacy level. Baseline and follow-up assessments must fit the research objectives and be consistent with treatment duration and expected survival or disease progression rates. Potential problems with administering the HRQoL instruments and the data collection timing and methods need to be anticipated and possible solutions must be worked out before the study is started. Finally, sufficient personnel and data management resources need to be provided to ensure that it is possible to implement and monitor the HRQoL protocol in the clinical centers.

Data collection forms

The data collection forms should be attractive and professional in appearance, using fonts that are large enough to ensure readability (e.g., 12-point characters or greater). For example, cognitive laboratory procedures have been used to improve the formatting of HRQoL questions and response scales (Mullin *et al.* 2000). Two-sided forms should not be used since patients will often not look on the back of the page and, if forms are copied at the sites, there is a high probability that only the front side will be copied (Hopwood *et al.* 1997). Care must be taken when the HRQoL forms for data collection are prepared and printed to ensure that all the instrument's items are included to avoid subsequent problems with incomplete study forms.

Study personnel and training

The clinical center person responsible for administering the HRQoL forms should be clearly identified and their roles and responsibilities need to be clearly delineated (Gotay *et al.* 1992; Cella 1995; Hopwood *et al.* 1997). Depending on the size of the study and expected subject recruitment, it is also advisable to identify at least one back-up research staff member to fill in when the primary person is unavailable. The responsibilities of the research coordinator include, in addition to the usual responsibilities associated with the clinical trial, knowing when the patient will arrive, making sure the patient receives the questionnaire prior to undergoing diagnostic or therapeutic procedures, having a quiet place for the patient to complete the assessment, reviewing completed HRQoL forms, and implementing follow-up procedures when the patient is not available as expected. At the time of the first HRQoL assessment, this key person should emphasize the importance of obtaining the patient's perspective, reviewing the instructions with the subjects, emphasizing that there are no correct or incorrect responses, encouraging subjects to provide the best answer they can to every question, and reminding them that follow-up assessments will be completed over the course of the study (if applicable). The study coordinator may have the responsibility of reviewing the forms for missing item responses, but care must be taken to balance confidentiality with the need to minimize missing data. If the HRQoL assessment is administered as an interview, sufficient trained research personnel to schedule and conduct the interviews are required.

Education and training of study center personnel is an important part of minimizing missing data (Gotay *et al.* 1992; Cella 1995; Hahn *et al.* 1998; Moinpour and Lovato 1998; Fayers and Machin 2000). Training must begin at the investigator level and include research support staff (often nurse researchers) as well as the patient. Training of center investigators and research support staff can be accomplished through group meetings and/or through individual site meetings. The education and training of clinical center staff includes information on the protocol (with strong justifications for importance of the HRQoL assessments), written study manuals, and video study manuals. Videos may be valuable as training vehicles both for research staff and patients. While there are often face-to-face training sessions at the initiation of a study, research personnel can change over time. Training manuals and videotapes directed toward research personnel can deal with procedures in more detail than is possible in the protocol. Examples would include how to handle a patient who is unable to fill in the questionnaire and not letting family or friends assist in the completion of the HRQoL questionnaires, and what to do if the person requires assistance. Training tapes are especially useful for providing positive ways of approaching the patient. For example, instead of referring to participation as burdensome, the assessment can be placed in a positive light (Cella *et al.* 1993). Rather than 'We have a lot of forms that you need to fill out', a better approach is:

> We want to know more about the quality of life of people as they go through this treatment and the only way to know is to ask you, so we're asking you to complete this brief questionnaire. It usually takes about 10 minutes.

Hopwood *et al.* (1997) noted that, in three trials for lung and head and neck cancer, the most commonly cited factor affecting the distribution of questionnaires was the staff's judgment that the patient was too ill to complete a HRQoL assessment. Patient refusal was the least frequently indicated problem. It is understandable that study personnel may be reluctant to approach patients when they appear to be feeling ill. To minimize the bias from selecting out these patients, all subjects should be asked to complete the questionnaire. There are ways of encouraging ill patients, specifically by providing conditions that make it as easy as possible for them to complete the questionnaire. However, when a patient refuses, that refusal must be respected.

Patient information sheets that explain the rationale behind the assessments will minimize missing data. These fact sheets can contain messages about the importance of the patient's perspective, that there are no 'correct' answers, and reasons why it is important to respond to every question and to complete the follow-up questionnaires.

In addition to the persuasive information, patients should be informed that they can refuse without affecting their treatment or relationship with their doctor.

Study management and quality control procedures

Another key to a successful study is a system that identifies when patients are due for assessments (Cella 1995). This may include preprinted orders in the patient's chart that identify which assessments should be administered at each clinic visit, or modifying data collection forms to remind research staff to collect the HRQoL data (Cella 1995). A central data management office where calendars and expectation notices are generated can support this process. Stickers on patients' charts identifying them as part of a study, flow sheets, study calendars, and patient tracking cards (Moinpour *et al.* 1989) may all be helpful in ensuring that HRQoL assessments are completed when scheduled.

Data monitoring and quality control procedures need to be developed and implemented to identify problems with the collection of the HRQoL data early in the clinical trial. In this way, interventions to correct identified problems can be implemented early to minimize missing data. Central statistical or coordinating centers can implement quality assurance and enhancement systems to monitor activities associated with the quality of HRQoL data collection and the continued education and training of site research staff. For example, as patients are randomized into the clinical trial, the coordinating center can generate a HRQoL data collection schedule documenting the target dates and acceptable assessment windows for all HRQoL assessments.

Explicit procedures for follow-up

A practical schedule with assessments linked to planned treatment or follow-up visits can decrease the number of missing assessments. When possible, it is important to link HRQoL outcomes with other study-related clinical assessments. The availability of the patient at the center increases the likelihood that the assessment will be completed. Staff may be more likely to remember when the assessment is scheduled if the timing is linked to clinical or laboratory follow-up. Finally, it is possible to link clinical events and laboratory values to the assessments. Less frequent assessment decreases patient burden slightly, but may introduce confusion about the schedule and lead to missed assessments. If more frequent assessments are specified in the design, strategies for obtaining the additional assessments must be identified. If the duration of assessment continues after therapy is discontinued, this procedure should be clearly stated, and protocol flow charts for treatment and assessment schedules should clearly reflect the difference.

The protocol and training materials should include specific procedures to minimize missing data. These study-related documents should clearly state the acceptable windows for each assessment and whether follow-up by telephone or mail is allowed (Cella 1995; Young *et al.* 1999; Fayers and Machin 2000). Documentation of the reasons for missing assessments can be combined with other questions about the conditions under which the HRQoL assessment was administered. For example, 'What was the site and mode of administration?', 'Was any assistance given and, if so, by whom?' or 'What about having interviewers available to administer survey in non-English languages?'

Secondary prevention

Secondary prevention of missing HRQoL data consists of gathering information useful in the analysis and interpretation of the results, including collection of data on factors that contribute to missing assessments and data that are likely to predict the missing data. When constructing the set of possible reasons for missing data, the options should differentiate whether the non-response was likely to be related to the patient's HRQoL. For example, categories such as 'Patient refusal' do not clarify this, but reasons such as 'Patient refusal due to poor health' and 'Patient refusal unrelated to health' are informative. A hypothetical form for recording information on the reasons for missing HRQoL assessments is included in Table 3.2.1. The systematic collection of information on the reasons for missing HRQoL form data will inform the statistical analysis and interpretation of these data.

Secondary prevention may include gathering concurrent data on toxicity, evaluations of health status by the clinical staff, or assessments from a caregiver. There are a number of examples of missing data reporting forms that have been used in previous clinical trials (Bernhard *et al.* 1998; Osoba and Zee 1998; Fayers *et al.* 1997; Fayers and Machin 2000). While it is possible to collect some information on the health status of the patient from caregivers or other proxy respondents, appropriate caution must be taken when using this information in analyses. Several studies have demonstrated that patient self-reported data on HRQoL is often poorly correlated with reports from

Table 3.2.1 Hypothetical Study Form for Recording Reasons for Missing HRQoL Assessment Data

Was the scheduled HRQoL assessment completed by the patient?
Yes
No (if no, record the primary reason below)
◆ Patient missed scheduled assessment visit
◆ Patient refused due to poor health
◆ Patient refused unrelated to health
◆ Study staff felt patient was too ill
◆ Administrative failure
◆ Other, please specify: _____

caregivers or clinicians (Rothman *et al.* 1991; Sprangers and Aaronson 1992; Sneeuw *et al.* 1997; Wu *et al.* 1997). Proxy respondents provide ratings that are most strongly correlated with patient self-assessments for observable domains such as physical functioning and activities of daily living. However, proxy data may be useful in interpreting whether any observed differences in HRQoL may be associated with the missing HRQoL form data (Simes *et al.* 1998).

Summary

Missing HRQoL item and form data is a source of selection bias and compromises the power of clinical trials to detect treatment differences. Many sources of missing HRQoL data are preventable, and careful attention to the rationale and motivation for the study, the research design, instrument selection, and data collection schedule will help minimize missing data rates. Education and training of investigators and study coordinators, including how to deal with potential issues associated with the HRQoL data collection, is critically important. Some missing HRQoL is inevitable, especially in clinical trials in advanced disease, so methods of secondary prevention should be implemented in all clinical studies. Effective strategies for minimizing missing HRQoL data are available and can be systematically incorporated in clinical studies.

References

Bernhard, J., Cella, D. F., and Coates, A. S., *et al.* (1998). Missing quality of life data in cancer clinical trials: serious problems and challenges. *Statistics in Medicine*, **17**, 517–532.

Bernstein, D., Kleinman, L., Barker, C., Revicki, D., and Green, J. (2002). Relationship of health-related quality of life to treatment adherence and sustained response in chronic hepatitis C patients. *Hepatology*, **35**, 704–708.

Cella, D. F. (1995). Methods and problems in measuring QOL. *Supportive Care in Cancer*, **3**, 11–22.

Cella, D. F., Skeel, R. T., and Bonomi, A. E. (1993). *Policies and Procedures Manual*. Boston, MA: Eastern Cooperative Oncology Group Quality of Life Subcommittee.

Curran, D., Molenberghs, G., Fayers, P. M., and Machin, D. (1998). Incomplete quality of life data in randomized trials: missing forms. *Statistics in Medicine*, **17**, 697–710.

Fairclough, D. L. (1998). Comparison of several model-based methods for analyzing incomplete quality of life data in cancer clinical trials. *Statistics in Medicine*, **17**, 781–796.

Fairclough, D. L. (2002). *Design and Analysis of Quality of Life Studies in Clinical Trials*. Boca Raton: Chapman & Hall/CRC.

Fairclough, D. L. (in press). Practical considerations in outcomes assessment for clinical trials. In J. Lipscomb, C. Gotay and C. Snyder (eds.) *Outcomes Assessment in Cancer: Findings and recommendations of the Cancer Outcomes Measurement Working Group*. Cambridge: Cambridge University Press.

Fairclough, D. L. and Cella, D. F. (1996). A cooperative group report on quality of life research: lessons learned. Eastern Cooperative Oncology Group (ECOG). *Journal of the National Cancer Institute*, **40**, 73–75.

Fayers, P. M., Curran, D., and Machin, D. (1998). Incomplete quality of life data in randomized trials: missing items. *Statistics in Medicine*, **17**, 679–696.

Fayers, P. M., Hopwood, P., Harvey, A., Girling, D. J., Machin, D., and Stephens, R. (1997). Quality of life assessments in clinical trials –guidelines and a checklist for protocol writers: the UK MRC experience. *European Journal of Cancer*, **33**, 20–28.

Fayers, P. M. and Machin, D. (2000). *Quality of Life: Assessment, Analysis and Interpretation*. New York: Wiley.

Ganz, P. A., Day, R., and Costantino, J. (1998). Compliance with quality of life data collection in the National Surgical Adjuvant Breast and Bowel Project (NSABP) Breast Cancer Prevention Trial. *Statistics in Medicine*, **17**, 613–622.

Gotay, C. C., Korn, E. L., McCabe, M. S., Moore, T. D., and Cheson, B. D. (1992). Quality of life assessment in cancer treatment protocols: research issues in protocol development. *Journal of the National Cancer Institute*, **84**, 575–579.

Hahn, E. A., Webster, K. A., Cella, D. F., and Fairclough, D. L. (1998). Missing data in quality of life research in Eastern Cooperative Oncology Group (ECOG) clinical trials: problems and solutions. *Statistics in Medicine*, **17**, 547–559.

Hopwood, P., Harvey, A., and Davies, J., *et al.* (1997). Survey of the administration of quality of life questionnaires in three multicentre randomized trials in cancer. *European Journal of Cancer*, **90**, 49–57.

Little, R. J. A. and Rubin, D. B. (1987). *Statistical Analysis with Missing Data*. New York: Wiley.

Moinpour, C., Feigl, P., and Metch, B., *et al.* (1989). Quality of life end points in cancer clinical trials: review and administration. *Journal of the National Cancer Institute*, **81**, 485–495.

Moinpour, C. and Lovato, L. (1998). Ensuring the quality of quality of life data: the Southwest Oncology Group experience. *Statistics in Medicine*, **17**, 641–651.

Mosconi, P., Torri, V., and Cifani, S., *et al.* (1998). The multi-centre assessment of quality of life: the Interdisciplinary Group for Cancer Care Evaluation (GIVIO) experience in Italy. *Statistics in Medicine*, **17**, 577–586.

Mullin, P. A., Lohr, K. N., Bresnahan, B. W., and McNulty, P. (2000). Applying cognitive design principles to formatting HRQOL instruments. *Quality of Life Research*, **9**, 13–27.

Nayfield, S. G., Ganz, P. A., Moinpour, C. M., Cella, D. F., and Hailey, B. J. (1992). Report from a National Cancer Institute (USA) workshop on quality of life assessment in cancer clinical trials. *Quality of Life Research*, **1**, 203–210.

Olschewski, M. (1998). Compliance with QOL assessment in multicentre German breast cancer trials. *Statistics in Medicine*, **17**, 571–575.

Osoba, D. (1992). The Quality of Life Committee of the Clinical Trials Group of the National Cancer Institute of Canada: organization and functions. *Quality of Life Research*, **1**, 211–218.

Osoba, D. and Zee, B. (1998). Completion rates in health-related quality-of-life assessment: approach of the National Cancer Institute of Canada Clinical Trial Group. *Statistics in Medicine*, **17**, 603–612.

Rothman, M. L., Hedricks, S. C., and Bulcroft, K. A., *et al.* (1991). The validity of proxy-generated scores as measures of patient health status. *Medical Care*, **29**, 115–124.

Rubin, D. B. (1976). Inference and missing data. *Biometrika*, **63**, 581–592.

Simes, R. J., Greatorex, V., and Gebski, V. J. (1998). Practical approaches to minimize problems with missing quality of life data. *Statistics in Medicine*, **17**, 725–737.

Sneeuw, K. C. A., Aaronson, N. K., and Osoba, D., *et al.* (1997). The use of significant others as proxy raters of the quality of life of patients with brain cancer. *Medical Care*, **35**, 490–506.

Sprangers, M. A. G. and Aaronson, N. K. (1992). The role of health care providers and significant others in evaluating the quality of life of patients with chronic disease: a review. *Journal of Clinical Epidemiology*, **45**, 743–760.

Troxel, A. B., Fairclough, D. L., Curran, D., and Hahn, E. A. (1998). Statistical analysis of quality of life with missing data in cancer clinical trials. *Statistics in Medicine*, **17**, 653–667.

Wu, A. W., Jacobson, D. L., and Berzon, R. A., *et al.* (1997). The effect of mode of administration on Medical Outcomes Study health ratings and EuroQol scores in AIDS. *Quality of Life Research*, **6**, 3–10.

Young, T., de Haes, J. C. J. M., Curran, D., Fayers, P. M., and Brandberg, Y. (1999). *Guidelines for Assessing Quality of Life in EORTC Clinical Trials*. Brussels: EORTC.

Young, T. and Maher, J. (1999). Collecting quality of life data in EORTC clinical trials-what happens in practice? *Psycho-Oncology*, **8**, 260–263.

3.3

Analysing studies with missing data

Diane L. Fairclough

Introduction

Missing data are inevitable in any longitudinal study; over an extended period of time patients will potentially experience morbidity or mortality due to disease or its treatment. As described in Revicki's chapter (3.2), missing data may be unrelated to the patient's quality of life (QoL) and result from administrative problems such as staff forgetting to give the forms to the patient during a very busy time. Other reasons are directly related to the patient's quality of life, such as the patient being unable to complete the questionnaire because of severe toxicity or death.

Because QoL is assessed based on patient report, generally in the form of a multi-item questionnaire, there are two main types of missing data. *Item non-response* occurs when an individual fails to respond to one or more of the items (questions) of a QoL questionnaire. *Unit (questionnaire) non-response* occurs when an individual fails to complete any items in a questionnaire. This may occur intermittently throughout the clinical trial or because a subject drops out of the clinical trial. In rare cases, early assessments may be missing because the QoL assessments were added after the trials had begun.

Why do missing data matter?

Missing data present difficulties in clinical trials for several reasons. First is the loss of power to detect change over time or differences between groups as a result of a reduced number of observations. However, in many large trials, the sample size has been based on other clinical end points, and the power to detect meaningful differences in QoL measures is generally adequate. If not, increasing the sample size of the trial may be feasible, depending on patient and economic resources.

Second is the potential for bias of the estimates as a result of non-randomly missing data. For example, patients who are experiencing a negative impact of the disease or therapy on their lives may be less likely to complete the QoL assessments. In other settings, patients who have had an excellent response to therapy may feel that they no longer need to continue their participation in the treatment study. In either case, as will be illustrated below, a clear understanding of the reasons for missing assessments is a critical factor in the selection of the appropriate method of analysis for these longitudinal studies. Olschewski *et al.* (1994) describe a worst-case scenario where dropout in one arm occurs because the treatment is ineffective and the patient's health status deteriorates. In contrast, dropout in the other arm is minimal despite some toxicity because the treatment is effective. They point out that the ineffective treatment may appear better because the QoL is being reported only by a selected group of subjects who have not yet deteriorated because of their disease.

Missing items

It is not uncommon to have a small proportion (1 to 2 per cent) of the items skipped in a QoL questionnaire. The frequency of missing items has been observed to be higher among elderly individuals (Kosinski *et al.* 2000) and those who are more ill (Hopwood *et al.* 1994). If the responses from selected patients are excluded from analysis because of missing items, there is a danger of biasing the results. Sometimes skipping an item is inadvertent, but it may also occur because a question is not applicable for that subject. Questions about sexual function or relationship with spouse/partner are good examples of questions that are likely to be skipped by some subjects. It is also possible that a particular item will be missing because of a problem with the wording of a question or the responses, the structure of the questionnaire, problems with translations, culture-related difficulties with interpretation, or exhaustion. These problems are rare for well-developed and validated instruments. However, when a particular item is missing for more than 3–4 per cent of patients, the cause of the problem should be investigated. The exception occurs for questions that are asked only if relevant to the individual; missing data for those items can be quite high.

To avoid missing subscale scores because of one or two missing responses, most scales specify exactly how to score the question in the presence of missing items. When a strategy is specified for a particular instrument, it should be used unless there is a strong justification for an alternative scoring system. Use of the standard facilitates interpretation and comparisons across studies.

These strategies for missing responses to individual questions may have different implications for analysis of data to assess outcomes of interventions versus analyzing psychometric properties (factor analysis, item-scale correlations) of scales. In the first case, the objective is to obtain unbiased estimates of the scale or subscale scores. In the second case, the methods examine the correlations within the scale. In theory, regression methods may have a tendency to overestimate the correlations involving the missing item. But if the proportion of missing responses for any individual question is small, this potential disadvantage may be outweighed by the advantages of including all of the subjects in the analyses.

Treat the score for the scales as missing

One strategy for handling a missing item is to treat the scores based on that item as missing. This strategy is rarely recommended for QoL questionnaires. Typically, in most studies, between 0.5–2 per cent of the items in QoL questionnaires will be missing. This would not seem a concern, but if a questionnaire had 30 items a rate of 1 per cent missing items could result in missing scale scores for as many as 30 per cent of the subjects. The problem is exacerbated because subjects who are feeling poorly either physically or emotionally are more likely to have missing items; thus, the scores on the remaining subjects are a biased sample of the subjects.

Simple mean imputation

The most typical strategy, sometimes referred to as the *half rule*, is to substitute the mean of the answered questions for that specific subscale for the missing responses as long as at least half the questions were answered. Less typically, imputation using any available information, not requiring half or more items in a scale, is also used, though much less often. Use of the mean of the available items works well for scales where there is no particular ordering of the *difficulty* of the questions (Fairclough and Cella 1996) and the difficulty of the question does not have a wide range across the subscale items.

Simple mean imputation should be used cautiously when the questions have a hierarchy, as when physical functioning is assessed through the ability to do certain activities. The physical functioning scale of the SF-36 is a good example of a scale where the individual items have some hierarchical structure. If individuals are *limited a lot* in moderate activities, it is clear that they are also limited a lot in strenuous activities. Similarly, if subjects respond that they can walk a mile without limitations, they will also be able to walk several blocks. Special strategies may need to be specified for these types of questions (Kosinski *et al.* 2000). However, simple mean imputation works surprisingly well, generally resulting in a value that is not very different from the obvious response, and handles all cases including those where the appropriate response is not obvious.

Other options

There are a number of other possibilities for imputation, including the mean of the item responses provided by other subjects or regression of the missing item on the remaining items of the scale. A limitation of these other options is that the values imputed will differ from study to study, and could also differ from analyst to analyst within the same study if different subsets of subjects are used to estimate the missing value. The later might occur if one analyst chose to stratify on treatment and another on disease severity. Interestingly, these other options rarely perform better than the half rule approach describe above (Fairclough and Cella 1996). The relative performance of different methods will depend on the sample size, where the regression-based methods will perform poorly in smaller studies.

Missing questionnaires

There are three classes of missing data that determine which methods of analysis are appropriate for longitudinal studies (Little and Rubin 1987). Briefly, if the reasons for missing assessments are completely unrelated to the patient's QoL, then we consider the data to be missing completely at random (MCAR). If the probability of a missing assessment only depends on the observed measures of QoL and other explanatory factors, we consider the data to be missing at random (MAR). Finally, missing data are considered to be not missing at random (MNAR) or non-ignorable if the probability that an observation is missing depends on the value of the missing observation. Formal definitions and further discussion of these three types of missing assessments are presented in Appendix I.

Various formal approaches to testing the assumption of MCAR versus MAR exist (Little 1988; Diggle 1989; Schluchter 1990; Ridout 1991; Park and Davis 1993). Common sense and historical evidence suggest that this assumption will not be true in most clinical trials and it is rare to observe completely random missingness in QoL assessments. When this does occur, it is usually the result of preventable administrative errors. It would be helpful if a formal test of the assumptions of MAR versus MNAR were possible, however, we need the data that we are missing to perform these tests. Informal evidence of non-ignorable missingness may, however, be obtained through careful documentation of the reasons for missing assessments or correlations with other outcomes that may act as surrogates for QoL. For example, it is reasonable to assume that missingness is non-random when assessments are documented as missing because the subject feels too ill or is physically/cognitively unable to complete the assessments. Similarly, one would expect QoL to have worsened in subjects who drop out due to the progression of their disease.

Imputation-based approaches for missing questionnaires

One approach for handling missing data due to missing assessments occurring in clinical trials with extended longitudinal assessments uses the strategy of imputation to estimate the missing data (Little and Rubin 1987; Rubin and Schenker 1986; Crawford *et al.* 1995; Lavori *et al.* 1995). The motivation for this approach is that simple complete data methods can be used to analyze the imputed data sets. If thoughtfully implemented, using information about the reasons for missing data and other clinical outcomes, this approach has great promise. However, these methods also have the potential for obscuring the problem when not properly implemented. When choosing the method for imputation the analyst should consider the missing data mechanism. For example, methods such as regression models or hot-deck imputation assume that the data are MAR. When that assumption is not correct, the results will be biased. A few of the possibilities, including both single and multiple imputation using both model-based and sampling methods for imputation, follow.

Last observation carried forward

A popular approach is to use the last observation (or value) carried forward (LOCF or LVCF), where the patient's last available assessment is substituted for each of the missing assessments. This approach has limited utility (Heyting *et al.* 1992) and should be employed with great caution. For example, in a study where QoL is decreasing over time, a treatment with early drop out could possibly look better than a treatment where tolerance to the therapy was better. If employed, the assumptions should be explicitly stated and examined. If it is likely that the values for those dropping out due to lack of efficacy or to side-effects will be lower than for those remaining on the study, LOCF is a poor choice. If there is a strong argument for LOCF, it is wise to plan for a QoL assessment at discontinuation as well as documentation of the reason for discontinuation.

Single mean or predicted value imputation

Single imputation methods include *mean imputation* and *predicted value (regression) imputation*. In mean imputation, the average value of the measure of QoL from subjects with non-missing data is substituted for the missing observations. The assumption is that the missing values are random within the group of subjects used to estimate the missing value. If the questionnaire is missing for administrative reasons, this is a reasonable assumption. But if it is missing because the patient feels to ill to complete the questionnaire, the results will be biased.

In regression imputation, the predicted value of the measure of QoL estimated using a regression model is substituted for the missing assessments. The assumption is relaxed slightly so that missingness is random for patients with the same characteristics. The dilemma is that even when important explanatory variables are included in the model, there remains the concern that the sicker subjects are not responding.

When the concern about bias can be overcome, there still remains an important criticism of the single imputation methods. Specifically, most methods of analysis treat imputed values just like observed values in the analysis and underestimate the uncertainty by ignoring the measurement error, among-subject variability, and the incomplete knowledge of the reason for non-response.

Hot-deck imputation

Hot-deck imputation involves selecting a score at random from subjects with observed data. This reduces the inflation of test statistics associated with simple mean imputation. This approach assumes that the data are randomly missing in the group of subjects from which the new score is sampled. The procedures may involve very elaborate schemes for selecting responses for substitution, or the identification of one or two key variables to stratify upon to reduce the complexity. Lavori *et al.* (1995) propose a strategy based on a 'propensity score' for the probability of drop out. The idea is to find a univariate score that summarizes the multiple variables defining the history of each patient, stratify patients using the quintiles of the score, and then use an approximate Bayesian bootstrap (Rubin and Schenker 1986) to select the responses for substitution within each of the strata. This approach assumes that, conditional on the propensity score, the missing data are missing at random. A multi-step process is used to compute the score for each of the planned observation times. As the number of assessments increases with multiple causes for missing data, these strategies quickly become very complex.

Multiple imputation

Multiple imputation (Rubin and Schenker 1986; Little and Rubin 1987) retains many of the advantages of single imputation, but rectifies the problem of underestimation of the variance of estimates and the resulting inflation of test statistics. The basic strategy of multiple imputation is to impute 3 to 10 sets of values for the missing data that incorporate both sampling variability and the uncertainty about the reasons for non-response. Methods of sampling can include explicit models such as a fully normal regression model, Markov chain Monte Carlo procedures (Schafer and Olsen 1998) or implicit models such as approximate Bayesian bootstrap (Rubin and Schenker 1991). Each set of data is then analyzed using complete data methods and the analyses are combined in a way that reflects the extra variability due to missing data (Rubin and Schenker 1991). As with all the previous methods, if the analyst includes patient characteristics and outcome measures that fully explain the missing values, the results will be unbiased. However, this is difficult to do as the most important information that would allow prediction of the missing QoL measure is often also missing (Crawford *et al.* 1995).

Non-parametric analysis using ranked data

Gould (1980) describes a practical method for the analysis of clinical trials with withdrawal. If there is adequate documentation concerning the reasons for missing assessments, it may be possible to determine a reasonable ordering (or ranking) of QoL among the subjects. For example, it would be reasonable to assign patients who withdraw because of disease progression, excessive toxicity, or death a rank that is lower than that observed for patients remaining on the study. The advantage of this approach is that we do not have to impute the specific value. Heyting *et al.* (1992) identifies some limitations, including multiple reasons for drop out that are not clearly ordered. Methods for non-parametric analysis of repeated measures are proposed by Wei and Johnson (1985).

Imputation associated with death

Ware *et al.* (1996) in a study of four-year health outcomes as part of the Medical Outcomes Study, defined three outcome groups: improved, stable and declined. Patients who died during the interval were classified as having declined. Diehr *et al.* (1995) explored a number of methods for handling deaths, including ignoring deaths, assigning an arbitrary value (0 on a 0–100 point scale) and probabilities of remaining healthy or alive in two years. They note that strategies that gave less influence to death tended to show more favorable changes in health status over time and therefore favored the group that had more deaths. The strategies that gave more influence to death favored the group with fewer deaths.

Maximum-likelihood based methods

Analysis of complete cases (MCAR)

Multivariate analysis of variance (MANOVA) or growth curve models that only include data from patients who have completed *all* of the scheduled assessments (Complete Cases) is the least desirable approach and increasingly less common. These methods were popular because they are taught in most intermediate statistical courses and are available in almost every statistical analysis package. If the proportion of subjects with any missing assessments is very small (< 5 per cent of the cases), these methods may be reasonable. However, in many studies with extended follow-up and patients who may be experiencing morbidity and/or mortality, these methods could easily exclude more than half the subjects from the analysis. More critically, these approaches are based on the very strong assumption of MCAR; if that assumption is untrue then the results may be seriously biased.

To illustrate this concept, consider a longitudinal study conducted by the International Breast Study Group (IBCSG) (Hurny *et al.* 1996) of 1475 premenopausal breast cancer patients. Figure 3.3.1 presents the available scores from the Perceived Adaptation to Chronic Illness Scales (PACIS) (Hurny *et al.* 1992) for patients who did not experience disease progression during the first 18 months of follow-up. The relationship of missing assessments to the QoL measured during the non-missing assessments is demonstrated by the higher scores reported by the 344 patients who completed all seven assessments, with the scores dropping for the 403 patients who missed one or two assessments, and the lowest scores for the 224 patients who completed only one to four assessments. Thus, even after excluding patients with missing assessments due to disease progression, the probability that an observation is missing does depend on the QoL that the patient is experiencing. Thus, an analysis of the complete cases (the 344 patients with all seven assessments) would overestimate the PACIS score and not be representative of the patients who are disease-free.

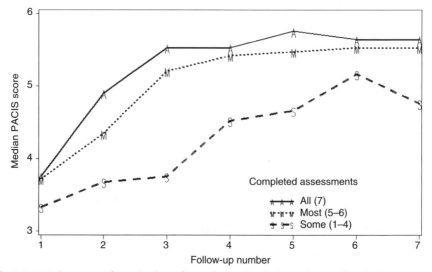

Fig. 3.3.1 Median scores from the (transformed) Perceived Adaptation to Chronic Illness Scale (PACIS) (Hurny *et al.* 1992) for patients who completed 1–4 (N = 224), 5–6 (N = 403) or all seven of the scheduled assessments. Patients who experience disease progression are excluded. Scores are transformed so that higher scores indicate better QoL. Reproduced with permission from Fairclough, D. L. (1998), Chapter 13, *Quality of Life Assessment in Clinical Trials: Methods and Practice* (1st edn), M. J. Staquet, R. D. Hays, and P. Fayers (eds). Oxford University Press, New York.

Analysis of all available data (MAR)

The assumption that data are MCAR, required in the analysis of complete cases, can be relaxed to the assumption that data are missing at random (MAR) (Anonymous 1987) or ignorable (Laird 1988). In this situation, the probability that an observation is missing may depend on observed data and covariates, but still must be independent of the value of the missing observation(s) after adjustment for the observed data and covariates. Likelihood-based methods (Dempster *et al.* 1977; Jennrich and Schluchter 1986) which use all the available data, result in unbiased estimates when the data are MAR. These methods are available in most major statistical software packages.

One approach to understanding the assumption of MAR is to consider a study where the assumption is incorrect. In this observational study (Hwang *et al.* 1996), 68 patients with metastatic or progressive disease completed an assessment of QoL every 3–6 weeks. When the data are analyzed using a model that assumes the data are MAR, there is only a small insignificant decrease in the estimates of QoL over time (Figure 3.3.2). However, when stratified by the duration of follow-up (or survival), patients who died earlier experienced a rapid rate of decline in QoL over time (Figure 3.3.3). The counterintuitive results displayed in Figure 3.3.2 are the consequence of the MAR assumption. In this setting, the estimates obtained from the MAR models describe the average QoL of the surviving patients rather than the entire population.

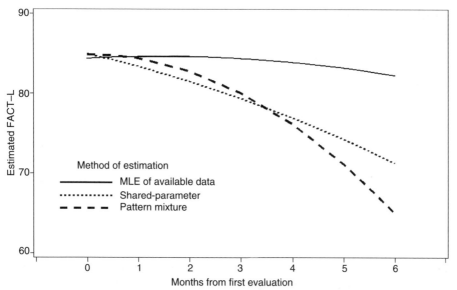

Fig. 3.3.2 Functional Assessment of Cancer Therapy-General (FACT-G) assessments in terminal cancer patients. Estimated FACT-G scores from three different methods of analyses. MLE (mixed-effects model) of available data assuming data are missing at random, Shared-parameter (joint) model for non-ignorable drop out and mixture model for non-ignorable drop out.

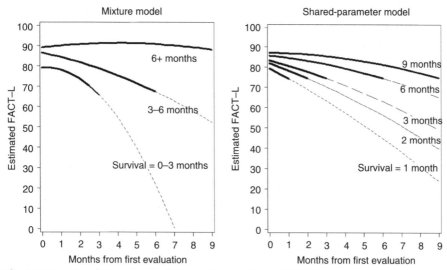

Fig. 3.3.3 Functional Assessment of Cancer Therapy-General (FACT-G) assessments in terminal cancer patients. Estimated FACT-G scores by length of survival for pattern-mixture and shared parameter models. Dashed lines indicate extrapolation of scores after death. Reproduced with permission from Fairclough, D. L. (1998), Chapter 13, *Quality of Life Assessment in Clinical Trials: Methods and Practice* (1st edn), M. J. Staquet, R. D. Hays, and P. Fayers (eds). Oxford University Press, New York.

Methods for non-ignorable missing data (NMAR)

Little (1995) describes two general classes of models, selection and pattern mixture. The choice between the two classes depends partially on whether the missing data mechanism is viewed to be solely a 'nuisance' or not. In contrast to the selection models, the pattern mixture models do not require the specification of a particular model for the missing data mechanism. The large number of potential patterns of missing data and the difficulties of estimating parameters in the underidentified models for some of the missing data patterns counterbalances this advantage. Shared parameter models bridge these two classes of models and can be expressed as mixture models or as selection models. The following sections describe examples of these classes of models in more detail.

Pattern mixture models

The basic concept behind the pattern mixture models described by Little (1994) is that the distribution of the measures of QoL, Y_i, may differ across the K different missing data patterns, having different means, $\mu^{(k)}$, and variance, $\Sigma^{(k)}$. For example, patients who die earlier (with missing data due to death) may have lower QoL scores (different means) and also may have more or less variability in their scores (different variance) than patients who survive longer. The true distribution of the measures of QoL for the entire group of patients will be a mixture of the distributions of each of the K groups of patients. The general method of analysis is to stratify the patients by the missing data patterns. Then the mean and variance parameters ($\hat{\mu}^{(k)}$, $\Sigma^{(k)}$) are estimated within each stratum. Weights are determined by the number of subjects within each of the K missing data patterns ($w_k = n_k/N$). The population estimates are the weighted average of the estimates from the K missing data patterns ($\hat{\mu} = \Sigma w_k \hat{\mu}^{(k)}$). The advantage of these models is that one does not have to define a model for the missing data mechanism. One of the difficulties of this approach is the large number of missing data patterns that occur in actual studies where there may only be a few subjects with some patterns. But more critically, for all but the one pattern where there are no missing observations, the model may be under-identified. Specifically, it may not be possible to estimate all the parameters of the model without making additional assumptions. The most obvious example of an under-identified model occurs for the pattern where all the observations are missing. The assumptions that allow for estimation of all the model parameters are often difficult to communicate and cannot be validated because they depend on the values of the missing data.

The pattern mixture model is one example of a mixture model. Others include mixture models for random effects-dependent drop out (Little 1995) and time-dependent drop out. Wu and Bailey (1989) describe a conditional linear model where the rate of change in an individual is modeled as a polynomial function of the time to drop out.

An application of a mixture model is illustrated using the previously described study of terminal cancer patients. In this study, each patient had a unique pattern of observations and the number of patterns is almost equal to the number of patients. So to simplify the problem, the patients are stratified into three groups based on their duration of survival or follow-up: less than three months ($n_1 = 24$), 3–6 months ($n_2 = 19$), and greater than 6 months ($n_3 = 25$). A mixed-effects model was used to estimate the parameters in each of the three strata (Figure 3.3.3). The assumption in this application is that the quadratic model used to estimate the changes in the FACT-G over the first three months for the first group could be extrapolated to estimate the unobserved QoL during the second three months. Using this method, the estimated FACT-G scores, decline approximately 20 points over a six-month period (Figure 3.3.2). These results are much more consistent with the expected changes in QoL based on clinical observation than those resulting from the MAR analysis.

Selection models

In selection models, a statistical model is specified for the missing data mechanism. In addition to adjusting the estimates for the missing data, these models allow the investigator to make inferences about the relationship of QoL and other explanatory factors causing missing observations. This might be particularly interesting, for example, if death or disease progression was the cause of drop out. Selection models for the analysis of studies with non-ignorable missing data include models where the change in QoL over time is functionally related to the time of death, disease progression, or study drop out.

Wu and Carroll (1988) proposed a probit model for the probability of drop out, which depends on the linear change in QoL over time. The most well-known of the selection models was proposed by Diggle and Kenward (1994). They proposed that the probability of drop out could be a function of subject characteristics (covariates), the past history (previous observations), and the current value of the outcome. The ability to estimate the relation of drop out to the value of the QoL measure at the time of drop out depends entirely on the distribution that is specified for the outcome score. While initially appearing to have great promise, this model has been extensively criticized because of the sensitivity of the results to this assumption. This may be particularly relevant for QoL measures. In many studies, QoL scores are skewed with longer tails for lower scores. If subjects with poorer QoL are more likely to be missing, the non-missing scores will have a roughly normal distribution. If the scores are assumed to be normal, the most common assumption, the drop outs will appear to be random when in fact they are non-random.

Shared-parameter models

An example of a shared parameter model is the proposed extension of the random effects or two-stage mixed-effects model by Schluchter (1992) and DeGruttola and Tu (1994). In this joint model of both the longitudinal QoL scores and the duration of survival, the time of censoring (or death) is incorporated into the model by allowing the time of censoring to be correlated with the random effects of the longitudinal model for QoL.

Returning to the previous example of the study of 68 terminal cancer patients, it might be reasonable to assume that the rate of decline in the FACT-G over time, and possibly the baseline values, are correlated with the time of death in these patients. Using this model, the estimated correlations of the random intercept and slope terms with the log of the survival times was 0.38 and 0.89, respectively. Thus, patients who died earlier had both lower initial values of the FACT-G and a more rapid rate of decline in their FACT-G scores (Figure 3.3.3). Further, there was a significant decline in the estimated mean FACT-G score for the entire study population over a six-month period (Figure 3.3.2).

Sensitivity analyses

Given the numerous potential methods of analysis, how do we choose between different strategies? In some cases, we will have information such as the reason for missing assessments or a clearly defined objective that will determine the 'best' approach. But in general, while certain approaches may be eliminated from consideration, we will be left with several possibilities. A sensitivity analysis in which the effect of the different methods of analysis is examined may be informative. There are two likely outcomes of the sensitivity analysis. The first is that the conclusions are consistent regardless of the approach. An example of this is a sensitivity analysis of four methods of handling missing data in a clinical trial of two adjuvant therapies for breast cancer (Fetting *et al.* 1998). In both arms, 9 per cent of the patients were missing the assessment that occurred during therapy. The end point was the change in QoL (during–before therapy) as measured by the BCQ (Levine *et al.* 1988). In a non-parametric two-sample comparison (Wilcoxon rank-sum test), the four strategies considered included (1) analysis of available data, (2) assigning the lowest rank when missing data occurred in patients discontinuing treatment because of toxicity or relapse, (3) simple imputation of the missing data using regression, and (4) assigning the lowest rank when missing data occurred regardless of the reason. The medians, interquartile ranges, and p-values associated with the treatment comparisons are displayed in Figure 3.3.4 (Fairclough *et al.* 1999). Regardless of the approach taken, medians and interquartile ranges were similar and the treatment differences were statistically significant.

The alternative outcome of a sensitivity analysis is that the conclusions are dependent on the method of analysis or the summary measure selected. When this occurs, the methods should be examined to ascertain the reason for the discrepancy. For example, in the study of the 68 terminal cancer patients (Figure 3.3.2), there was a dramatic difference in the estimates of change over time between the analysis that assumed the missing data was missing at random and the two that considered non-random patterns. In a second example, an Eastern Cooperative Oncology Group trial of three regimens of chemotherapy for patients with advanced non-small cell lung cancer (NSCLC), two summary statistics were considered. The first was the change in QoL (measured by

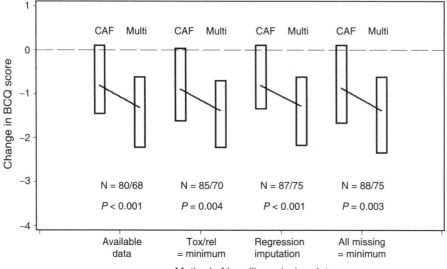

Fig. 3.3.4 Comparison of four methods of analysis (See text for detailed description). Scores represent the difference between BCQ scores measured prior to and during therapy. The vertical boxes show the interquartile ranges (25–75 percentiles) of the distribution of scores and the horizontal lines connect the median scores for the two treatment groups. P-values correspond to the Wilcoxon Rank Sum test for the treatment comparisons. Reproduced with permission from Fairclough, D. L. (1998), Chapter 13, *Quality of Life Assessment in Clinical Trials: Methods and Practice* (1st edn), M. J. Staquet, R. D. Hays, and P. Fayers (eds). Oxford University Press, New York.

the Functional Assessment of Cancer Therapy – Lung [FACT-L]) (Cella *et al.* 1995) over a six-month period and the second was the AUC under the QoL vs. time curve for the same period. In the sensitivity analysis, three different analysis models were considered (Fairclough *et al.* 1998), including an analysis of complete cases (MCAR), all available data (MAR), and a shared-parameter model (NMAR) (Schluchter 1992). The results, summarized in Table 3.3.1, demonstrate both the sensitivity of the estimates to the method of analysis and the choice of the summary measure. Specifically, analyses that assume the missing data are ignorable (either MCAR or MAR) underestimate the six-month change in QoL and overestimate the AUC in all three treatment arms relative to the analyses that assume the missing data are not random (NMAR). This result was expected in this trial of patients with advanced disease, and is consistent with other information obtained from this trial concerning the reasons that QoL assessments were missing. The most striking result was that tests of treatment differences were sensitive to the summary measure selected. Specifically, the tests were non-significant for the change over time, but significant for the AUC. Further examination indicated that baseline and follow-up scores where consistently higher in one of the treatment groups (Taxol only). As a result, the average AUC for that treatment group was higher despite

Table 3.3.1 Sensitivity analysis of non-small cell lung cancer (NSCLC) trial

Treatment Arm[#]	Assumption/ analysis	VP-16		Taxol		Taxol+G-CSF		p-value*
		Estimate	S.E.	Estimate	S.E.	Estimate	S.E.	
Summary statistic: Change over 6 months								
MCAR	Complete case analysis	−1.8	2.7	−5.2	2.1	−5.0	2.2	NS
MAR	MLE of available data	−8.0	2.3	−6.7	2.1	−6.0	2.0	NS
MNAR	Shared parameter model	−14.5	1.6	−11.7	1.4	−12.3	1.4	NS
Summary statistic: Area under the curve								
MCAR	Complete case analysis	53.8	1.1	56.8	0.9	53.2	0.8	0.01
MAR	MLE of available data	50.3	0.7	52.8	0.7	51.1	0.7	0.03
MNAR	Shared parameter model	49.1	0.5	51.3	0.5	49.4	0.5	<0.01

* H_0: Likelihood ratio test of equality of three treatment groups.

[#] Patients received either cisplatin and etoposide (VP-16), cisplatin and paclitaxel (Taxol), or cisplatin, paclitaxel and filgrastin (Taxol+G-CSF).

similar rates of change for all three groups. In this trial, the explanation for the discrepant results was clear, and the results were reported using the selection model for the analysis of the change in QoL over six months.

Summary

The impact of missing data in QoL studies should be carefully evaluated. Non-ignorable missing data are likely in QoL studies where there is drop out due to toxicity, disease progression, or even therapeutic effectiveness. Studies with this type of missing data are also the most difficult to analyze. The primary reason is that there are numerous potential models, and it is impossible to verify statistically the 'correctness' of any model because the data required to distinguish between models are missing. In practice, current application of methods (selection, pattern mixture, and shared-parameter models) for non-ignorable missing data is limited by several factors. The first is the large number of subjects that will be required to distinguish between alternate models. The second is the restriction of some assumptions such as linear changes over time and the inability of many techniques to deal with both dropout and intermittent missing data. In addition, the sophisticated programming required for these methods and the lack of generally available software are barriers to implementation. However, the most significant barrier may be the difficulty of presenting these complicated models in a manner that is readily interpretable in the clinical literature.

References

Cella, D. F., Bonomi, A. E., Lloyd, S. R., Tulsky, D. S., Kaplan, E., and Bonomi, P. (1995). Reliability and validity of the Functional Assessment of Cancer Therapy-Lung (FACT-L) quality of life instrument. *Lung Cancer*, **12**, 199–220.

Crawford, S. L., Tennstedt, S. L., and McKinlay, J. B. (1995). A comparison of analytic methods for non-random missingness of outcome data. *J Clin Epidemiol*, **48**, 209–219.

DeGruttola, V. and Tu, X.M. (1994). Modeling progression of CD-4 lymphocyte count and its relationship to survival time. *Biometrics*, **50**, 1003–1014.

Dempster, A. P., Laird, N. M., and Rubin, D. B. (1977). Maximum likelihood from incomplete data via the EM algorithm. *Journal of the Royal Statistical Society (B)*, **39**, 1–38.

Diehr, P., Patrick, D., Hedrick, S., Rothman, M., Grembowski, D., Raghunathan, T. E., and Beresford, S. (1995). Including deaths when measuring health status over time. *Med Care*, **33**, AS164–AS172.

Diggle, P. and Kenward, M. G. (1994). Informative drop-out in longitudinal data analysis. *Appl Stat*, **43**, 49–93.

Diggle, P. J. (1989). Testing for random dropouts in repeated measurement data. *Biometrics*, **45**, 1255–1258.

Fairclough, D. L. and Cella, D. F. (1996). Functional Assessment of Cancer Therapy (FACT-G): non-response to individual questions. *Qual Life Res*, **5**, 321–329.

Fairclough, D. L., Fetting, J. H., Cella, D., Wonson, W., and Moinpour, C. M. (1999). Quality of life and quality adjusted survival for breast cancer patients receiving adjuvant therapy. Eastern Cooperative Oncology Group (ECOG). *Qual Life Res*, **8**, 723–731.

Fairclough, D. L., Peterson, H. F., Cella, D., and Bonomi, P. (1998). Comparison of several model-based methods for analysing incomplete quality of life data in cancer clinical trials. *Stat Med*, **17**, 781–796.

Fetting, J. H., Gray, R., Fairclough, D. L., Smith, T. J., Margolin, K. A., Citron, M. L., Grove-Conrad, M., Cella, D., Pandya, K., Robert, N., Henderson, I. C., Osborne, C. K., and Abeloff, M. D. (1998). Sixteen-week multidrug regimen versus cyclophosphamide, doxorubicin, and fluorouracil as adjuvant therapy for node-positive, receptor-negative breast cancer: an Intergroup study. *J Clin Oncol*, **16**, 2382–2391.

Gould, A. L. (1980). A new approach to the analysis of clinical drug trials with withdrawals. *Biometrics*, **36**, 721–727.

Heyting, A., Tolboom, J. T., and Essers, J. G. (1992). Statistical handling of drop-outs in longitudinal clinical trials. *Stat Med*, **11**, 2043–2061.

Hopwood, P., Stephens, R. J., and Machin, D. (1994). Approaches to the analysis of quality of life data: experiences gained from a medical research council lung cancer working party palliative chemotherapy trial. *Qual Life Res*, **3**, 339–352.

Hurny, C., Bernhard, J., Coates, A. S., Castiglione-Gertsch, M., Peterson, H. F., Gelber, R. D., Forbes, J. F., Rudenstam, C. M., Simoncini, E., Crivellari, D., Goldhirsch, A., and Senn, H. J. (1996). Impact of adjuvant therapy on quality of life in women with node- positive operable breast cancer. International Breast Cancer Study Group. *Lancet*, **347**, 1279–1284.

Hurny, C., Bernhard, J., Gelber, R. D., Coates, A., Castiglione, M., Isley, M., Dreher, D., Peterson, H., Goldhirsch, A., and Senn, H. J. (1992). Quality of life measures for patients receiving adjuvant therapy for breast cancer: an international trial. The International Breast Cancer Study Group. *Eur J Cancer*, **28**, 118–124.

Hwang, S.S., Chang, V.T., Fairclough, D.F., Hoch, K., Latorre, M., and Corpion, C. (1996). Longitudinal measuremnt for quality of life and symptoms in terminal cancer patients. *Proceeding of the American Society for Clinical Oncology* (Abstract).

Jennrich, R. I. and Schluchter, M. D. (1986). Unbalanced repeated-measures models with structured covariance matrices. *Biometrics*, **42**, 805–820.

Kosinski, M., Bayliss, M., Bjomer, J. B., and Ware, J. E. Jr. (2000). Improving estimates of SF-36 Health Survey Scores for respondents with missing data. *Monitor: Med Outcomes Trust*, **5**, 8–10.

Laird, N. M. (1988). Missing data in longitudinal studies. *Statistics in Medicine,* **7,** 305–315.

Lavori, P. W., Dawson, R. and Shera, D. (1995). A multiple imputation strategy for clinical trials with truncation of patient data. *Stat Med,* **14,** 1913–1925.

Levine, M. N., Guyatt, G. H., Gent, M., De Pauw, S., Goodyear, M. D., Hryniuk, W. M., Arnold, A., Findlay, B., Skillings, J. R., and Bramwell, V. H., *et al.* (1988). Quality of life in stage II breast cancer: an instrument for clinical trials. *J Clin Oncol,* **6,** 1798–1810.

Little, R. J.A. (1988). A test of missing completely at random for multivariate data with missing values. *J Am Stat Assoc,* **83,** 1198–1202.

Little, R. J.A. (1994). A class of pattern-mixture models for normal incomplete data. *Biometrika,* **81,** 471–483.

Little, R. J.A. (1995). Modeling the drop-out mechanism in repeated-measures studies. *J Am Stat Assoc,* **90,** 1112–1121.

Little, R. J.A. and Rubin, D. B. (1987). *Statistical Analysis with Missing Data.* New York: John Wiley & Sons.

Olschewski M., Schulgen G., Schumacher M. and Altman D. G. (1994). Quality of life assessment in clinical cancer research. *Br J Cancer,* **70,** 1–5.

Park, T. and Davis, C. S. (1993). A test of the missing data mechanism for repeated categorical data. *Biometrics,* **49,** 631–638.

Ridout, M. S. (1991). Testing for random dropouts in repeated measurement data. *Biometrics,* **47,** 1617–1621.

Rubin, D. B. (1987). *Multiple Imputation for Nonresponse in Surveys.* New York: John Wiley and Sons.

Rubin, D. B. and Schenker, N. (1986). Multiple imputation for interval estimation from simple random samples with ignorable nonresponse. *J Am Stat Assoc,* **81,** 366–374.

Rubin, D. B. and Schenker, N. (1991). Multiple imputation in health-care databases: an overview and some applications. *Stat Med,* **10,** 585–598.

Schafer, J. L. and Olsen, M. K. (1998). Multiple imputation for multivariate missing-data problems: A data analyst's perspective. *Multivariate Beh Res,* **33,** 454–471.

Schluchter, M. D. (1992). Methods for the analysis of informatively censored longitudinal data. *Stat Med,* **11,** 1861–1870.

Schluchter, M.D. (1990). BMDP 5V: Unbalanced Repeated Measures Models with Structured Covariance Matrices. In W.J. Dixon (ed.) *BMDP Statistics Software,* pp. 1207–1244. Berkeley, CA: University of California Press.

Ware, J.E., Bayless, M.S., Rogers, W.H., Kosinski, M., and Tarlov, A.R. (1996). Differences in 4-year health outcomes for elderly and poor, chronically ill patients treated in HMO and fee-for-service systems. Results from the Medical Outcomes Study. *Journal of the American Medical Association,* **276,** 1039–1047.

Wei, L. J. and Johnson, W. E. (1985). Combining dependent tests with incomplete repeated measurements. *Biometrika,* **72,** 359–364.

Wu, M. C. and Bailey, K. R. (1989). Estimation and comparison of changes in the presence of informative right censoring: conditional linear model. *Biometrics,* **45,** 939–55.

Wu, M. C. and Carroll, R. J. (1988). Estimation and comparison of changes in the presence of informative right censoring by modeling the censoring process. *Biometrics,* **44,** 175–88.

The role and use of differential item functioning (DIF) analysis of quality of life data from clinical trials

Mogens Groenvold and Morten Aagaard Petersen

Introduction

When using a multi-item scale as an end point in a clinical trial we assume that the scale provides a correct description of the level of the construct (e.g. pain) it is supposed to assess. However, in some cases the use of a multi-item scale may lead to incorrect conclusions.

Differential item functioning (DIF) analysis (previously called item bias analysis) investigates how a multi-item scale performs in specific analytic situations. For example, when used to compare groups in a trial, does the score from a multi-item scale yield a correct representation of the information in its items?

The EORTC QLQ-C30 cognitive function scale consists of two items, one asking about difficulties concentrating, and one about memory problems (Aaronson *et al.* 1993). In a study of breast cancer patients, some were treated with chemotherapy, others were not (Groenvold *et al.* 1995). An analysis of the cognitive function scale in relation to the variable 'chemotherapy' showed DIF. In other words, the two items did not perform in the same way in relation to the variable 'chemotherapy'. There was a strong association between chemotherapy and concentration difficulties whereas there was no or only a very weak association with memory problems.

The DIF in this scale could lead to either a false negative or a false positive conclusion if used in a trial of chemotherapy versus no treatment. A false negative conclusion could be that there was no impact of chemotherapy on cognitive function. This could be the case if the sample size was modest and the effect on concentration difficulties was diluted by the lack of effect on memory, with the result that no overall significant difference was found. A false positive result could be found in a trial with greater power (larger sample size) if it were concluded that chemotherapy affected 'cognitive function' (i.e. concentration *and* memory) even though the trial had in fact shown an effect on concentration difficulties but no effect on memory.

DIF analysis is extensively described in the literature (Nunnally and Bernstein 1994; Holland and Wainer 1993). In particular, DIF analysis has been used in educational testing to investigate whether some test items are more difficult for specific subgroups, e.g. whether students from ethnic minorities have more difficulties with these items even though they have the same abilities. Despite the adoption of much of the thinking and methodology of modern psychometrics by the HRQoL field, the knowledge and use of DIF analysis in this area is still limited.

DIF in multi-item scales distorts measurement. The solution to this problem is not to use single items instead of multi-item scales (unless this is preferable for other reasons) but to examine multi-item scales for DIF when they are used for important analyses. As shown in this chapter, testing for DIF requires that an additional procedure be added to the analysis plan. DIF may be related to any subgrouping of a population. Therefore, testing for DIF cannot be left to scale developers or to specific validation studies; it is an ongoing and integrated part of the analysis of multi-item scales in a study. This chapter defines DIF, gives examples of DIF, reviews ways to examine for DIF, and discusses how to interpret and act on findings of DIF in clinical trials.

Definition of DIF

The question asked in DIF analysis is 'Do all the items of a multi-item scale behave in the same way in relation to a particular variable?' The particular variable could be the one defining the groups in a clinical trial, and the question is then whether the items perform in the same way for each of the groups compared in the trial. In the example given above, the two items had different associations (a strong association, and no or a weak association, respectively) with the grouping variable, chemotherapy, and therefore the scale score was not a sufficient representation of the information in the two items.

The following definition will be used: absence of DIF in a multi-item scale requires that all persons at a given level of the construct measured (i.e. at a given scale score) have the same probability of answering an item in a given way regardless of their group membership as to sex, age, or other subgrouping (modified from Osterlind 1983 and Groenvold *et al.* 1995).

The items of a multi-item scale are expected to be unidimensional, that is, to elucidate a common construct like fatigue, depression, or physical functioning. The assumption of unidimensionality is traditionally tested using psychometric methods like multitrait scaling or factor analysis (Fayers and Machin 2000). These methods do not take variables outside the questionnaire into account. In contrast, DIF analysis tests the unidimensionality of scales in relation to other variables. There is no simple relationship between unidimensionality *within* a scale and unidimensionality in relation to other variables (absence of DIF). A scale can be perfectly unidimensional according to traditional tests but may still not be unidimensional as to its relationship with other variables, i.e. has DIF.

Examples of DIF

Imagine that we have conducted a clinical trial investigating a new drug against pain. Pain was measured by a three-item pain scale. Contrary to expectations, the analysis of the multi-item scale shows that the new drug does not lead to significantly better pain relief than standard treatment. The DIF analysis shows that the multi-item scale exhibits DIF in relation to treatment. Better pain relief is found in one of the three items of the pain scale only. The two other items show an inferior effect of the new drug. The interpretation of this finding could be that the item showing a difference favouring the new treatment covers a kind of pain (e.g. neuropathic pain), which is particularly responsive to the new treatment. In contrast, the new pain treatment had inferior effect on the type of pain measured by the two other items. The items 'behaved' differently in relation to the grouping variable, treatment. When pooling the disparate effects in the scale score, we may incorrectly conclude that the new treatment is similar to the standard treatment (if the opposite effects sum up to no significant difference). The DIF analysis reveals a more complicated reality.

In the pain treatment example, we hypothesize that there were true, opposite effects on the items. However, if we had found these results in the analysis of the primary end point of a clinical trial, we would have to report the results of the multi-item scale specified in the protocol, e.g. that there was no difference between treatments. We could also report the results of the DIF analysis, but as these are unexpected results from a secondary analysis, our finding of differential effects must be viewed as a hypothesis needing confirmation in new data.

The pain drug example shows how the simple analysis of a clinical trial having a multi-item scale as end point may be supplemented by a DIF analysis in order to investigate whether any additional information is hidden in the items constituting the scale. The DIF analysis was carried out in relation to the variable defining the trial, i.e. the treatment group. *In the analysis of clinical trials, treatment group is usually the most important variable to include in the DIF analysis.*

However, other relevant variables could be sex, age, diagnosis, etc. If we examine for DIF in relation to sex, we find out whether the three pain items behave in the same way in men and women. A hypothetical pain item could be 'Do you feel pain in your arm when using a hair-drier?' If none (or only a few) of the men in the trial were ever using a hair-drier, this item would be unrelated (or very weakly related) to the level of pain in men, whereas it might be a good measure of arm pain in women. If used in a pain scale this item would result in underestimation of the level of pain in men compared to women (DIF in relation to sex). And if used in a pain trial in men, this item would dilute the true effect of pain treatment. Furthermore, if used in a trial where treatment groups were unbalanced as to men and women, the DIF could directly influence the outcome of the trial.

In randomized clinical trials background characteristics like sex, age, diagnosis, etc. are usually evenly distributed between the treatment groups and even strong DIF in relation to these variables may therefore not directly change the conclusions regarding treatment effects. However, the DIF may reflect that items have reduced responsiveness in certain subgroups (e.g. the hair-drier item); this may lead to an underestimation of the true effect, which in some cases may mean that a true effect is overlooked.

Of course, by this we do not mean that one should use the DIF analysis to select items showing maximal effect in a study. DIF results must be interpreted in relation to the nature of the items and the research questions. As for any other unexpected finding, results of DIF analysis must be confirmed in independent data before important actions are taken.

Another application of DIF analysis is to investigate whether imperfect translations of one or more items in a multi-item scale lead to systematically higher or lower scores in some countries than in others, even though the true levels were the same (Petersen *et al.* 2003). An example of this is given in the section on analysis methods below.

How to test for DIF

Several statistical methods for DIF analysis are available (Holland and Wainer 1993). Three groups of frequently used methods will be presented here: three-way contingency table methods, logistic regression analysis, and item response theory (IRT)-based methods. All three groups of methods investigate the fundamental requirement that patients at the same level of the construct, measured by the scale, have the same probability of answering an item in a given way regardless of which subgroup they belong to. The methods have different advantages and disadvantages. The choice of method depends on the data, the planned methods for the primary analysis of the trial, and the software and expertise available.

Contingency table methods

This is the simplest of the three groups of methods. Contingency table methods have few requirements of the data, and in general they are the most robust of the DIF methods. A three-way table of item response, group variable, and scale score is constructed. Item response is tested for independence of group membership when controlling for scale score. A significant test indicates that the item performs differently across groups (DIF). A three-way table (and a DIF test) is made for each combination of item and grouping variable. Therefore, testing a four-item scale for DIF in relation to two grouping variables (e.g. the grouping variable of the trial and gender) involves eight tables.

A number of statistical tests can be used to test for DIF in three-way tables. When two groups are compared the Mantel–Haenszel approach (Holland and Thayer 1988) is commonly used to test for DIF. Alternatively the partial gamma coefficient can be used (Davis 1967). The gamma coefficient takes values between −1 and 1, with values significantly different from zero indicating DIF. The gamma coefficient can be used to test for DIF between any number of ordered groups (e.g. age groups or stages of disease). Furthermore, the gamma coefficient has the advantage that software for fast estimation of exact p-values is available (Kreiner 1989, 2003) (*http://www.biostat.ku.dk/research-reports/2003/rr-03–10.doc*). Exact p-values are preferable when having tables with few observations (<5) in many cells because in such cases the usual asymptotic p-values are questionable (Kreiner 1987). Because of the strong association between item response and scale score, tables for DIF analysis are often sparse.

We recently evaluated nine translations of the four items of the EORTC QLQ-C30 (Aaronson *et al.* 1993) emotional functioning (EF) scale by testing for DIF between each translation and the original English version (Petersen *et al.* 2003). DIF in the Swedish translation was found for item 21 'feel tense' (gamma = 0.52, $P < 0.001$) and item 24 'feel depressed' (gamma = −0.58, $P < 0.001$). Guidelines for interpretation of the magnitude of gammas and Mantel–Haenszel odds ratios are given in (Bjorner *et al.* 1998). According to these guidelines gammas smaller than −0.31 or larger than 0.31 indicate moderate to large DIF. The negative gamma for item 24 reflected that Swedes reported feeling more depressed (lower item scores) than subjects *with the same EF score* answering the English version. This finding is evident when inspecting the three-way table of item responses by language stratified by EF scale scores (Table 3.4.1). At each level of EF score (each score stratum), Swedes had lower mean scores (more symptoms) on the item than subjects answering the English version.

In the Swedish version depressed is translated into '*nedstämd*', which means something like 'being down'. It is likely that more people rate themselves as *nedstämd*/being down than feeling 'depressed'. This probably explains the DIF. The DIF for the other item ('tense') was judged to be 'pseudo-DIF'. Due to the close association between item responses and scale score, DIF in one item can produce correspondingly significant 'DIF' findings in other items. That is, the DIF finding for item 21 (tense) was probably an artifact caused by the DIF in item 24 (depressed). Pseudo-DIF is also discussed in the section on interpreting findings in DIF.

DIF can be divided into *uniform* and *non-uniform* DIF. If the difference in item scores between groups is the same for all levels of the scale the DIF is called uniform. Table 3.4.1 is an example of uniform DIF. If the difference differs across scale scores it is called non-uniform DIF. A disadvantage of the contingency table methods is that they test for uniform DIF only. In particular, if the direction of DIF differs across the scale scores: that is, if one subgroup has lower item scores for low scale scores but higher for high scale scores relative to another subgroup, the contingency table methods may not detect the DIF.

Logistic regression

Logistic regression has the advantage that it is straightforward to test for both uniform and non-uniform DIF. Furthermore, logistic regression analysis can be performed with most statistical packages. In DIF analysis with logistic regression the item is the

Table 3.4.1 DIF table of the EORTC QLQ-C30 item 24 'Did you feel depressed?' by language stratified by scale score (English (UK), N = 986; Swedish (S), N = 1060)

Scale score*	Language	Responses to item 24 'depressed'				Item mean score	N
		0 Very much (%)	1 Quite a bit (%)	2 A little (%)	3 Not at all (%)		
1	UK	9 (82)	2 (18)	–	–	0.18	11
	S	18 (95)	1 (5)	–	–	0.05	19
2	UK	7 (47)	6 (40)	2 (13)	–	0.67	15
	S	18 (62)	11 (38)	0 (0)	–	0.38	29
3	UK	13 (48)	11 (41)	2 (7)	1 (4)	0.67	27
	S	12 (39)	18 (58)	1 (3)	0 (0)	0.65	31
4	UK	4 (14)	17 (61)	6 (21)	1 (4)	1.14	28
	S	11 (18)	49 (79)	2 (3)	0 (0)	0.85	62
5	UK	5 (12)	16 (38)	20 (48)	1 (2)	1.40	42
	S	7 (10)	51 (72)	13 (18)	0 (0)	1.08	71
6	UK	4 (6)	18 (27)	40 (60)	5 (7)	1.69	67
	S	2 (3)	39 (53)	32 (43)	1 (1)	1.43	74
7	UK	2 (3)	13 (17)	54 (70)	8 (10)	1.88	77
	S	1 (1)	23 (26)	61 (70)	2 (2)	1.74	87
8	UK	1 (1)	5 (3)	150 (84)	22 (12)	2.08	178
	S	1 (1)	18 (10)	162 (88)	4 (2)	1.91	185
9	UK	1 (1)	8 (5)	77 (47)	78 (48)	2.41	164
	S	2 (1)	7 (4)	123 (79)	24 (15)	2.08	156
10	UK	–	2 (1)	44 (21)	161 (78)	2.77	207
	S	–	3 (2)	97 (59)	65 (39)	2.38	165
11	UK	–	–	17 (10)	153 (90)	2.90	170
	S	–	–	60 (33)	121 (67)	2.67	181

Partial gamma = –0.58, $P < 0.001$.

The scale score is the sum of the scores on the four items transformed as shown to 0, 1, 2, 3.

dependent variable and the group variable and scale score are the explanatory variables. Again, the principle is that when we control for scale score (hypothesizing that the scale score is a sufficient measure of the information in items) there should be no significant association between the group variable and item score. A significant effect of group indicates uniform DIF. Non-uniform DIF can be tested for by adding the interaction term of group variable and scale score to the model. A significant interaction term indicates non-uniform DIF. The scale score may be used as a continuous variable or as a categorical variable. If used as categorical, observations having extreme scales scores (which are non-informative in DIF analyses because all respondents have the same scores on items) should be deleted to avoid problems in the model estimation.

In the study mentioned above examining translations the contingency table method and logistic regression were compared (Petersen *et al.* 2003). Comparing the Swedish translation with English using logistic regression identified uniform DIF for item 21 (beta = 1.08, $P < 0.001$) and item 24 (beta = -1.18, $P < 0.001$). Using the same guidelines as discussed in relation to contingency tables, betas lower than -0.64 or higher than 0.64 correspond to moderate to large DIF (Bjorner *et al.* 1998; Petersen *et al.* 2003). There were no indications of non-uniform DIF. That is, using the contingency table method and logistic regression method resulted in exactly the same conclusions. With a few exceptions, the two methods also identified the same cases of DIF for the other eight translations. The logistic regression analysis identified a few cases of non-uniform DIF. The contingency table method found uniform DIF in these analyses. Whether the DIF was uniform or non-uniform was not important in these cases. However, the distinction between uniform and non-uniform DIF may be important in other cases.

Item response theory (IRT) based methods

As described elsewhere in this book (Chapter 1.5), several IRT models are available. Common for all IRT models is that they assume that there exists a latent (unobservable) variable describing the 'true' level of the construct, e.g. the level of symptoms or well-being of the respondent. IRT models have a set of location parameters describing how 'difficult' the items are. Some models also include slope parameters describing how well the items discriminate. When IRT models are used for DIF analysis, it is investigated whether the item parameters are equal across groups. If a slope parameter for an item is significantly different across groups, it indicates non-uniform DIF. Uniform DIF is indicated if the location parameter differs among the groups but the slopes are similar. Further descriptions of DIF analysis using IRT are given by, among others, Thissen *et al.* (1993) and Muraki (1999).

IRT based methods are the most complex and demanding of the three types of DIF analysis methods discussed here. Several assumptions underlie IRT, and IRT analysis requires large sample sizes (Muraki and Bock 1996). In our experience, a minimum of 50–100 observations per group (to be tested for DIF) is needed for the Rasch (one-parameter) model and 250–500 observations per group are needed for the more generalized models. If the model assumptions are not fulfilled or if sample sizes are small, the simpler and more robust contingency table methods or logistic regression are generally preferable. However, if the assumptions are valid and sample sizes are sufficient, the IRT methods are probably the most powerful of the DIF analysis methods. In such cases, and when the sufficient expertise is available, IRT based DIF analysis methods may be preferred, especially if IRT is to be used in subsequent analyses.

Comparing the Swedish and English versions of the EORTC QLQ-C30 EF items using the generalised partial credit model (an IRT model) and the software program PARSCALE (Muraki and Bock 1996) confirmed the finding of uniform DIF (different locations) for item 24 ($P < 0.001$) (corresponding to the contingency table approach shown in Table 3.4.1). However, whereas the two other DIF methods had suggested uniform DIF for item 21, the IRT analysis indicated non-uniform DIF for this item ($P < 0.001$). If the interpretation that the DIF for item 21 is 'pseudo-DIF' caused by the DIF in item 24 is correct this difference is of no practical importance.

How to interpret findings of DIF

As for any statistical test, significant findings of DIF have to be interpreted. A finding of significant DIF may have several causes (Figure 3.4.1, adapted from Petersen *et al.* 2003).

As for any statistical test, the finding of significant DIF may arise *purely by chance*. DIF analysis involves multiple testing when several items are tested for DIF in relation to several variables. The method of cross-validation (i.e. that the sample is divided into two, and only analyses which are significant in both samples are interpreted) may be

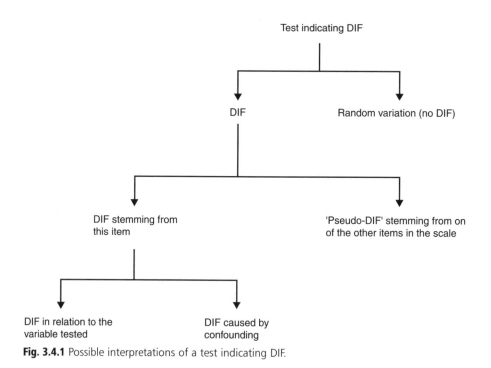

Fig. 3.4.1 Possible interpretations of a test indicating DIF.

useful to limit the number of false positive findings (Groenvold *et al.* 1995). A conservative Bonferroni-corrected p-level may also be appropriate to help reduce the number of findings of DIF with minimal clinical importance; thus Groenvold *et al.* (1995) used $P < 0.001$.

If the DIF is not random variation, it may stem either from the item investigated or from another item in the same scale. As mentioned above, '*pseudo-DIF*' is an artifact, which may result from the use of the scale score to control for the level of the construct measured by the scale. The scale score is the sum (or mean) of the individual item scores, and therefore the DIF tests are not independent. In particular, when there are few items in the scale, it can be difficult to know which item(s) cause the observed DIF. In a two-item scale, as the most extreme example, DIF results for the two items will by definition be similar but in opposite directions, and cannot be used to determine which item causes the DIF. When DIF is found for more than one item in a scale, some of the findings are often pseudo-DIF. This points out that, ideally, DIF analysis should be made using another variable than the scale score to control for the true level of the construct. When a contingency table method or logistic regression is used to test for DIF *and* a golden standard measuring the construct is available, the problem of pseudo-DIF can be removed by using the golden standard instead of the scale score.

Even if the DIF does stem from the particular item, there is still the possibility that the DIF reflects confounding from another variable. For example, DIF in relation to age may be misinterpreted as DIF related to diagnosis in a clinical trial data set where age and diagnosis are associated. Approaches to DIF like logistic regression, which allow for multivariate analysis (i.e. testing for DIF in relation to more than one variable at a time) reduce the risk of misinterpretation of DIF due to confounding from other variables.

Finally, the finding of significant DIF may be real. This leads to considerations as to how this should be handled, as discussed in the next section.

How to act on findings of DIF

When significant DIF has been found and it has been established that it *is* DIF with regard to the particular item and variable (see the preceding section), the issue is to determine whether the DIF significantly affects results. In a clinical trial it is important to distinguish between DIF in relation to the grouping variable of the trial and DIF in relation to any other variable. If the DIF concerns a variable other than the primary grouping variable of the trial (treatment), it need not have any impact on the trial outcome. The DIF may have been 'neutralized' either by randomization (non-treatment factors will usually be reasonably well balanced) or by controlling for the variable in the statistical analyses (e.g. analysis of covariance). However, the DIF may indirectly affect the outcome of the trial if the DIF results in reduced responsiveness in some groups, e.g. as in the pain example, and thus leads to underestimation of the true effect.

One solution to the finding of potentially important DIF is to construct a 'DIF-free' scale by removing the items showing DIF from the multi-item scale. Results using this new DIF-free scale can be compared to the full scale. If the results from the two scales differ significantly, the results for the DIF-free scale should probably be viewed as most correct. This is primarily a solution in case of longer scales, and, in particular, when it is clear which items should be included in the DIF-free scale. Results using both the original scale and the modified scale should be reported to elucidate the effect of DIF and to allow comparison with studies using the original scale.

Even if DIF analysis shows strong evidence that the multi-item scale used as the primary end point in a trial is problematic due to the DIF, the 'rules' related to clinical trials dictate that only the analyses pre-specified in the protocol may be reported as the outcome. However, a description of the consequences of DIF should be added.

Alternatively, analyses at the single-item level can be added. Comparing the results obtained with the single items to the full-scale score will elucidate the impact of DIF, as illustrated in the examples with the cognitive function and the pain scales. If there are no clinically relevant differences in the conclusions drawn from the items as compared to the scale score, then the scale score can be used as intended and the DIF can be ignored. Otherwise, results on the single item level can be added when reporting the trial.

In some cases it is possible to adjust directly for the effect of DIF. For example, our analyses of translations of the EORTC QLQ-C30 emotional scale suggested that the DIF related to the Swedish version of the item on depression results in mean scale scores, which are approximately two points lower on a 0–100 scale than if there had been no DIF (Petersen *et al.* 2003). DIF of this magnitude plays little role in most studies but if confirmed in other studies, adjustment for this effect could be built into scoring programs or taken into account when mean scores are estimated.

If IRT scoring of the scale is used it is possible to adjust the scores taking the DIF into account (Reise *et al.* 1993). However, common IRT models assume that the scale is unidimensional. Therefore, if the DIF is caused by multidimensionality as in the example with the pain scale, these models cannot be used to adjust for the DIF.

In summary, when DIF is found, and it is not thought to result from random variation, and IRT methods are not used to adjust for the DIF, its impact on the results should be investigated by comparing results from the single item level or a modified scale to those obtained with the original scale. If clinically important differences between approaches are found, all results should be reported. Otherwise, results using the multi-item scale only can be reported, accompanied with a statement that DIF was detected but was found to have no importance.

The role of DIF analysis

It is unusual to include DIF analysis in the reporting of a clinical trial with HRQoL outcomes. This chapter has reviewed several reasons for doing so. Should DIF analysis be part of the recommended standard analysis of HRQoL multi-item scales in clinical trial?

In our view, the question is similar to whether one should include possible confounding variables in epidemiological analyses. Often, there is good argument for testing for confounding but it is not always possible or feasible, and in many cases it will not change conclusions. Our point of view is that DIF analysis is relevant as an integral part of the analysis of any multi-item measure. This applies widely beyond the use of HRQoL multi-item scales in clinical trials, for example to any aggregated measure used in epidemiology.

Carrying out DIF analysis and interpreting the results clearly takes time and effort. However, compared to the other work required to conduct and analyse a clinical trial, this extra work is minimal, especially once the research group has performed DIF analyses a few times. Still, it is highly understandable if some clinical trialists who do not have HRQoL assessment as their main interest react:

> First they argued that we had to assess quality of life, then they said that we had to spend time validating questionnaires, and now they say that we have to add another layer of analysis to the already extremely complicated analysis of HRQoL results.

At present, the main problem with DIF analysis is probably not the doing of the analytic work. The larger problem is that DIF analysis is still little known in the context of HRQoL research in clinical trials. Many editors and reviewers of clinical journals have no knowledge of DIF analysis. Therefore, researchers adding their DIF analysis results to their papers (and realizing the problems with finding space for explaining this within word count restrictions) may not be met with appreciation but with confusion or negative reactions.

There is no simple solution to this dilemma. However, if DIF analysis shows no problems, one may choose to report the methods and results very briefly.

If important findings of DIF are made it is more difficult. In selected cases, the DIF problems may be reported as part of a methodologically-oriented paper, possibly dealing with other aspects of validity as well. In other cases, mainly when clinically relevant findings are made, one should report the methods and results even in a clinically oriented paper. With time, this will increase knowledge of the usefulness of DIF analysis.

Which variables should be included in DIF analysis? As in epidemiology, where the question is 'which variables should be included as possible confounders?', it is not possible to give specific answers. The choice of group variables for DIF analysis is determined by the research question and data. In clinical trials, this translates into 'the relevant clinical and sociodemographic variables', for example age, sex, diagnosis, disease stage, treatment, etc.

In the context of randomized clinical trials, one can argue that 'randomization group' is the only relevant variable because the randomization should lead to a balanced distribution of the variables in relation to which the multi-item scale might have DIF. This variable is clearly the most important, as the main issue for DIF analysis is to check that the outcome of the trial is not affected by DIF, as in the examples given earlier. However, there are good reasons for carrying out additional DIF analyses in relation to the basic clinical and sociodemographic characteristics of the trial sample.

Furthermore, such analyses are relevant prior to any subgroup analyses of the trial data since, of course, these analyses do not benefit from the randomization.

In our view, it is difficult to dispute the potential relevance of DIF analysis to clinical trial data. At present there is insufficient experience with DIF analysis in relation to HRQoL data to determine its role more precisely. In relation to which variables will DIF analysis most often produce clinically important findings? Will important DIF be found more frequently in some domains of HRQoL than others, or more often in some types of questionnaires than others? Will some approaches to DIF analysis prove more useful than others? These questions will be elucidated as more experience accumulates.

Even though DIF analysis is clearly relevant in important analyses of multi-item scales, it is not always realistic or necessary to do so. DIF analysis is of particular relevance:

- in analyses of great clinical importance (to make sure that the conclusions as to content are correct)
- if the unidimensionality of the scale is questionable, e.g. scales covering broad domains of HRQoL
- if DIF has previously been detected in the scale in relation to the variable
- in analyses focusing on variables, which may be associated with DIF, e.g. ethnicity or sociodemographic variables like sex and age
- in studies using questionnaire versions in more than one language

Concerning the choice of methods, a major consideration is to choose methods depending on the expertise and software available. For those who are familiar with multivariate logistic regression this is probably the simplest solution. Contingency tables are simpler for non-statisticians, and when the software is available it is an advantage to be able to make exact tests in large, sparse tables. IRT models are the most complicated but, when these are used in the analysis for other reasons, the DIF analysis is part of the typical analytic process because absence of DIF is a basic assumption of these models.

One reaction to the discussion of the possible problems with DIF in multi-item scales could be that one should use single-item outcome measures. Here, we will not review the discussion of the trade-offs between single-item measures and multi-item scales. But if we have a research question where a multi-item scale seems preferable, in most cases using a single item scale instead to avoid potential DIF is inappropriate. In the pain drug example discussed above, the DIF analysis of the three-item scale showed that the answer was not a simple superior/inferior dichotomy, but rather a differential impact of the new drug on the various aspects of pain assessed by the three items. A single item would provide a simple answer (superior or inferior), but we would not have seen that the reality was more complicated than anticipated. Switching from a multi-item scale to a single item in order to avoid DIF analysis corresponds to dropping confounder analysis in epidemiological studies to avoiding making things messy.

Similarly, the problem of DIF in relation to translations of questionnaires cannot be avoided by using single items instead of multi-item scales: the problem is the translation process, not the multi-item scales. It is a major advantage of multi-item scales that DIF analysis can detect these problems, which would remain unknown and undetectable in single item measures. This issue is of particular relevance when data from clinical trials are used to explore cross-cultural differences, e.g. whether there are differences in the impact of various diseases on HRQoL between patients in different countries. If different translations of a questionnaire are used in the countries being compared, even minor translation errors may affect the results and be misinterpreted as an effect of culture (country). When possible cross-country comparisons should be based on multi-item scales rather than single items, and DIF analysis should be used to test whether the translations are equivalent.

Given that analyses at the single item level can be used to elucidate the consequences of DIF in a multi-item scale, one could ask whether one could replace DIF analysis with simple analyses of the single items in relation to the treatment variable of the trial and other variables. This alternative is attractive because of its analytical simplicity, but cannot be recommended. Analyses of multi-item scales at the single item level increase the problems of multiple significance testing, and the results may be difficult to handle in a stringent way. Furthermore, such analyses are less likely to produce knowledge, which can be used to improve multi-item scales or to increase our understanding of their strengths and weaknesses.

DIF analyses can be seen as an extended method of construct validation, taking variables outside the questionnaire into account. Besides serving as a validation of the findings of specific analyses (e.g. clinical trials) it increases our understanding of the constructs measured by the multi-item scale and the associations between these constructs and important variables. Thus, DIF analysis extends the psychometric analyses from focusing on the questionnaire to investigating the use of the questionnaire.

In summary, DIF analysis investigates whether the items of multi-item scales perform in a consistent way in relation to other variables. In clinical trials these other variables may be the treatment group (usually the most important) or other clinical or sociodemographic variables. Significant DIF means that the scale score distorts the information in the items of the scale and may therefore affect the outcome of a clinical trial using the multi-item scale as end point. DIF analysis tests whether this is the case, and serves as a validation of the use of the scale.

References

Aaronson, N. K., Ahmedzai, S., and Bergman, B., *et al.* (1993). The European Organization for Research and Treatment of Cancer QLQ-C30: a quality-of-life instrument for use in international clinical trials in oncology. *Journal of National Cancer Institute,* **85**, 365–376.

Bjorner, J. B., Kreiner, S., Ware, J. E., Damsgaard, M. T., and Bech, P. (1998). Differential item functioning in the Danish translation of the SF-36. *Journal of Clinical Epidemiology,* **51**, 1189–1202.

Davis, J. A. (1967). A partial coefficient for Goodman and Kruskal's gamma. *Journal of the American Statistical Association,* 174–180.

Fayers, P. M. and Machin, D. (2000). *Quality of Life – Assessment, Analysis and Interpretation.* Chichester: John Wiley and Sons Ltd.

Groenvold, M., Bjorner, J. B., Klee, M. C., and Kreiner, S. (1995). Test for item bias in a quality of life questionnaire. *Journal of Clinical Epidemiology,* **48,** 805–816.

Holland, P. W. and Thayer, D. T. (1988). Differential item performance and the Mantel–Haenszel procedure. In H. Wainer and H. Brain (eds). *Test Validity,* pp. 129–145. Hillsdale, NJ: Lawrence Erlbaum Associates.

Holland, P. W. and Wainer, H. E. (1993). *Differential Item Functioning.* Hillsdale, NJ: Lawrence Erlbaum Associates.

Kreiner, S. (1987). Analysis of multidimensional contingency tables by exact conditional tests: techniques and strategies. *Scandinavian Journal of Statistics,* **14,** 97–112.

Kreiner, S. (1989). *User Guide to DIGRAM – a program for discrete graphical modelling.* Copenhagen: Statistical Research Unit, University of Copenhagen.

Kreiner, S. (2003). *Introduction to Digram.* Copenhagen: Department of Biostatistics, Institute of Public Health, University of Copenhagen.

Muraki, E. (1999). Stepwise analysis of differential item functioning based on multiple-group partial credit model. *Journal of Educational Measurement,* **36,** 217–232.

Muraki, E. and Bock, R. D. (1996). *PARSCALE – IRT based Test Scoring and Item Analysis for Graded Open-ended Exercises and Performance Tasks.* Chicago, IL: Scientific Software International, Inc.

Nunnally, J.C. and Bernstein, I. H. (1994). *Psychometric Theory.* New York: McGraw-Hill Inc.

Osterlind, S. J. (1983). *Test Item Bias.* Beverly Hills, CA: Sage.

Petersen, M. A., Groenvold, M., and Bjorner, J. B., *et al.* (2003). Use of differential item functioning analysis to assess the equivalence of translations of a questionnaire. *Quality of Life Research,* **12,** 373–385.

Reise, S. P., Widaman, K. F., and Pugh, R. H. (1993). Confirmatory factor analysis and item response theory: two approaches for exploring measurement invariance. *Psychological Bulletin,* **114,** 552–566.

Thissen, D., Steinberg, L., and Wainer, H. (1993). Detection of differential item functioning using the parameters of item response models. In P. W. Holland and H. Wainer (eds) *Differential Item Functioning,* pp. 67–113. Hillsdale, NJ: Lawrence Erlbaum Associates Inc.

3.5

Reporting analyses from clinical trials

Dennis A. Revicki

Introduction

The methods and findings of health-related quality of life (HRQoL) outcomes from clinical trials have been reported over the past 50 years. Well-designed and implemented studies, with relevant, psychometrically sound and sensitive measures and appropriate statistical analyses are important for understanding the effectiveness of health care interventions on patient functioning and well-being. Equally important are well written reports and articles that provide sufficient information so that readers understand the rationale for and objectives of the study, the research design and methods, HRQoL measures, and the results and interpretation of these results. Several authors have provided guidelines for preparing articles summarizing the methods and findings of HRQoL studies (Staquet *et al.* 1996; Fayers and Machin 2000). Recent reviews of the HRQoL research literature demonstrate considerable variability in reporting quality on the methods and measures used in clinical studies (Kong and Gandhi 1997; Sanders *et al.* 1998; Lee and Chi 2000; Efficace and Bottomley 2002).

This chapter extends these guidelines and also takes into account more recent CONSORT guidelines on reporting on randomized clinical trials (Begg *et al.* 1996; Moher *et al.* 1995, 2001a,b; Altman *et al.* 2001). Attention to these guidelines may assist investigators completing systematic reviews and meta-analyses (see Fayers and Scott, Chapter 6.4) and readers of the HRQoL clinical trial literature. Articles and reports on clinical trials incorporating HRQoL end points need to clearly and completely summarize the key methods, measures, data analyses, and results to inform clinicians and other health care decision makers about the impact of treatment on HRQoL outcomes.

Reporting clinical trials involving HRQoL end points

Reports and articles on clinical trials incorporating HRQoL as primary or secondary end points should conform to existing guidelines for reporting any randomized clinical trial (Begg *et al.* 1996; Moher *et al.* 1996; Moher *et al.* 2001a,b; Egger *et al.* 2001; Altman *et al.* 2001). Table 3.5.1 contains a summary of key aspects for reporting the methods and results of clinical trials.

Table 3.5.1 Key aspects for reporting randomized clinical trials

Section	Summary Description
Title	Include HRQoL (or other patient-reported outcome) and how subjects were allocated to treatment (i.e., randomized or randomly assigned)
Abstract	Include HRQoL (or other patient-reported outcome) and how subjects were allocated to treatment (i.e., randomized or randomly assigned)
Introduction	
Background	Scientific background for study, including rationale and importance of HRQoL outcomes
Objectives	Specific objectives and study related hypotheses
Methods	
Subjects	Study settings and inclusion/exclusion criteria for study subjects
Interventions	Sufficient detail on the interventions and administration of these interventions for each treatment group
Outcomes	Clearly defined primary and secondary clinical and HRQoL outcome measures and summary of psychometric characteristics of HRQoL measures
Data collection	Timing and mode of administration of all outcome measures
Sample size	Justification for sample size and how determined
Randomization	Methods, procedures and responsibilities for random allocation of subjects to treatment groups
Blinding	Whether or not subjects, investigators and outcome assessors were blinded to treatment group assignment
Statistical Methods	Sufficient detail on statistical analysis methods used to compare treatment groups on primary and secondary outcomes and any additional analyses (i.e., subgroup analyses, sensitivity analyses)
Results	
Subject flow	Detail on subject flow and completion status throughout course of study (a structured diagram is recommended). By treatment group, report number randomized, receiving treatment, completing protocol, and analyzed
Recruitment	Dates defining periods of subject recruitment and follow-up
Baseline data	Baseline demographic, clinical and HRQoL data by treatment group
Numbers analyzed	Number of subjects by treatment group included in statistical analyses and whether analyses were intent to treat
Outcomes and estimation	For primary and secondary outcomes, summary of results by treatment group and estimated effect size and variability (i.e., 95% confidence interval, standard deviation, standard error)
Additional analyses	Report summary of results for any additional or secondary analyses (e.g., sensitivity analyses to address missing data, subgroup analyses, etc.)
Adverse events	Summarize all adverse events by treatment group

Continued

Table 3.5.1 (*Continued*) Key aspects for reporting randomized clinical trials

Section	Summary Description
Discussion	
Interpretation	Interpretation of the results, taking into account study hypotheses, sources of potential bias or imprecision in outcome measures or methods, and study limitations. Guidance for readers in interpreting clinical significance of HRQoL results
Generalizability	Generalizability (external validity) of the clinical trial results
Overall Evidence	General interpretation of the findings of the study in the context of current research evidence

Source: Staquet *et al.* (1996); Moher *et al.* (2001a,b).

Title

The title needs to clearly describe that the study is a randomized clinical trial and that it incorporates HRQoL, or other patient-reported outcomes, such as symptom assessment, treatment satisfaction or other end point. Accurate delineation of the HRQoL outcomes within a clinical trial context will assist interested readers and others completing literature reviews in identifying clinical trials with HRQoL end points.

All authors and their institutional affiliations need to be included, and information as to funding sources needs to be reported.

Abstract

Within the abstract it is important to clearly identify that the study is a randomized clinical trial and in the methods section of the abstract that HRQoL outcomes, or other patient reported measures, are included as important primary or secondary end points in the clinical study. Structured abstracts for many peer-reviewed medical journals require clear specification of the study design and the important outcome measures. Studies have found that structured abstracts are often of higher quality than descriptive abstracts (Taddio *et al.* 1994) and that the structured abstracts enable readers to more easily locate information (Hartley *et al.* 1996).

Introduction

The introduction for the report provides the scientific rationale and background for the study and includes the main objectives and/or research questions that represent the main focus of the study. For HRQoL studies, it is necessary to provide support for the importance of measuring HRQoL for the disease and for understanding the effectiveness of the treatments under study. How do the HRQoL end points add to the understanding of the impact of disease and the treatment from the patient's perspective?

Why is the HRQoL useful to clinicians in understanding treatment outcomes and in making treatment decisions? The clinical trial may be explanatory or pragmatic (Revicki and Frank 1999), and the introduction should be structured to address the different research focus of these types of studies. This information provides the overall context for the importance and potential application of the findings of the clinical trial. The introduction should summarize previously completed research, both clinical and HRQoL focused. Information, based on research evidence, needs to be supplied as to the importance of the problem and as to how the current study addresses the research problem.

The introduction needs to describe the overall objectives and the main research questions or clinical and HRQoL hypotheses for the clinical trial. This information helps orient the reader as to the purpose of the study. The HRQoL-related research objectives and hypotheses should be specified in the data analysis plan. This section of the report should identify the primary and secondary HRQoL end points and associated hypotheses. Research objectives and questions should be stated as comparisons. For example, in a study of the HRQoL outcomes in a clinical trial comparing treatments for schizophrenia (Revicki *et al.* 1999), the research objective was stated as follows: 'The overall research objective was to compare the clinical and HRQoL effects of olanzapine compared to haloperidol in the treatment of schizophrenia and other psychotic disorders.' Particular care must be taken in identifying the primary and secondary HRQoL end points for the statistical analysis. The selection of two to five primary HRQoL end points is recommended (Fayers and Machin 2000; Revicki *et al.* 2000) as a way to deal with multiplicity (see below) in the statistical analyses. The disease indication, population characteristics, and effects of treatment should guide the selection of the primary HRQoL end points on patient functioning and well-being.

Methods

Study population and subjects

Clinical trials address a research question relevant to a particular population with some disease of interest. Within the context of randomized clinical trials, this potential patient population is restricted by inclusion and exclusion criteria and is conducted within selected clinical centers. The clinical trial report requires careful description of the study subjects and these criteria so that readers can evaluate the external validity (generalizability) of the results of the clinical trial. The study eligibility criteria need to be described clearly and concisely and the method of subject recruitment needs to be included.

The location and settings where the subjects were recruited and the data were collected needs to be described. For example, a clinical trial comparing HRQoL outcomes associated with antidepressant therapy may be conducted in specialty psychiatry settings or in primary care settings. Despite that fact that subjects enrolled into either clinical trial are required to meet DSM-IV diagnostic criteria for major depressive disorder, there will likely be differences between the study populations in terms of severity of depressive symptoms or in exposure to previous antidepressant treatments. The study report should provide sufficient information for the clinician or other reader to determine whether the findings of the clinical trial are relevant to their setting.

Interventions

The health care interventions received by each treatment group need to be described in detail, including how and when they were administered. It is important to summarize how the interventions were actually administered. Information about the placebo condition (if relevant) needs to be described. For example in a randomized clinical trial comparing HRQoL and other outcomes of arthroscopy with debridement or lavage, a placebo arthroscopy group was included (Moseley *et al.* 2001). The placebo group subject's knees were prepped and draped, three incisions were made in the skin, the surgeon requested instruments and manipulated the knee, saline was splashed to simulate lavage and the subject was kept in the operating room for the usual amount of time for arthroscopic surgery. Clearly, this 'placebo' surgery was necessary to mask the control intervention from the study subjects randomly assigned to this group. If the treatment is given in combination with other therapies or 'usual care', these treatments should be described clearly and concisely in the treatment intervention section of the article. Details on the timing and the duration of all interventions need to be provided in this section.

HRQoL and other outcome measures

Clinical trials include several primary and secondary outcome end points, and few clinical trials are designed where the HRQoL outcomes are the primary end point. The primary outcome measure is the pre-specified end point of greatest importance and is usually the end point used to determine sample size (Altman *et al.* 2001). All outcome measures, clinical and HRQoL, should be identified and completely defined with sufficient detail so that the reader can fully understand the end points.

For the HRQoL measures, it is recommended to include information on the rationale for selecting the specific measures, the instrument's content and domain(s), relevant subscales, summary or total scores, a brief summary of the instrument's psychometric characteristics, and scoring range and direction (e.g., higher scores reflect greater physical functioning). Many studies fail to provide any rationale for including the HRQoL outcomes or for the selection of the instruments used to measure HRQoL outcomes. For recently developed measures, it is useful to provide more detail as to the development and psychometric characteristics (i.e., reliability, validity) of the measure, and it is useful to report internal consistency (or test–retest) reliabilities for all the HRQoL measures included in the clinical trial. If an existing HRQoL measure is modified for the study, information must be provided as to the rationale, specific changes, and evidence on the psychometric qualities of the modified measure. For multi-country clinical trials, information should be provided as to the methods applied to translating and culturally adapting the HRQoL for the different countries and languages included among the clinical study subjects.

Citations for the HRQoL instruments are required, and these references should direct the interested reader to the main published articles or instrument manuals for the measures. Clearly, clinical trials including HRQoL outcomes should utilize previously developed measures with sufficient information on reliability and validity, and evidence needs to be provided to the reader that the measures used met current standards for instrument measurement quality (Medical Outcome Trust 2002; Hays and Revicki, Chapter 1.3).

Data collection procedures

The timing and mode of administration of all the study outcome measures needs to be described. HRQoL measures can be administered through self-completed questionnaires, computer administered or web-based questionnaires, in-person or telephone interviewer administered, interactive voice recognition program administered, or through daily paper or electronic diaries. In some studies, proxy assessments are used to measure HRQoL and other outcomes, and in these cases, details must be provided as to how the proxy assessments were completed. Details need to be provided about how the HRQoL measures were given to subjects and whether there were any procedures put in place to enhance the reliability and validity of the measurements. The timing of the HRQoL, and clinical, end point data collection over the course of the study needs to be summarized. For example, in many oncology clinical trials, the collection of the HRQoL data is often organized according the schedule of these chemotherapy treatments. The study report therefore needs to provide information as to when the HRQoL were administered relative to the planned chemotherapy cycles. In addition, if the interviewers were blinded to the subject's treatment group, this information should be supplied. Often within clinical trials, research staff at the clinical centers are instructed to administer the HRQoL measures before the subject interacts with the study clinicians, or before the subject receives any information on laboratory tests, to minimize bias.

Sample size

Some justification needs to be documented as to the sample size within the clinical trial. Also, the methods used to determine sample size should be reported. This is important for studies where HRQoL end points may be secondary, and where a primary clinical outcome was used to select the sample size for the treatment groups. It is recommended that information be included about the statistical power for detecting clinically meaningful differences in the HRQoL outcomes included in the clinical trial (Sprangers *et al.* 2002). Ideally, the clinical trial should have large enough group sample sizes to have reasonable power for detecting a clinically relevant difference in the HRQoL end points between the treatment groups, if this difference exists. Post hoc power calculations, once the results for the HRQoL outcomes are known, have little merit, and confidence intervals may be more useful in this situation (Goodman and Berlin 1994).

Randomization

The methods and procedures used for the random allocation of subjects to the treatment conditions needs to be delineated in the study report. Authors need to report the randomization ratio, especially in situations where subjects are allocated to treatment conditions in unequal numbers. Specifics regarding and restrictions in randomization, such as blocking or stratification, need to be described. Enough information should be provided to allow the readers to evaluate the methods used to generate the random allocation sequence and the possibility of bias in subject assignment to groups.

Blinding

The authors should provide information as to whether or not the study subjects, clinical investigators, and health outcomes evaluators were blinded (or masked) to treatment group assignment. The statisticians performing the HRQoL data analysis may also be blinded to treatment group. Blinding is important for minimizing several sources of bias in randomized clinical trials, and the effectiveness of masking treatment group is important to examine, where possible. Not all HRQoL studies are double-blinded and readers need to know whether the subjects or the study clinicians knew the treatment assignment. For example, in a pragmatic clinical trial comparing tricyclic antidepressant and fluoxetine treatment for primary care patients with depression, both subjects and their physicians were not blinded to treatment; however, the outcomes assessors were blinded to treatment group (Simon *et al.* 1996).

Statistical methods

The statistical analysis and methods section of the report should specify the planned statistical models and tests that were used for the treatment comparisons to evaluate the stated study hypotheses. These statistical models should be specified in detail for the primary and secondary HRQoL end points. There are number of relatively simple and complex statistical techniques that can be used to model HRQoL data collected in clinical trials. The number of HRQoL end points, number of assessments over time and duration of the clinical trial, number of treatment groups, rates of missing data, and inclusion of pre-treatment covariates should guide the selection of a statistical model. The data analysis section must also specify how center or geographic regional effects will be incorporated into the statistical analyses. Guidelines for reporting statistical analyses are available (Bailar and Mosteller 1988; Fayers and Machin 2000).

The statistical methodology should be clearly specified and described. Procedures for handling anticipated problems of multiplicity in HRQoL end points, longitudinal data structure, and missing data need to be discussed. There are a number of statistical models available for handling HRQoL data, ranging from t-tests and analysis of variance or analysis of covariance for repeated measures to mixed-model analysis of variance, pattern-mixture models, joint survival models, and hierarchical models (Fayers and Machin 2000; Fairclough 2002, Mesbah *et al.* 2002; Fairclough, Chapter 3.1, this book). Care should be exercised in selecting the statistical models for analyzing HRQoL data and attention must be paid to the statistical model's underlying assumptions. The data analysis plan should provide information on the exact statistical models selected for testing the study hypotheses related to the primary and secondary HRQoL end points. The data analysis section should describe, in detail, the planned statistical models and tests. Enough detail should be provided to enable another statistician or researcher to repeat the data analysis if the full data set was provided. The statistical analysis section should include detailed information for executing the statistical analysis of the primary and secondary HRQoL end points.

Results

Subject Flow

The initial part of the results section needs to provide details as to subject recruitment and flow through the study. Detail is needed on subject flow and completion status throughout course of the study, and the use of a structured diagram is recommended (Altman *et al.* 2001; Moher *et al.* 2001a; Egger *et al.* 2001). An example of a flow diagram for a hypothetical study comparing antidepressant therapies is summarized in Figure 3.5.1. Authors should report details on the numbers of subjects randomized, and the number receiving treatment, completing the protocol, and analyzed. Information on the percent of missing HRQoL data by treatment group should be reported. In addition, it is often useful to compare the baseline demographic, clinical and HRQoL characteristics of those subjects with complete versus those with missing HRQoL data to evaluate extent and direct of bias in the resultant HRQoL data analyses. Since health care interventions and systems change over time, it is also recommended that clinical trial reports include information on the dates of subject recruitment and study follow-up.

Baseline characteristics

The pre-intervention demographic, clinical and HRQoL characteristics of each treatment group needs to be reported using relevant descriptive statistics, such as means, medians and standard deviations for continuous variables and number and percentages for categorical variables. Table 3.5.2 summarizes the baseline characteristics for a hypothetical clinical trial comparing two-combination highly active antiretroviral

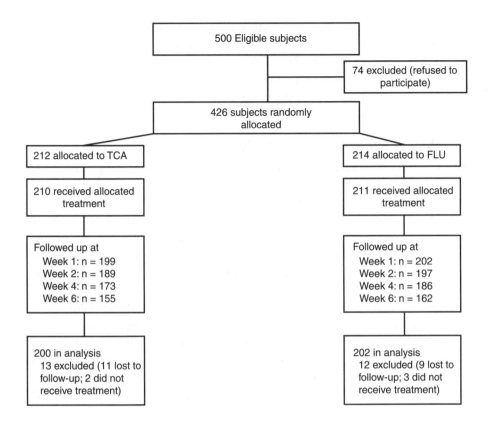

Fig. 3.5.1 Flow diagram for hypothetical antidepressant clinical trial.

Table 3.5.2 Baseline demographic and clinical characteristics

	HAART-1	HAART-2
N	312	324
Mean (SD) age, years	37.0 (9.3)	36.3 (8.8)
Male, n (%)	268 (86)	275 (85)
White, n (%)	275 (88)	298 (87)
Previous ZDV therapy, n (%)	61 (20)	71 (22)
Mean (SD) HIV RNA, log10 copies/ml	5.1 (0.7)	4.9 (0.7)
Mean (SD) CD4 counts cells/mm3	201 (95)	199 (91)
Mean (SD) Karnofsky performance status score	87.8 (7.2)	86.9 (6.9)

Source: hypothetical data.

treatments for patients with symptomatic human immunodeficiency virus. Although there are cautions expressed about the appropriateness of statistical comparisons of baseline characteristics (Altman and Dore 1990; Fayers and Machin 2000), these comparisons are very common. Post hoc covariance adjustment for detected baseline differences are likely to bias the estimated treatment effects and should be avoided (Altman 1998).

Number of subjects in data analyses

Often, because of missing data, the number of subjects per treatment group included in the statistical analyses of HRQoL outcomes may vary. Information needs to be provided as to the number of subjects in each treatment group included in each analysis of HRQoL or clinical end points. This is important for determining whether the completed data analysis conformed to intention-to-treat principles. Although some of this information may be included in the subject flow diagram, the number of subjects with non-missing HRQoL outcomes may vary. In HRQoL data analyses, the analytic sample is often restricted to those subjects with a baseline and at least one completed follow-up assessment. For some studies, the analysis of clinical and HRQoL end points may be restricted to subjects who fulfill protocol requirements of minimal treatment exposure and follow-up. These analyses are referred to as 'on-treatment' or 'per protocol' analyses and should be clearly specified in the description of results, including the number of randomized subjects included in the per protocol analyses. Complete disclosure is necessary for readers to judge whether or not the statistical analysis was truly intention to treat.

Outcomes and estimation

The results section of the HRQoL study report should include the complete summary of specified primary and secondary outcomes (both clinical and HRQoL) for each treatment group. The results should include the estimated effect, such as means over time or baseline to end point change in HRQoL scores, and some indication of its precision (either standard errors or standard deviations or 95 per cent confidence intervals). If 95 per cent confidence intervals are reported, they should be around the contrast between treatment groups. Many medical journals strongly recommend the use of 95 per cent confidence intervals (International Committee of Medical Journal Editors 1997). Effect sizes can also be used to quantify the comparison of HRQoL outcomes between treatment groups. Results should be provided for all planned primary and secondary outcomes, and not just for those comparisons that were statistically significant.

Results of the HRQoL data analyses may be best summarized in tables or figures. Fayers and Machin (1998) provide a useful summary of different graphical methods for displaying HRQoL data from clinical trials. Selection of the most relevant method for summarizing the results depends on the number of primary or important secondary end points, the longitudinal structure of the outcome data, and the complexity of the statistical analysis. For example, figures may best display mean HRQoL scores over time in clinical trials where there are three or more post-baseline assessments. Tables with rows and rows of statistics may be difficult for readers to understand and interpret. The intent of the results section is to summarize the main study findings as clearly and comprehensively as possible. Therefore, the judicious use of results described in the text, tables and figures can best accomplish this communication objective.

Additional and exploratory analyses

In many clinical trials, one or more secondary or sensitivity analyses are planned, either to examine the impact of missing HRQoL data on the treatment comparisons or to examine treatment effects across important subgroups of participants. A clear distinction needs to be made between those secondary analyses that were pre-specified and those that were post hoc exploratory analyses. For example, in the Bernstein *et al.* (2002) clinical trial on HRQoL outcome differences between pegylated interferon alfa-2a and interferon alfa-2a in patients with chronic hepatitis C, a planned secondary analysis examined the relationship between changes in HRQoL scores and viral response and discontinuation from treatment. Although the overall comparisons showed no statistically significant differences between the treatments, the authors did demonstrate that increases in fatigue symptoms, reduced vitality and reduced physical function were associated with treatment discontinuation.

Adverse effects

For clinical trials comparing pharmaceutical, surgical or other health care interventions, all adverse events and side effects of treatment should be reported by treatment group. These data are important for readers to understand the undesirable effects of the medical interventions, as well as the clinical effectiveness, including any HRQoL benefits associated with the interventions. At minimum, the authors should provide a summary of the frequency of the main adverse events and the reasons for treatment discontinuation separately for each treatment group (Altman *et al.* 2001). Serious adverse events (deaths, hospitalizations, etc.) should be reported for the treatment groups involved in the clinical trial.

Discussion

The discussion section is important for providing an interpretation of the main study findings within the context of other published research on the treatment interventions and known information about the HRQoL impact of the targeted disease or the treatments. This section of the HRQoL study report should include an interpretation of the results, taking into account the specified clinical trial hypotheses, sources of potential bias and imprecision, and any limitations attributable to missing data or multiplicity in end points. Because of inconsistencies in the quality of discussion sections, some medical journals encourage the authors to provide more structure in the discussion of findings (Annals of Internal Medicine 2003; Docherty and Smith 1999).

The Annals of Internal Medicine (2003) recommends that authors structure the discussions section by including: (1) a brief synopsis of key study findings; (2) consideration of possible mechanisms and explanations for the results; (3) comparisons with relevant results from published studies or meta-analyses; (4) delineation of study limitations including how these limitations were handled; and (5) a brief section that summarizes the clinical and research implications of the study. These recommendations seem useful for structuring discussion sections for HRQoL reports, with attention to providing explanations for the main observed HRQoL findings in relationship to the interventions and, where possible, the clinical effects of the interventions.

The discussion of any study limitations associated with the HRQoL part of the clinical trial is very important in understanding the results. For example, missing data is often a problem for analyzing HRQoL end points, and most missing HRQoL data is missing at random or missing not at random (see Fairclough, Chapter 3.3). Often the more impaired subjects are more likely to discontinue from the clinical trial, resulting in some bias introduced into the treatment comparisons. Understanding the extent and direction of these potential biases is important for evaluating the quality of the statistical methods applied and the findings of these analyses. Other potential study limitations associated with HRQoL components of clinical trials include poor implementation of the HRQoL data collection by clinical centers, and unblinding of subjects or disclosure of clinical end points.

Generalizability

The generalizability, or external validity, of the clinical trial results is dependent of the study inclusion and exclusion criteria and study setting. The discussion section needs to address the generalizability of the study findings on clinical and HRQoL outcomes. It is important to discuss whether the results are relevant to patient groups that are dissimilar to those entered in the clinical trial with regard to gender, age, severity of disease or comorbid conditions or other practice settings. The generalizability of a clinical trial is largely a matter of judgment, but some discussion of whether the results observed in the study can be generalized to other clinical settings or patient populations is useful for assisting clinical readers in interpreting the findings for their own practice setting and individual patients.

Overall evidence

It is useful to end the discussion section with a paragraph that summarizes the general interpretation of the results of the study within the context of other published literature, and any clinical implications. Areas for future research should be mentioned and included in this summary. Any overall conclusions should be delineated in this section.

Summary

Describing the results of any analysis of HRQoL data requires attention to the rationale for the study, relevant health outcome and medical literature, the study design and methods, HRQoL measurements, and the statistical methods. These results must also be interpreted within the context of clinical practice and the existing knowledge base on the treatments, underlying disease, and HRQoL research. More attention needs to be focused on interpreting minimal important differences or changes and clinical relevance of HRQoL research, whether within a clinical trials or observational clinical study. Complete and clear descriptions of the research methods, HRQoL and other end point measures, the results, and the clinical and health policy implications of these results may increase the use of HRQoL study data in clinical decision-making.

References

Altman, D. G. (1998). Adjustment for covariance imbalance. In P. Armitage, T. Colton (eds) *Encyclopedia of Biostatistics*, pp. 1000–1005. Chichester: John Wiley.

Altman, D. G. and Dore, C. J. (1990). Randomisation and baseline comparisons in clinical tirals. *Lancet*, **335**, 149–153.

Altman, D. G., Schultz, K. F., and Moher, D., *et al.* (2001). The revised CONSORT statement for reporting randomized trials: explanation and elaboration. *Annals of Internal Medicine*, **134**, 663–694.

Annals of Internal Medicine. (2003). Information for authors. Available at *www.annals.org*. Accessed October 23, 2003.

Bailar, J. C. and Mosteller, F. (1988). Guidelines for statistical reporting in articles for medical journals: amplifications and explanations. *Annals of Internal Medicine*, **108**, 266–273.

Begg, C., Cho, M., and Eastwood, S., *et al.* (1996). Improving the quality of reporting of randomized controlled trials: the CONSORT statement. *Journal of the American Medical Association*, **276**, 637–639.

Bernstein, D., Kleinman, L., Barker, C., Revicki, D., and Green, J. (2002). Relationship of health-related quality of life to treatment adherence and sustained response in chronic hepatitis C patients. *Hepatology* **35**, 704–708.

Doherty, M. and Smith, R. (1999). The case for structuring the discussion of scientific papers (editorial). *BMJ*, **318**, 1224–1225.

Efficace, F. and Bottomley, A. (2002). Health related quality of life assessment methodology and reported outcomes in randomized controlled trials of primary brain cancer patients. *European Journal of Cancer*, **38**, 1824–1831.

Egger, M., Juni, P., and Bartlett, C. (2001). Value of flow diagrams in reports of randomized controlled trials. *Journal of the American Medical Association*, **285**, 1996–1999.

Fairclough, D. L. (2002). *Design and Analysis of Quality of Life Studies in Clinical Trials*. Boca Raton, FL: Chapman and Hall/CRC.

Fayers, P. M. and Machin, D. (1998). Summarizing quality of life data using graphical methods. In M. J. Staquest, R. D. Hays, P. M. Fayers (eds) *Quality of Life Assessment in Clinical Trials: Methods and Practice*. Oxford: Oxford University Press.

Fayers, P. and Machin, D. (2000). *Quality of Life: Assessment, Analysis and Interpretation*. Chichester: John Wiley and Sons.

Fayers, P. and Scott, N. (in press). Combining clinical trials – meta analysis. In P. Fayers, R. D. Hays (eds) *Quality of Life Assessment in Clinical Trials, 2nd edn*. New York: Oxford University Press.

Goodman, S. N. and Berlin, J. A. (1994). The use of predicted confidence intervals when planning experiments and the misuse of power when interpreting results. *Annals of Internal Medicine*, **121**, 200–206.

Hartley, J., Sydes, M., and Blurton, A. (1996). Obtaining information accurately and quickly: are structured abstracts more efficient? *Journal of Information Science*, **22**, 349–356.

Hays, R. D. and Revicki, D. A. (in press). Reliability and validity. In P. Fayers, R. D. Hays (eds) *Quality of Life Assessment in Clinical Trials, 2nd edn*. New York: Oxford University Press.

International Committee of Medical Journal Editors (1997). Uniform requirements for manuscripts submitted to biomedical journals. *Annals of Internal Medicine*, **126**, 36–47.

Kong, S. X. and Gandhi, S. K. (1997). Methodologic assessments of quality of life measures in clinical trials. *The Annals of Pharmacotherapy*, **31**, 830–836.

Lee, C. W. and Chi, K. N. (2000). The standard of reporting on health-related quality of life in clinical trials. *Journal of Clinical Epidemiology*, **53**, 451–458.

Medical Outcome Trust (2002). Assessing health status and quality-of-life instruments: attributes and review criteria. *Quality of Life Research*, **11**, 193–205.

Mesbah, M., Cole, B. F., and Lee, M. L.T (eds) (2002). *Statistical Methods for Quality of Life Studies: Design, measurements and analysis*. Dordecht, The Netherlands: Kluwer.

Moher, D., Jadad, A. R., and Nichol, G., *et al.* (1995). Assessing the quality of randomized controlled trials: an annotated bibliography of scales and checklists. *Controlled Clinical Trials*, **16**, 62–73.

Moher, D., Schultz, K. F., and Altman, D. G. (2001a). The CONSORT statement: revised recommendations for improving the quality of reports of parallel group randomized trials. *Annals of Internal Medicine*, **134**, 657–662.

Moher, D., Shultz, K. F., and Altman, D. G. (2001b). The CONSORT statement: revised recommendations for improving the quality of reports of parallel group randomized trials. *Journal of the American Medical Association*, **285**, 1987–1991.

Moseley, J. B., O'Malley, K., and Petersen, N. J., *et al.* (2001). A controlled trial of arthroscopic surgery for osteoarthritis of the knee. *New England Journal of Medicine*, **347**, 81–88.

Revicki, D. A. and Frank, L. (1999). Pharmacoeconomic evaluation in the real world: effectiveness versus efficacy studies. *Pharmacoeconomics*, **15**, 423–434.

Revicki, D. A., Genduso, L. A., Hamilton, S. H., Ganozcy, D., and Beasley, C. M. (1999). Olanzapine versus haloperidol in the treatment of schizophrenia and other psychotic disorders: quality of life and clinical outcomes from a randomized clinical trial. *Quality of Life Research*, **8**, 417–426.

Revicki, D. A., Osoba, D., and Fairclough, D., *et al.* (2000). Recommendations on health-related quality of life research to support labeling and promotional claims in the United States. *Quality of Life Research*, **9**, 887–900.

Sanders, C., Egger, M., Donovan, J., Tallon, D., and Frankel, S. (1998). Reporting on quality of life in randomized controlled trials: bibliographic study. *British Journal of Medicine*, **317**, 1191–1194.

Simon, G. E., VonKorff, M., and Heiligenstein, J. H., *et al.* (1996). Initial antidepressant choice in primary care: effectiveness and cost of fluoxetine versus tricyclic antidepressants. *Journal of the American Medical Association* **275**, 1897–1902.

Sprangers, M., Moinpour, C., Moyniham, T., Patrick, D., and Revicki, D. (2002). Assessing meaningful change over time in quality of life: a user's guide. *Mayo Clinic Proceedings*, **77**, 561–571.

Staquet, M., Berzon, R. A., Osoba, D., and Machin, D. (1996). Guidelines for reporting results of quality of life assessments in clinical trials. *Quality of Life Research*, **5**, 496–502.

Taddio, A., Pain, T., and Fassos, F. F., *et al.* (1994). Quality of nonstructured and structured abstracts of original research articles in the British Medical Journal, the Canadian Medical Association Journal and the Journal of the American Medical Association. *Canadian Medical Association Journal*, **150**, 1611–1615.

Interpreting QoL in individuals and groups

4.1

Individualized quality of life

Ciaran A. O'Boyle, Stefan Höfer and Lena Ring

Introduction

Despite the burgeoning use of quality of life (QoL) as an outcome in health care, there is still little agreement on the definition of the construct or on the most appropriate ways to measure it (Joyce *et al.* 2003). Most instruments that purport to measure QoL adopt an operational definition and many, measuring as they do symptoms and functioning, would be better described as health status measures. One problem is that what is measured is predetermined and therefore cannot represent the free choice of the individual. Also, implicit in measures of *health-related quality of life* is the assumption that a specific subset of domains, usually chosen by the investigator, accounts for most of the variance (Gill and Feinstein 1994). The implication is that QoL means the same thing to everyone and can be defined and measured in general terms using fixed questions that may not reflect the perspective of the individual. Scoring also presents problems, since the answers to each question or section are often given equal weight on the assumption that there is a commonality of importance for different life areas for all individuals. Alternatively, weights may have been predetermined and standardized using a normative sample, but will be meaningless for a particular individual. This assumption is challenged by empirical findings showing that the definition of QoL is highly individual and that patients vary significantly in the importance they attach to different aspects of their lives (Joyce *et al.* 1999). It cannot even be guaranteed that a seriously ill patient will nominate health as an important feature, let alone the most important determinant of their QoL (Waldron *et al.*1999).

The fundamental issue is that externally defined normative categories may have little meaning for individuals. Many people would consider their QoL to be based on such matters as:

'having one's individual needs and desires fulfilled to a reasonable degree; a belief that life is offering or lacking the right balance of challenges and successes in those areas that are of personal salience; happiness and satisfaction that life is delivering all or most of what is expected or desired.'

(Dijkers 2003)

Even if the domains included in a particular measure were those that patients considered critical, 'data are gathered on the level of functional limitation, symptom distress or global well-being, without fully understanding the *meaning* that these terms carry for each patient' (Rapkin *et al.* 1994).

If an individual's perspective is to be validly captured, he or she must be permitted to influence each step of the assessment. The issues addressed should be those that the individual holds to be important and they should be able to assess the level of functioning and/or satisfaction in each of these areas and indicate the relative importance of each. The true complexity and challenge in measurement can be further appreciated when one considers that an individual's assessment may have important unconscious components and, further, that all of the parameters outlined are likely to change with time (response shift is discussed in Chapter 4.4 by Schwartz *et al.*). Over the past decade, a number of measures have been developed that seek to capture the unique perspective of the individual.

Approaches to individualized measurement

Individualized QoL (IQoL) measures are designed to increase respondents' discretion in selecting the areas of life (domains) that are most important and/or determining the relative importance of these domains. We can consider the degree of individualization on a continuum, at one end of which are those measures in which the respondent is given neither the option to select the salient domains nor to indicate their relative importance (Dijkers 2003). Traditional HRQoL instruments such as the SF-36 fall into this category. In contrast, individualized measures such as the Patient Generated Index (PGI) (Ruta *et al.* 1994) and the Schedule for Evaluation of Individual Quality of Life (SEIQoL) (O'Boyle *et al.* 1992) allow the respondent to nominate or select the important domains, rate their level of functioning/satisfaction with each and determine the relative importance (weight) of each. Other instruments can also be categorized along this continuum (see Table 4.1.1).

Investigator nominates domains; investigator weights domains

Some researchers have attempted to develop IQoL measures using Kelly's psychology of personal constructs and its associated methodology, the repertory grid (Kelly 1955). Kelly believed that 'every man is his own scientist' and that, in order to make sense out of our universe, out of ourselves and out of particular situations we encounter, we invent and reinvent implicit theoretical frameworks called personal constructs. Two groups have attempted to apply this methodology to the measurement of IQoL. One approach is the Individual Quality of Life Interview (IQoLI), described later. Another is the SmithKline Beecham Quality of Life Index (SBQoL), which has a low level of individualization (Dunbar *et al.* 1992). Rather than allowing respondents to describe their own unique QoL elements and constructs, the SBQoL provides ten predefined domains such as physical well-being, mood and sexual function for assessment. These domains are further divided into 28 subdomains, on which the patient can rate his or

Table 4.1.1 Selective review of the development of IQoL measures and their application in clinical studies

Instrument	Type of Instrument	Population used in Development of Instrument	Sample Application	Sample Application Outcome
Investigator nominates domains; investigator weights domains				
SmithKline-Beecham Quality of Life Index (SBQoL) (Dunbar et al. 1992)	Interview or computerized Generic based on Repertory Grid	Affective disorder	Longitudinal (pre-post) pilot study to investigate applicability and validity of SBQoL in manic-melancholic patients (n = 23) (Thunedborg et al. 1995)	The computerized SBQoL had an adequate applicability and internal validity and seemed to be able to predict recurrence of depression
Investigator nominates domains; subject weights domains				
The Ferrans and Powers Quality of Life Index (QLI) (Ferrans and Powers 1985)	Questionnaire Disease-specific versions (cancer, cardiac)	Cancer, ischemic heart disease	Longitudinal comparison (preoperative and 6-month postoperative) of lung cancer patients undergoing lung cancer resection (n = 139) with a healthy age-matched control population (Handy et al. 2002)	The analysis of preoperative and postoperative scores revealed no significant differences in the QoL or subscales for the study group as a whole
The Flanagan Quality of Life Scale (QoLS) (Flanagan 1978)	Questionnaire Generic		Randomized controlled trial in women with stress incontinence (n = 59) (Bo et al. 2000)	Pelvic floor muscle exercise showed some effect on disease-specific quality of life and sex-life variables, but not on QoLS
Subjective Quality of Life Profile (SQLP) (Dazord et al. 1994)	Questionnaire Generic	Psychiatry, Diabetes	Study of different forms of insulin delivery in patients with diabetes type I (n = 743) (Dazord et al. 1998)	SQLP was sensitive to increased satisfaction in patients adopting a simplified insulin injection regimen

Continued

Table 4.1.1 (*Continued*) Selective review of the development of IQoL measures and their application in clinical studies

Instrument	Type of Instrument	Population used in Development of Instrument	Sample Application	Sample Application Outcome
Audit of Diabetes Dependent Quality of Life (ADDQoL) (Bradley 1994)	Questionnaire Disease specific	Diabetes	Randomized study in adults with type I diabetes, taught flexible intensive insulin treatment immediately or acting as waiting list controls (n = 169) (DAFNE 2002)	Training leads to significant improvements in treatment satisfaction, psychological well-being and QoL.
Renal-Dependent Quality of Life (RDQOL) (Bradley 1997)	Questionnaire Disease specific	Dialysis, haemodialysis, and transplant patients	Study to design an individualized questionnaire to measure the impact of renal disease (n = 40) (Bradley 1997)	Face and content validity is established for adult renal patients
Wisconsin Quality of Life Index (W-QLI) (Becker et al. 1993)	Questionnaire	Psychiatric disorders (schizophrenia)	Longitudinal study assessing the impact of phase-specific treatment of first episode of psychosis (n = 41) (Malla et al. 2001).	A significant improvement of Quality of Life over one year with a phase-specific comprehensive treatment was found. This improvement was independent of changes in symptoms.
Quality of Life Inventory (QoLI) (Frisch et al. 1992)	Questionnaire	Psychological disorders, physical disability, community-wide social problems	Longitudinal study comparing two different marital enrichment programs with a control group (Burchard et al. 2003)	Hope-focused marital enrichment program significantly improved QoL, and improvement after a forgiveness-based program approached significance.
Quality of Life Systemic Inventory (QLSI) (Duquette et al. 1994)	Interview Goal attainment measure	Cardiac patients, psychological disorders	Cross sectional clinical study comparing psychological distress and adaptational problems associated with discontinuation of benzodiazepines (n = 60) (O'Connor et al. 1999)	High neuroticism, lower education level, and lower quality of life were associated with higher levels of distress during withdrawal.

Investigator nominates domains; subject elaborates domains; no weighting

Measure	Type	Condition	Study	Findings
Disease Repercussion Profile (DRP) (Carr 1996)	Questionnaire Disease specific	Rheumatoid arthritis	Study of the management of non-surgical referrals in patients with severe osteoarthritis (n = 81) (Carr 1999)	Patients reported handicap in functional and social activities, relationships, socio-economic status, emotional well-being and body image
Individual Quality of Life Interview (IQoLI) (Thunedborg et al. 1993)	Interview Repertory Grid	Anxiety disorder	Randomized controlled trial, comparing three treatments in patients with generalized anxiety (n = 33) (Thunedborg et al. 1993)	IQoLI based on repertory grid is acceptable to patients and gives quantifiable and interpretable individual results.
Idiographic Functional Status Assessment (IFSA) (Rapkin et al. 1994)	Interview Generic Goal Attainment	AIDS	Study to assess the psychometric properties of the Idiographic Functional Status Assessment (IFSA) and examine its usefulness as a quality of life/functional status measurement in comparison with other standard measures (n = 224) (Rapkin et al. 1994)	IFSA showed good temporal stability and correlated well with other subjective measures

Investigator nominates domains; subject elaborates domains; subject weights domains

Measure	Type	Condition	Study	Findings
McMaster Toronto Arthritis Patient Preference Disability Questionnaire (MACTAR) (Tugwell et al. 1987)	Interview Disease specific	Arthritis	Randomized controlled trial in rheumatoid arthritis patients (n = 210) comparing clinical nurse specialist intervention, inpatient and day patient team care (Tijhuis et al. 2002)	QoL and functional status improved significantly in all three groups with no significant differences between treatment groups

Continued

Table 4.1.1 (*Continued*) Selective review of the development of IQoL measures and their application in clinical studies

Instrument	Type of Instrument	Population used in Development of Instrument	Sample Application	Sample Application Outcome
Patient-Specific Index (PASI) (Wright and Young 1997; Wright et al. 2000)	Questionnaire Disease specific	Arthritic hip problems	Longitudinal clinical study (pre-post design) assessing hip arthroplasty (Wright and Young, 1997)	Authors conclude that PASI is reliable, valid and responsive
Subject nominates domains; subject provides implicit weighting				
Schedule for the Evaluation of Individual Quality of Life (SEIQoL) (O'Boyle et al. 1992)	Interview Generic	Hip replacement, healthy elderly, gastroenterology	Longitudinal intervention study in hip replacement patients (n = 20) (O'Boyle et al. 1992)	Quality of life measured by the SEIQoL increased significantly following surgery, compared to control.
Measure Yourself Medical Outcome Profile (MYMOP) (Paterson 1996)	Questionnaire Generic	General practice	Quasi-randomised pilot study, of acupuncture or homeopathy versus normal GP care in patients with dyspepsia (n = 60) (Paterson et al. 2003)	Mean MYMOP scores improved in all groups up to 6 months, then reached a plateau with no significant difference between the groups.
Subject nominates domains; subject provides explicit weights				
Schedule for the Evaluation of Individual Quality of Life – Direct Weighting (SEIQoL-DW) (Hickey et al. 1999)	Interview Generic	Hip replacement, healthy elderly, gastroenterology	Randomized controlled trial in HIV-1 patients comparing Chinese medicinal herbs and placebo (n = 68) (Weber et al. 1999)	The Chinese herbs did not improve QoL, clinical manifestations, plasma virus loads, or CD4 cell counts.

Measure	Method	Population	Study	Findings
Patient Generated Index (PGI) (Ruta et al. 1994)	Interview Generic	Low back pain, cancer, general practice, other diseases	Longitudinal clinical study (Pre-post) in patients with rectal cancer (n = 33) (Camilleri-Brennan et al. 2002)	Quality of life measured by the mean PGI score showed significant improvement 3 months following surgery. The PGI was found to be more responsive to change than the SF-36, the QLQ-C30 or the QLQ-CR38.
Personal Strivings approach (Emmons 1986)	Interview Generic Goal Attainment	Students	Longitudinal study in undergraduates (n = 82, 177 and 159) (Elliot and Sheldon 1998)	Avoidance goals predicted symptom reports in each of the three studies, and across studies.
Global measures				
Satisfaction with Life Scale (SWLS) (Diener et al. 1985)	Questionnaire Generic Global	Haemodialysis patients	Prospective, longitudinal, multicenter study in urban haemodialysis patients (n = 295) (Kimmel et al. 1998)	SWLS was not a predictor of mortality. But there was a non-significant trend towards association of increased satisfaction with life scores with improved survival.
The Gottschalk–Lolas Approach (Content Analysis) (Gottschalk and Lolas 1992)	Interview Generic Global Content analysis		No clinical studies found	
Duggan–Dijkers Approach (Dijkers et al. 1998)	Interview Generic Global	Spinal cord injuries	Study describing the impact of the nursing home environment on the quality of life of patients with spinal cord injury (n = 6) (Duggan et al. 2002)	Self-rated QoL was at a low shortly after injury, rose during the rehabilitation stay, declined by the first nursing home interview, and improved somewhat thereafter.

her current status by using a computerized visual analogue scale. The gap between *current QoL* and *ideal QoL* reflects the QoL of the individual. One problem here is that if a patient marks the maximum possible for their ideal QoL, which is highly likely, it becomes redundant to collect this information. A computerized version of the SBQoL has been shown to be valid in a pilot study in depressed patients receiving antidepressant medication (Thunedborg *et al.* 1995).

Investigator nominates domains; subject weights domains

The Quality of Life Index (QLI) was developed to measure morbidity in ill and healthy populations and it is based on the assumption that QoL is the sum of satisfactions derived from important life domains (Ferrans and Powers 1985). It provides the respondent with the opportunity to apply subjective preferences for QoL in various domains. Two persons may have the same physical capacity, for example, but because of different aspirations (different calibration), they may differ significantly in their levels of satisfaction. Even if their level of satisfaction with a particular domain were the same, the impact on their overall QoL might be different because of the relative importance of that domain (different prioritization). The QLI uses six-point Likert scales to measure the level of satisfaction with, and the importance of, 32 items representing four underlying domains: socio-economic, psychological/spiritual, health and functioning and family. Sixteen subdomains are covered including health care, physical health and functioning, occupation, personal faith, life goals and self-acceptance. Overall happiness and satisfaction are also measured. Although the authors reported the reliability and validity of the QLI to be appropriate, extensive psychometric testing was not undertaken (Ferrans and Ferrell 1990). The measure has been applied in a study of surgical resection in lung cancer patients (Handy *et al.* 2002) and in a number of clinical trials.

Other IQoL scales in this category are the Flanagan Quality of Life Scale (QoLS) (Flanagan 1982) the Subjective Quality of Life Profile (SQLP) (Dazord *et al.* 1994) and the Audit of Diabetes Dependent Quality of Life (ADDQoL) (Bradley 1997). The Wisconsin Quality of Life Index (W-QLI) (Becker *et al.* 1993) represents a new development, as it combines the perspectives of the patient, family and physician.

Investigator nominates domains; subject elaborates domains; no weighting

The Disease Repercussion Profile (DRP) was designed as a clinical tool allowing patients with rheumatoid arthritis to specify their most important problems and needs (Carr 1996). It combines open questions and graphic rating scales to measure perceived handicap on an individual basis. The authors provide six domains: functional activities, social activities, socio-economic status, relationships, emotional well-being and body image. In addition, patients can specify particular handicaps they are currently experiencing, but there is no option for the patient to prioritize the assessed domains. It was designed for routine clinical settings to assist individualizing treatment, but is not recommended for comparing the effectiveness of clinical interventions or for assessing longitudinal disease outcome.

Another approach is the Individual Quality of Life Interview (IQoLI) which is based on the repertory grid technique, as is the SBQoL described earlier. The IQoLI was developed using patients with generalized anxiety disorder to provide measures of 'self before treatment', 'self now' and 'ideal self' (Thunedborg et al. 1993). The study established the applicability of the method in a clinical trial, but the authors did not report treatment outcomes.

A related approach focuses on personal goals. The Ideographic Functional Status Assessment (IFSA) is a semi-structured interview in which up to 15 personal goals and their associated goal attainment activities are elicited (Rapkin et al. 1994). Five types of goals are identified: (i) the main things the respondent wants to accomplish; (ii) the problems facing the respondent which they want to solve; (iii) the things the respondent wants to prevent or avoid; (iv) the things the respondent wants to keep the same; (v) the commitments the respondent wants to relinquish. These goals are then grouped into eight categories and patients describe the activities they have carried out to achieve their goals and which goals they have been unable to pursue due to health problems over the last month. Although the IFSA is individual in its focus, allowing the individual to identify relevant goals, it does not provide the opportunity to prioritize (weight) the elicited areas.

Investigator nominates domains; subject elaborates domains; subject weights domains

The McMaster Toronto Arthritis Patient Preference Disability Questionnaire (MACTAR) is an individualized measure, requiring trained interviewers, designed to assess changes in physical disabilities as well as the effects that an individual patient would most like to see improved by treatment (Tugwell et al. 1987). First, patients are asked to nominate problems spontaneously. Then the interviewer lists domains expected to be relevant and the patient personalizes these by adding their own particular problems to each domain. Patients are then asked to identify their five most important problems and rank these in the order they would prefer to see them improved (prioritization). The MACTAR has been shown to be sensitive to clinical intervention in a number of patient populations (Tijhuis et al. 2002).

Another approach is to attempt to individualize questionnaires. Here the investigator provides domains and/or items and respondents select and/or choose or add items that they perceive to be important (Lacasse et al. 1999). The Chronic Respiratory Disease Questionnaire, for example, allows the patient to personalize the measurement of dyspnoea, and this has been found to increase the sensitivity of the measure to pharmacological intervention (Guyatt et al. 1989).

Subject nominates domains; subject provides implicit weights

The Schedule for the Evaluation of Individual Quality of Life (SEIQoL) assumes that QoL is defined as 'what the individual determines it to be' (O'Boyle *et al.* 1993). Individuals are first asked to nominate and describe those five areas of their lives (cues) that they consider to be the most central to their QoL. Next they assess their current status or level of satisfaction/functioning on each cue using a visual analogue scale. In the third stage they rate their current overall QoL on a visual analogue scale. The weighting procedure then follows and is designed to examine the importance attached by the individual to each cue. The procedure is based on Judgment Analysis, a method derived from Social Judgment Theory (Hammond *et al.* 1975), and it makes use of multiple regression analysis to model the structure of an individual's 'judgment policy' by quantifying the weight s/he gives to each cue in judging the QoL associated with 30 hypothetical cases. By examining its importance, this step quantifies the relative contribution of each cue to the individual's judgment of his or her overall QoL. Since the individual is not explicitly asked to rank the importance of each cue, the derived values incorporate implicit ('unconscious') elements into the weighting procedure. Where grouped data are needed, a single score (the SEIQoL Index score) can be derived by multiplying each cue weight by its corresponding level and summing the products across the five cues. The SEIQoL is sensitive to interventions such as hip replacement surgery (O'Boyle *et al.* 1992) and the treatment of leg ulcers (Vandongen 1997) and it has been used successfully in terminally ill patients (Waldron *et al.* 1999).

Subject nominates domains; subject provides explicit weights

The Schedule for the Evaluation of Individual Quality of Life: Direct Weighting (SEIQoL-DW) was derived from the SEIQoL to provide a less complex method of determining cue weights (Hickey *et al.* 1996). It consists of a pie-chart containing five overlapping discs, each of which represents one QoL cue nominated and rated by the respondent. The individual is requested to allocate 100 points to indicate the relative importance of each cue. While it is simple to use and is becoming increasingly popular, the SEIQoL-DW cannot provide the depth of information provided by the full SEIQoL. Furthermore, it is clear that the two methods are not interchangeable, as the SEIQoL-DW clearly elicits explicit conscious weights (Waldron *et al.*1999). Neudert*et al.* (2001) found that amyotrophic lateral sclerosis patients rated the SEIQoL-DW as more valid than the SIP and the SF-36 in measuring their QoL. Not all studies have found changes in SEIQoL-DW scores following intervention (Smith *et al.* 2000) although Ramstrom *et al.* (2000) found increased QoL in patients using pre-constituted disposable infusion devices for antibiotic administration compared with patients who were required to reconstitute the drugs themselves. In one study, the SEIQoL DW was itself used as an intervention and its addition to counselling in alcoholics was associated with more favourable outcomes (Cheyne and Kinn 2001). Another well-developed measure in this category is the Patient Generated Index (PGI)

(Ruta *et al.* 1994), that has been applied in patient populations including a randomized trial of acute post-stroke care (Ahmed *et al.* 2003).

Global measures

A number of global measures have been developed and applied to the measurement of QoL. Global measures of QoL can either employ one single item that requires an evaluation of quality of life taking all domains of life together in an overall judgment, or multiple items that require a number of judgments considering all of life. An example of the first approach is the question 'What is your overall quality of life?' , while the Satisfaction with Life Scale (SWLS) follows the latter approach. The SWLS consists of five items requiring the subject to provide a global evaluation of his or her life (Diener *et al.* 1985). More complex measures include verbal content analysis (Gottschalk and Lolas 1992) and in-depth qualitative interviews (Dijkers *et al.* 1998). These two measures make it possible for the insiders' perspective to be revealed by allowing (implicit) nomination and weighting of domains. Neither of these more complex measures allows any summing of the scores to form a single score or index. They also require trained interviewers, and this together with their complexity poses challenges to their routine use in clinical trials. However, they may prove particularly useful in exploring the phenomenology of QoL.

Preference-based measures

Many of the preference based measures, designed to assist in the economic analysis of interventions, incorporate individualized judgements. Although beyond the scope of this chapter, techniques such as rating scales, time trade-off or standard gamble used for eliciting utilities essentially recognize the individual nature of such judgments. These approaches are described by Feeny in Chapter 6.2.

Clinical trials and methodological challenges

IQoL measures are not yet widely used in clinical trials and those that have been used are at the lower end of the continuum of individualization. The use of IQoL measures presents a number of challenges, including the potentially long administration time and the increased resources and expertise needed. More efficient computer-administered versions might solve this problem. A computerized version of the SBQoL (Thunedborg *et al.* 1995) and a pilot version of SEIQoL using a touch screen (Lindblad *et al.* 2003) have been tested. A further significant issue is the 'apples and oranges' problem that arises when an individual can choose his or her domains. Is it valid to combine individual scores if they are based on different domains for different persons or to compare scores over time for one person, if the domains change? Although some measures such as the SEIQoL allow combination of scores to obtain a single summary score (the SEIQoL Index score), the outcome from IQoL measures is usually best represented as a profile for each individual. A related problem with some IQoL measures is that the effects of a disease, treatment or intervention on a specific QoL area can be assessed only for those patients who nominate that area as important. One approach to overcome this is to add investigator-generated domains of particular interest to those nominated by the patient. Another approach would be to use IQoL measures together with health status measures to provide a broader picture of the patient's QoL and functioning.

One challenge to the use of some IQoL measures in randomized controlled trials (RCTs) is that their outcomes are best represented as profiles rather than as summary scores. Obviously there is trade-off between simplicity (ease of use) and validity (broad representation) when using summary scores and profiles scores. While the latter provides a better measure of the components of quality of life for a given individual, summary scores while losing information, are easier to manage when applying group-based statistical methods.

Traditional concepts of validity and reliability may be less relevant in the case of IQoL measures. There is no agreement of how best to establish the validity of individualized measures, since the individual determines their content and the absence of concurrent validity in the form of high correlations with HRQoL measures is to be expected and valued, since they measure different things. Establishing test–retest reliability also presents challenges since it is increasingly clear that individuals adapt to their circumstances using a variety of cognitive strategies, a phenomenon increasingly referred to as response shift. One definition of response shift states that when individuals undergo a change in health state, they may change their internal standards (recalibration), their values (reprioritization), and/or their conceptualization of QoL (re-conceptualization); this is discussed by Schwartz *et al.* in the chapter on response shift (Chapter 4.4). IQoL measures like the SEIQoL and the PGI, may prove to be particularly useful in tracking response shift. The SEIQoL, for example, administered on subsequent occasions could detect re-conceptualization if the respondent's nominated cues changed between the time points. Reprioritization would be reflected in changes in cue weights (O'Boyle *et al.* 2000). By applying IQoL instruments, the researcher could implicitly or explicitly try to detect and/or control for response shift. This may be especially important in clinical trials, where the assessment of change over time in response to a treatment is the ultimate goal. A further possible application is that IQoL measures might be used to help patients achieve appropriate response shifts, since response shift might be considered as one outcome of adaptation/coping. This might, for example, be achieved by providing QoL feedback to patients to support a positive directed adaptation.

The interpretability of QoL instruments, particularly the clinical significance of the results, is important if QoL measures are to be widely used as outcome assessments. Indicators of clinical significance include, for example, effect size, content-based interpretation tables, norm and reference values and anchor based scores: these methods are described in the chapter on meaningful differences, by Osoba and King in Chapter 4.2.

In addition, subjective transition questions can be used. These involve asking patients to evaluate the size of the change or asking them to evaluate the importance or impact of the change. Such an approach may prove to be particularly relevant for interpreting change when using IQoL measures and in factoring in the contribution of response shift to such changes.

Clinical applications of IQoL measures

Many types of outcome measure may be applied to the assessment of a disease, its likely impact on the patient and the likely impact of curative or palliative treatment (Table 4.1.2). Pathological processes are reflected in biological markers such as tumour volume or MRI scans which provide objective evidence of disease status. Some symptom assessments are concerned with objective indicators (e.g. vomiting) and some with subjective indicators (e.g. pain). Whereas curative treatment is aimed at stopping or reversing the pathological process, which in turn will result in decreased symptoms, palliative treatments are usually focused on minimizing symptoms, even in the presence of advancing disease. Health status measures or HRQoL measures are concerned with the broad impact of the disease and its symptoms on the physical, emotional psychological and social functioning of the patient. These measures may be generic or disease-specific, and the relationship between pathological processes and health status is highly complex and likely to be influenced by a variety of biological, psychological and social processes. In our formulation, the IQoL approach provides more valid measures of the individual's QoL than do HRQoL measures or QoL measures based on group foundations. It is likely to be influenced in part by the disease process, but this is not inevitable, and the exact contribution of health to IQoL is likely to vary from one person to another and to be influenced by the particular meaning of the condition for the individual. The relationships between these different levels of outcome are highly complex and are likely to change with time and with disease progression. IQoL measures introduce a new level of assessment and set the outcomes from the other levels of measurement in a phenomenological context.

QoL measures are increasingly important in assessing new treatments and in comparing existing treatments with one another (Revicki *et al.* 2000), but they are rarely used routinely in clinical practice. The amount of communication in a clinical consultation devoted to QoL is limited, and decisions are more likely to be based on clinical signs such as tumour progression (Detmar *et al.* 2002). Patients and physicians might wish to discuss QoL during the consultation, but they are often more comfortable discussing the physical aspects of the condition (Detmar *et al.* 2000). Intervention studies in cancer have shown that providing patient-specific QoL information to the doctor and the patient before an appointment results in better communication. More issues are addressed and more actions are taken by the clinician during the consultation (Detmar *et al.* 2002). QoL assessment in clinical practice requires good measures

Table 4.1.2 IQoL measures in the context of other outcomes – cancer as an example

Level of Outcome	Examples of Measure	Disease Progression	Curative Treatment	Palliative Treatment
Individual QoL	SEIQoL; PGI	Likely decrease but with adaptation could stay constant or even increase	Aim to achieve pre-level or new integration	Aim to maximize
HRQoL				
Health status: generic	SF36	Likely decrease	Aim to increase	Aim to increase
Health status: specific	EORTC scales	Likely decrease	Aim to increase	Aim to increase
Cost	Treatment cost QALY cost?			
Side-effects	Self-report scale	–	Aim to minimize	Aim to minimize
Symptoms	McGill pain scale	Likely increase	Aim to minimize	Aim to minimize
Pathological process/signs	Tumour volume CAT/MRI scan	Increase	Decrease	Little impact

that must to be easy to use, reliable, clinically relevant (valid) and sensitive to change: criteria not always met by many currently available instruments. IQoL measures may be particularly useful in day-to-day practice since they provide a patient-centred framework for improved communication and decision-making. They may help to empower patients as partners in the clinical process, and provide a means of individualizing care and thereby improving treatment outcomes.

Conclusion

QoL measures range from simple global questions through complex utility measures and questionnaires to individualized interviews. The early stages of most new research disciplines usually produce a somewhat confusing array of constructs and methods, and it is only as a discipline develops that greater refinement and clarity emerge. The field of QoL research is crucial to modern health care, and it is important that we begin to create sound theoretical foundations to underpin it. Researchers should be precise about the aims and objectives of their research and should select outcome measures with great care at the outset. They should at least consider whether the methods they choose are based on a sound theoretical formulation and are true indicators of QoL. The French biologist Rene Dubois once said that we must be careful in our scientific endeavours that the measurable does not drive out the important. Many of the hundreds of so-called QoL scales now available certainly assist measurement. The challenge posed by the IQoL approach is to determine whether the outcomes from many of these scales could be said to address importance.

Acknowledgment

This chapter was completed while the authors Stefan Höfer and Lena Ring were EU Marie Curie Research Fellows at the Department of Psychology, Royal College of Surgeons in Ireland.

References

Ahmed, S., Mayo, N., Hanley, J., Wood-Dauphinee, S., and Cohen, R. (2003). Individualized Health-related Quality of Life (HRQL) post stroke: evaluation response shift. *Qual Life Res* 12, (7), 765. Abstract Issue, 10th Annual conference of ISOQoL.

Becker, M., Diamond, R., and Sainfort, F. (1993). A new patient focused index for measuring quality of life in persons with severe and persistent mental illness. *Quality of Life Research*, 2, 239–51.

Bo, K., Talseth, T., and Vinsnes, A. (2000). Randomized controlled trial on the effect of pelvic floor muscle training on quality of life and sexual problems in genuine stress incontinent women. *Acta Obstet Gynecol Scand*, 79, 598–603.

Bradley, C. (1994). *Handbook of Psychology and Diabetes: A guide to psychological measurement in diabetes research and management.* Switzerland: Harwood Academic Publishers.

Bradley, C. (1997). Design of a renal-dependent individualized quality of life questionnaire. *Adv Perit Dial*, 16, 116–120.

Burchard, G. A., Yarhouse, M. A., Kilian, M. K., Worthington, E. L., Berry, J. W., and Canter, D. E. (2003). A study of two marital enrichment programs and couples' quality of life. *Journal of Psychology and Theology*, 31, (3), 250–252.

Camilleri-Brennan, J. Ruta, D. A., and Steele, R. J. (2002). Patient generated index: new instrument for measuring quality of life in patients with rectal cancer. *World J Surg*, 26, 1354–1359.

Carr, A. J. (1996). Margaret Holroyd Prize Essay. A patient-centred approach to evaluation and treatment in rheumatoid arthritis: the development of a clinical tool to measure patient-perceived handicap. *Br J Rheumatol*, 35, 921–932.

Carr, A. J. (1999). Beyond disability: measuring the social and personal consequences of osteoarthritis. *Osteoarthritis Cartilage*, 7, 230–238.

Cheyne, A. and Kinn, S. (2001). A pilot study for a randomised controlled trial of the use of the schedule for the evaluation of individual quality of life (SEIQoL) in an alcohol counselling setting. *Addiction Research & Theory*, 9, 165–178.

DAFNE Group (2002). Training in flexible, intensive insulin management to enable dietary freedom in people with type 1 diabetes: dose adjustment for normal eating (DAFNE) randomised controlled trial. *BMJ*, 325, 746.

Dazord, A., Astolf, F., Guisti, P., Rebetez, M. C., Mino, A., Terra, J. L., and Brochier, C. (1998). Quality of life assessment in psychiatry: the Subjective Quality of Life Profile (SQLP) – first results of a new Instrument. *Community Mental Health Journal*, 34, 525–535.

Dazord, A., Gerin, P., and Boissel, J. P. (1994). Subjective quality of live assessment in therapeutic trials: presentation of a new instrument in France (SQLP: Subjective Quality for Life Profile and

First Results). In J. Orley and W. Kuyken (eds) *Quality of Life Assessment: International Perspectives.* pp. 185–195. Heidelberg: Springer.

Detmar, S. B., Aaronson, N. K., Wever, L. D., Muller, M., and Schornagel, J. H. (2000). How are you feeling? Who wants to know? Patients' and oncologists' preferences for discussing health-related quality-of-life issues. *J Clin Oncol,* **18,** 3295–3301.

Detmar, S. B., Muller, M. J., Schornagel, J. H., Wever, L. D., and Aaronson, N. K. (2002). Health-related quality-of-life assessments and patient-physician communication: a randomized controlled trial. *JAMA,* **288,** 3027–3034.

Diener, E., Emmons, R., Larsen, J., and Griffin, S. (1985). The Satisfaction With Life Scale. *J Personality Assessment,* **49,** 71–75.

Dijkers, M., Tate, D., and Duggan, C. (1998). Quality of life after spinal cord injury: development of a new measure. *Arch Phys Med Rehabil,* **79,** 1344.

Dijkers, M. P. (2003). Individualization in quality of life measurement: Instruments and approaches. *Arch Phys Med Rehabil,* **84,** S3–S14.

Duggan, C. H., Lysack, C., Dijkers, M., and Jeji T. (2002). Daily life in a nursing home: impact on quality of life after a spinal cord injury. *Topics in Spinal Cord Injury Rehabilitation,* **7,** (3), 112–131.

Dunbar, G. C., Stoker, M. J., Hodges, T., and Beaumont, G. (1992). The development of SBQoL – a unique scale for measuring quality of life. *British Journal of Medical Economics,* **2,** 65–74.

Duquette, R. L., Dupuis, G., and Perrault, J. (1994). A new approach for quality of life assessment in cardiac patients: rationale and validation of the Quality of Life Systemic Inventory. *Can J Cardiol,* **10,** 106–112.

Elliot, A. and Sheldon, K. M. (1998). Avoidance personal goals and personality – illness relationship. *Journal of Personality and Social Psychology,* **75,** 1282–1299.

Emmons, R. (1986). Personal strivings: an approach to personality and subjective well-being. *Journal of Personality and Social Psychology,* 1058–1068.

Ferrans, C. E. and Powers, M. J. (1985). Quality of life index: development and psychometric properties. *Ans Advances in Nursing Science,* **8,** 15–24.

Ferrans, C. and Ferrell, B. (1990). Development of a quality of life index for patients with cancer. *Oncology Nursing Forum,* 15–19 (Suppl.).

Flanagan, J. (1978). A research appraoch to improving our quality of life. *American Psychologist,* **12,** 347–354.

Flanagen, J. (1982). Measurement of quality of life: current state of the art. *Arch Phys Med Rehabil,* **63,** 56–59.

Frisch, M. B., Cornell, J. Villaneueva, M., and Retzlaff, PJ. (1992). Clinical validation of the quality of Life Inventory. A measure of life satisfaction for use in treatment planning and outcome assessment. *Psychological Assessment,* **4,** 92–101.

Gill, T. M. and Feinstein, A. R. (1994). A critical appraisal of the quality of quality-of-life measurements. *JAMA,* **272,** 619–626.

Gottschalk, L. and Lolas, F. (1992). The measurement of quality of life through the content analysis of verbal behaviour. *Psychother Psychosom,* **58,** 69–78.

Guyatt, G. H., Townsend, M., Keller, J., Singer, J., and Nogradi, S. (1989). Measuring functional status in chronic lung disease: conclusions from a randomized control trial. *Respir Med,* **83,** 293–297.

Hammond, K. R., Stewart, T. R., Brehmer, B., and Steinmann, D. (1975). Social judgment theory. In M. F. Kaplan and S. Schwartz (eds) *Human Judgment and Decision Processes: Formal and mathematical approaches,* New York: Academic Press.

Handy, J. R. Jr, Asaph, J. W., Skokan, L., Reed, C. E., Koh, S., Brooks, G., Douville, E. C., Tsen, A. C., Ott, G. Y., and Silvestri, G. A. (2002). What happens to patients undergoing lung cancer surgery? Outcomes and quality of life before and after surgery. *Chest*, **122**, 21–30.

Hickey, A., O'Boyle, C., McGee, H., and Joyce, C. R. B. (1999). The schedule for the evaluation of individual quality of life. In C. R. B. Joyce, C. O'Boyle and H. McGee (eds) *Indivuidual Quality of Life: approaches to conceptualisation and assessment*, pp. 119–133. Netherlands: Harwood Academic Publishers.

Hickey, A. M., Bury, G., O'Boyle, C. A., Bradley, F., O'Kelly, F. D., and Shannon, W. (1996). A new short form individual quality of life measure (SEIQoL-DW): application in a cohort of individuals with HIV/AIDS. *BMJ*, **313**, 29–33.

Joyce, C. R., Hickey, A., McGee, H. M., and O'Boyle, C. A. (2003). A theory-based method for the evaluation of individual quality of life: the SEIQoL. *Qual Life Res*, **12**, 275–280.

Joyce, C. R. B., O'Boyle, C. A., and McGee, H. M. (1999). *Individual Quality of Life: Approaches to conceptualisation and assessment*. Amsterdam: Harwood Academic Publishers.

Kelly, G. A. (1955). *The Psychology of Personal Constructs*. New York: Norton.

Kimmel, P. L., Peterson, R. A., Weihs, K. L., Simmens, S. J., Alleyne, S., Cruz, I., and Veis, J. H. (1998). Psychosocial factors, behavioral compliance and survival in urban hemodialysis patients. *Kidney Int*, **54**, 245–54.

Lacasse, Y., Wong, E., and Guyatt, GH. (1999). Individualising Questionnaires. In C. R. B. Joyce, C. A. O'Boyle and H. M. McGee (eds) *Individual Quality of Life: Approaches to conceptualisation and assessment*, pp. 87–103. Amsterdam: Harwood Academic Publishers.

Lindblad, A. K., Ring, L., Jansson, R., Bendtsen, P,. and Gilmelius, B. (2003). Feasibility study of a computer-based version of the SEIQoL-DW in gastro-intestinal cancer patients. *Quality of Life Research*, **12**, (7), 781.

Malla, A. K., Norman, R. M. G., McLean, T. S., and McIntosh, E. (2001). Impact of phase-specific treatment of first episode of psychosis on Wisconsin Quality of Life Index (client version). *Acta Psychiatrica Scandinavica*, **103**, (5), 355–361.

Neudert, C., Wasner, M., and Borasio, G. D. (2001). Patients' assessment of quality of life instruments: a randomised study of SIP, SF-36 and SEIQoL-DW in patients with amyotrophic lateral sclerosis. *J Neurol Sci*, **191**, 103–109.

O'Boyle, C., McGee, H., and Browne, J. (2000). Measuring Response Shift with SEIQoL. In C. E. Schwartz and M. A. Sprangers (eds) *Adaptation to Changing Health: Response Shift in Quality-of-Life Research*, pp. 123–136. Washington, DC: American Psychological Association.

O'Boyle, C. A., McGee, H., Hickey, A., O'Malley, K., and Joyce, C. R. (1992). Individual quality of life in patients undergoing hip replacement. *Lancet*, **339**, 1088–1091.

O'Boyle, C. A., McGee, H., Hickey, A., O'Malley, K., and Joyce, C. R. B. (1993). *The Schedule for the Evaluation of Individual Quality of Life*. Dublin: Department of Psychology, Royal College of Surgeons in Ireland.

O'Connor, K., Belanger, L., Marchand, A., Dupuis, G., Elie, R., and Boyer, R. (1999). Psychological distress and adaptational problems associated with discontinuation of benzodiazepines. *Addictive Behaviours*, **24**, (4), 537–541.

Paterson, C. (1996). Measuring outcomes in primary care: a patient generated measure, MYMOP, compared with the SF-36 health survey. *BMJ*, **312**, 1016–1020.

Paterson, C., Ewings, P., Brazier, J. E., and Britten, N. (2003). Trating dyspepsia with acupuncture and homeopathy: reflections on a pilot study by researchers, practitioners and participants. *Complementary Therapies in Medicine*, **11**, 78–84.

Ramstrom, H., Erwander, I., Mared, L., Kornfalt, R., and Seiving, B. (2000). Pharmaceutical intervention in the care of cystic fibrosis patients. *J Clin Pharm Ther*, **25**, 427–434.

Rapkin, B. D., Smith, M. Y., Dumont, K., Correa, A., Palmer, S., and Cohen, S. (1994). Development of the Idiographic Functional Status Assessment: a measure of the personal goals and goal attainment activities of people with AIDS. *Psychology and Health*, **9**, 111–129.

Revicki, D. A., Osoba, D., Fairclough, D., Barovsky, I., Berzon, R., Leidy, N. K., and Rothman, M. (2000). Recommendations on health-related quality of life research to support labeling and promotional claims in the United States. *Qual Life Res*, **9**, 887–900.

Ruta, D. A., Garratt, A. M., Leng, M., Russell, I. T., and MacDonald, L. M. (1994). A new approach to the measurement of quality of life. The Patient-Generated Index. *Med Care*, **32**, 1109–1126.

Smith, H. J., Taylor, R., and Mitchell, A. (2000). A comparison of four quality of life instruments in cardiac patients: SF-36, QLI, QLMI, and SEIQoL. *Heart*, **84**, 390–394.

Thunedborg, K., Allerup, P., Bech, P., and Joyce C. R. B. (1993). Development of the reperatory grid for measurement of individual quality of life in clinical trials. *International Journal of Methods in Psychiatric Research*, **3**, 37–42.

Thunedborg K., Black, C., and Bech, P. (1995). Beyond the Hamilton depression scores in long/term treatment of manic/melancholic patients: prediction of recurrence of depression by quality of life measurements. *Psychother Psychosom*, **64**, 131–140.

Tijhuis, G. J., Zwinderman, A. H., Hazes, J. M., Van Den Hout, W. B., Breedveld, F. C., and Vliet Vlieland, T. P. (2002). A randomized comparison of care provided by a clinical nurse specialist, an inpatient team, and a day patient team in rheumatoid arthritis. *Arthritis Rheum*, **47**, 525–531.

Tugwell, P., Bombardier, C., Buchanan, W. W., Goldsmith, C. H., Grace, E., and Hanna, B. (1987). The MACTAR Patient Preference Disability Questionnaire: an individualized functional priority approach for assessing improvement in physical disability in clinical trial in rheumatoid arthritis. *J Rheumatol*, **14**, 446–451.

Vandongen, Y. K., French, D. J., and Stacey, M. C. (1997). Quality in life in patients attending a specialized leg ulcer clinic. *J Wound Care*, Conference Proceedings 18–12 November, 42–46.

Waldron, D., O'Boyle, C. A., Kearney, M., Moriarty, M., and Carney, D. (1999). Quality-of-life measurement in advanced cancer: assessing the individual. *J Clin Oncol*, **17**, 3603–3611.

Weber, R., Christen, L., Loy, M., Schaller, S., Christen, S., Joyce, C. R., Ledermann, U., Ledergerber, B., Cone, R., Luthy, R., and Cohen, M. R. (1999). Randomized, placebo-controlled trial of Chinese herb therapy for HIV-1-infected individuals. *J Acquir Immune Defic Syndr*, **22**, 56–64.

Wright, J. G. and Young, N. L. (1997). The Patient-Specific Index: asking patients what they want. *J Bone Joint Surg*, **79-A**, 974–983.

Wright, J. G., Young, N. L., and Waddell, J. P. (2000). The reliability and validity of the Self-Reported Patient-Specific Index for total hip arthroplasty. *Journal of Bone & Joint Surgery – American Volume*, **82A**, (6), 829–837.

Meaningful differences

David Osoba and Madeleine King

Introduction

The ultimate goal of health care is to improve, restore or preserve functioning and well-being related to health, that is, health-related quality of life (HRQoL). All health care endeavors, regardless of setting, are aimed directly or indirectly at achieving this goal. Whether immunizing against infectious diseases, screening for cancer, setting a broken bone, rehabilitating muscle strength after surgery, providing curative chemotherapy, or treating pain and dehydration in a palliative care setting, the intention is to restore an individual's previous level of functioning or preserve well-being, if restoration to the former level is not possible. These efforts may be directed at all or part of a general population (the macro level), at groups of individuals with identified health conditions (the meso level), or at individual patients (the micro level) (Osoba 2002).

At each of these levels there are many uses and users of HRQoL data (Table 4.2.1). Thus an important issue, when considering the meaning of differences or changes in HRQoL scores, is the perspectives of different users of HRQoL. Just as their perspectives differ, so do their reasons for assessing HRQoL, their uses of HRQoL data and the value they attach to differences in HRQoL. At the macro level, an economist or health policy decision-maker may argue that small differences in population HRQoL scores are important because attempts to modify population health on the basis of such scores can have a large economic impact. At the micro level, although a patient may perceive a given change over time as being meaningful, a physician may not think it sufficiently important to intervene. When monitoring an individual patient's care, a physician may wish to see a large difference to feel confident that a real change has occurred. Since the uses are as varied as are the perspectives of the users, it is not surprising that the results of HRQoL assessment are expressed in various ways, from qualitative discourses to quantitative summaries of sophisticated statistical analyses.

Despite a plethora of data and information, a satisfactory sense of the meaning of changes, or differences, in HRQoL scores is often lacking. When large samples of individuals are studied, at the macro or meso levels, differences in HRQoL scores that are very small in numerical terms may be highly significant in statistical terms. At the micro level, it is difficult to apply probability statements from group-based results to a

Table 4.2.1 Examples of users and uses of HRQoL information

User	Uses
Government policy-makers and advisors	Setting broad policy Allocating regional health care resources Monitoring population health Economic evaluations
Institutions, managed care organizations	Setting local policy Allocating local health care resources Economic evaluations
Epidemiologists	Understanding and explaining variations in health
Statisticians	Determining sample size for HRQoL component of clinical trials; drawing valid inferences from hypothesis tests in HRQoL analyses
Clinical trials groups	Evaluating group benefits
Health care professionals – physicians, nurses, social workers, psychologists, etc.	Evaluating, monitoring and advising individuals Decision-making re: values of interventions Communication
Patients	Communication, monitoring benefits of therapy
Families of patients	Communication, monitoring wellness and benefits

decision about an individual's treatment (Cella *et al.* 2002a). Given these difficulties, how should differences in HRQoL scores between two groups in a clinical trial or population survey be interpreted, either in cross-section or over time? Are the differences big or small, meaningful or trivial? What are the implications for peoples' individual concerns, clinical practice and health policy? At all levels, one needs to understand and explain HRQoL differences in ways that are relevant to the health care decision at hand and to the people involved in that decision.

Given the variety of perspectives of different users of HRQoL data, can the meaning of HRQoL results be captured in a manner that will satisfy all? Our thesis is that robust methodology may help to resolve some of the differences. In addition, robust methodology for determining meaningfulness has a value of its own, by providing various users a means for determining the relevance and value of HRQoL studies in their efforts to restore and preserve HRQoL.

Interpretability of HRQoL scores

Interpretability has been defined as 'the degree to which one can assign qualitative meaning – that is clinical or commonly understood connotations – to quantitative scores' (Lohr *et al.* 1996). It is an essential attribute of any HRQoL instrument, along with reliability and validity. Much like validity, interpretability is not established by a single psychometric manoeuvre; rather, it develops gradually as a body of evidence accumulates with repeated experience from a variety of perspectives (Ware and Keller 1996).

The interpretation of HRQoL scores poses a number of difficulties. First, HRQoL is a notion that may mean different things to different people at different times and in different contexts. For example, two people in the same apparent state of health (as viewed by an observer or by objective methods) may perceive their health states differently because of differences in their dispositions, experiences or circumstances (Wilson and Cleary 1995). Indeed, a person's perception of his/her health state may change over time even if the apparent state of health does not change from an observer's perspective (perhaps because the observer has incomplete information, or as a result of recall bias or response shift (see Chapter 4.4). Second, HRQoL measurement scales are in the strictest sense ordinal and their numeric values are arbitrary. Third, there are many HRQoL questionnaires or instruments, each with one or more different scales. This may be confusing to some users and it would be desirable to have a single method for standardizing differences in scores ('cross-walking') between different instruments (Gonin *et al.* 1996). Finally, HRQoL instruments and their scales are unfamiliar to many users of HRQoL data, with a resulting lack of accumulated experience and understanding of the significance of HRQoL scores as compared to more familiar outcomes such as survival or disease remission.

Despite these difficulties, many HRQoL instruments have been used in a wide range of health contexts, and in general, the resultant HRQoL scores seem to behave quite sensibly; for example, sick people and groups have lower HRQoL scores than do well people and groups. If the patterns of differences in HRQoL differences make sense, then these differences also must have some meaning at the various levels of health care.

Types of differences in HRQoL scores

Four types of differences in HRQoL scores arise in the provision of health care; each type has a different purpose and place in the provision of health care, and must be meaningful to the subjects who provide the scores and to the various users of the data.

Cross-sectional, individual-based differences

Differences in HRQoL scores between individuals may identify patients who have high levels of symptom experience or psychological problems—for example, screening for anxiety about prostate-specific-antigen testing (Cormier *et al.* 2002). Such individuals may be at risk for poor health outcomes and may benefit from targeted interventions.

Cross-sectional, group-based differences

Differences in HRQoL scores between two or more groups of people arise most commonly at the macro or meso levels of health care and are used to describe the health of different populations and subpopulations. These differences may be assessed by comparing means, medians, or the proportions of individuals with scores that fall within given ranges of the HRQoL scale. For example, decisions about resource allocation for groups with poor HRQoL may be informed by understanding the link between health status measures and health service utilization (Ware and Keller 1996). Also, a description of a cohort with a particular condition allows for a better understanding of the effect of the condition or its treatment on HRQoL. For example, patients with recurrent malignant gliomas have many HRQoL characteristics similar to patients with metastatic tumors, but they tend to have more cognitive problems and less pain (Osoba *et al.* 2000b).

Longitudinal, individual-based differences

Changes in the HRQoL scores of a person over time may be used to monitor the benefits and side-effects of treatment and to facilitate communication between the patient and clinician (Detmar *et al.* 2002; Taenzer *et al.* 2000; Velikova *et al.* 2002). The clinicians need to be confident that changes in scores over time reflect real changes in the individual's HRQoL. Thus, the precision of the instruments must be very high.

Longitudinal, group-based differences

Changes in the HRQoL scores of a group of people over time may be used at the macro level to monitor population health, but are most commonly used at the meso level, to determine the effectiveness of interventions for patients with particular health conditions. At the meso level, in contrast to the macro level, samples tend to be smaller and repeated measurement helps to increase the power of statistical tests of hypotheses about the effectiveness of interventions. Also, patients returning for repeated visits (for example, for treatment) make longitudinal follow-up feasible. Differences in scores are often expressed as the mean change over time within a group, or the difference in mean change between two groups, but may also be reported as median change. A result that clinicians find relevant to decision-making is the proportion of the sample whose scores have changed by given increments of the HRQoL scale. A study of the effectiveness of trastuzumab in the treatment of metastatic breast cancer used this approach to describe differences between the treated groups (Osoba *et al.* 2002). Patients in the trial were deemed to have an improvement in the HRQoL domains under study if their scores improved by at least 10 per cent from baseline in those domains. The proportions of patients achieving this change in each treatment arm of the trial were then compared with each other to determine which treatment was superior.

Making HRQoL differences meaningful

A number of approaches may be used to find meaning in HRQoL scores; some apply to individual differences and some to group differences, and some to both (Table 4.2.2).

Table 4.2.2 Approaches to interpretation of HRQoL differences and their applicability to individuals and groups

	Individuals		Groups	
	Cross-sectional	Longitudinal	Cross-sectional	Longitudinal
Internally-referenced approaches				
Content-based	✓	✓	✓	✓
Statistical significance			O	O
Effect size			✓	✓
Standard error of measurement	✓	✓		
Externally-referenced approaches				
Clinical known-groups			✓	✓
Norms and reference values	✓	✓	✓	✓
Global ratings of change		✓	✓	✓

✓ approach is useful

O approach is feasible but not appropriate

Blank cells indicate approach is not feasible, appropriate or useful.

These approaches can be grouped into two classes: internally-referenced and externally-referenced. We define internally referenced approaches as those that are derived solely from the HRQoL scores in the primary data set, that is, the observed distributions of HRQoL scores or related statistics, and from the instrument's known properties, such as it's content and reliability. Externally-referenced approaches compare the HRQoL data with information that is additional, or external, to the HRQoL data in the primary data set. Such information may include either well-established and understood variables familiar to the users of the HRQoL data that has been collected in parallel with the primary HRQoL dataset, or HRQoL scores of the same instrument measured in other well-defined and understood samples.

Our terms expand on the terms 'distribution-based' and 'anchor-based', described in the seminal paper by Lydick and Epstein (1993). We have chosen to introduce the new terms because they convey more simply and comprehensively the essential distinction between two broad types of approach to interpretation. The terms are also likely to be more transparent and less ambiguous across the many disciplines involved in HRQoL research.

Internally-referenced approaches to interpretation

Content-based interpretations

Ware and Keller (1996) defined content, construct and criterion-based interpretation methods. Their classification makes explicit the conceptual and empirical link between validation and interpretation. For example, an HRQoL scale can be referred back to the content of a questionnaire when interpreting its scores. The items illustrate the abstraction that the scale represents, and together with the item response scales, indicate the range of experience within the scale. However, content-based interpretation is complicated for multi-item scales because a particular score can be achieved by a myriad of combinations of item responses. For example, there are 2850 possible ways to obtain a score of 70 on the SF-36 physical functioning scale (McHorney and Tarlov 1995). Nevertheless, individual scale levels can be interpreted by using a single item from a scale to interpret scores across scale levels. For example, as the SF-36 physical function scale scores increase from 40 to 50, 18 per cent more people indicate they can walk one block without limitations (Ware *et al.* 1993).

For single items, literal interpretations of an individual's score can be derived from the item's content and its response options, and can be useful for the monitoring of individual patients over time in a clinical practice.

Statistical significance

The statistical significance associated with a hypothesis test does not indicate whether a difference is important clinically or not, but it is sometimes used that way. This misuse of statistical significance is compounded in HRQoL studies, where the multidimensional nature of HRQoL leads to multiple hypothesis testing and the associated danger of false–positive findings (Fayers and Machin 2000). For example, consider the following scenario: an innovative treatment (B) is developed in the hope that it will have a better effect on the HRQoL of patients than does current best treatment (A). A study is conducted and an appropriate statistical analysis is used to test the null hypothesis of no difference between the two treatments. The resultant p value is the probability of the observed HRQoL data if Treatment B truly is no better than Treatment A; a small p value provides evidence against the null. If the null hypothesis is rejected, we conclude that Treatment B is better than Treatment A. But how much better is it? How much better does HRQoL on Treatment B need to be than on Treatment A to convince patients, clinicians or policy makers to switch to B as the new best treatment? This difference is the 'clinically' important difference, and, to the extent possible, should be specified a priori to determine the appropriate sample size for the study to have the power to detect the alternative hypothesis.

Sample size is directly related to power. If the sample is too small, the study will not have the power to detect the smallest clinically important difference; the p value will be large, the confidence interval wide and the results inconclusive. Conversely, if the sample is very large, the study will have the power to detect effects so trivial that they do not warrant a change of health policy or patient management. The problem of over-powered comparisons is most common at the macro and meso levels, where large sample sizes are likely, such as in the Women's Health Initiative (Hays *et al.* 2003).

Thus, statistical significance is about the null hypothesis, and clinical importance is about the extent to which the null hypothesis is wrong. It is important to make clinical sense of the results of HRQoL studies in order to interpret the results in terms that are relevant to the uses and users of the HRQoL information.

Effect size

The effect size is an interpretation of the size of the observed effect, such as mean difference in HRQoL, in terms of the variability among individuals. This method has the advantage of requiring no information additional to the observed HRQoL scores; it is a signal-to-noise ratio. It is not a function of sample size, as are tests of statistical significance.

There are a number of effect size statistics, each one related to a particular statistical test (Cohen 1988). The effect sizes that are usually applied to HRQoL measures take the mean difference between the HRQoL scores of two independent groups divided by the standard deviation of the HRQoL scores in the two groups. Because the numerator (mean difference) and the denominator (standard deviation) are both in the same measurement units (HRQoL units of the particular scale used), the ratio is a standardized (unitless) measure. This allows comparison across HRQoL effects measured on different scales.

Cohen proposed operational definitions of 0.2, 0.5 and 0.8 as small, medium and large effect sizes, respectively. He described these as 'arbitrary conventions . . . recommended for use only when no better basis for estimating the effect size is available' (Cohen 1988, p. 12 and p. 25). The steady accrual of HRQoL data provides a better basis for understanding the meaning of effect sizes. For example, King (1996, 2001)and Osoba et al (1998) found that evidence-based effect sizes for the QLQ-C30 generally confirm Cohen's guidelines.

Effect sizes can be used to interpret both cross-sectional and longitudinal group-based differences, but they cannot be used to interpret individual-based differences. Specific interpretations rely on assumptions about the distributions of random variables. For example, for two normally distributed populations with equal sample size and equal variance, a 'small' effect size of 0.2 indicates that 85 per cent of the combined area of the two distributions overlaps, while an effect size of 0.5 indicates that 67 per cent of their combined area overlaps and an effect size of 0.8 indicates that 53 per cent of their combined area overlaps (Cohen 1988, pp. 25–26).

Standard error of measurement

When interpreting the change scores of individuals, the precision and reliability of the measurement is critical. Scales with a low internal consistency or with a relatively small number of possible scale values are imprecise measures of HRQoL, and are prone to measurement error. Determining a difference between two such measures, as when calculating a patient's change in HRQoL, adds to the measurement error.

The standard error of measurement (SEM), a function of both scale reliability and between-person variance (Anastasi and Urbina 1997), is useful for individual-level applications, because the SEM can be used to estimate a confidence interval around an individual score, indicating the smallest observed change that is likely to reliably reflect true change. However, opinion differs as to the reliable bounds of the SEM (Wyrwich *et al.* 1999); some authors use one SEM, others use 1.96 SEM, and the most conservative propose 2.77 or more SEM. The 1 SEM approach would yield confidence intervals (CI) that are smaller than the conventional 95 per cent CI, while 1.96 SEMs yield the conventional 95 per cent CI.

Applying the 95 per cent CI SEM approach to the SF-36 physical functioning scale, McHorney and Tarlov (1995) found that an individual change score must be greater than 14 points (in either direction, improved or deteriorated) to reliably reflect true change in physical functioning. This is noteworthy, given that this scale has 10 items and 21 possible scale values, and is certainly reliable enough for group-level research. Similar calculations for five commonly used health status instruments suggested that none of these instruments was sufficiently reliable to be useful in the monitoring and management of individual patients.

The SEM approach provides a useful guide to interpreting individual patient change, but it requires that end-users have access to suitable estimates of the between-person standard deviation and reliability for the scales they wish to use in order to calculate the SEM and its confidence intervals.

Externally-referenced approaches

To provide insights into the meaning of HRQoL scores, the external data with which differences in HRQoL scores will be compared should be easily understood and meaningful to the users of the HRQoL data, and be reasonably correlated with the HRQoL scores. For example, at the macro and meso levels, differences in HRQoL scores may be linked with health care utilization, job loss, ability to work, and other classifications related to the planning and provision of health care services. At the meso level, for hospitals, area health services and managed care organizations, linking with disease and diagnostic groups may be more relevant, since they are commonly used in the clinical management of patients. At the micro level, subjective, patient-specific links are appropriate (for example, the retrospective assessment of change in a patient's own health). A novel example of micro level application is the approach of having patients compare themselves with other patients (Redelmeier *et al.* 1996).

Known-groups comparisons

Clinical known groups Some of the most useful evidence for developing interpretations that are meaningful to clinicians comes from studies that report the HRQoL of patients grouped by established clinical criteria. (Aaronson *et al.* 1996). Such groups are 'known' in the sense that their characteristics are describable and understandable in clinical terms. These conventional, familiar measures are relevant to the purpose and users of HRQoL data and, thus, provide an external reference for interpretations of novel HRQoL scales.

The EORTC Quality of Life Group used the known-groups approach as an integral part of their strategy to develop and evaluate the cancer-specific QLQ-C30. Common grouping variables were performance status, weight loss, toxicity, extent or severity of disease. When patients were grouped according to various clinical indicators of disease or treatment, the patterns of the mean HRQoL scores were as would be expected. The set of mean scores underlying these patterns gave a sense of the relative size of means and of differences, and of the types of clinical groups which gave rise to them, thereby providing clinically-based benchmarks by which to interpret QLQ-C30 results (King 1996). For example, in the global QOL dimension, a mean of 70 (on a scale range of 0 to 100) was associated with asymptomatic patients with localized disease, while a mean of 55 was typical of a group of patients whose metastatic disease and treatment had reduced their performance status, caused considerable weight loss and toxicity. Thus, for the QLQ-C30 global dimension, a difference of 15 appears to be a relatively large difference. Such a difference derives its clinical relevance from knowledge of the patients' conditions that gave rise to the HRQoL scores. Indeed, the magnitude of this difference suggests that an improvement of about 10 in the global QOL dimension may be clinically worthwhile, representing considerable improvement in symptom control, and reduction or reversal of weight loss.

Normative and reference groups Comparison to normative data and reference values is a form of known-groups comparisons. The HRQoL scores are sampled from well-defined, large populations to provide normative data (that is, typical scores called norms, or reference values). Population norms are useful for generic instruments such as the SF-36 (Ware *et al.* 1993). For condition-specific instruments, samples with particular stages of disease or on particular treatments provide useful reference values, for example the cancer-specific QLQ-C30 (Fayers *et al.* 1998). Mean scores from a particular study or person may be compared to norms or reference values to give a sense of the impact of disease or treatment on HRQoL (Ware and Keller 1996). Because mean HRQoL scores vary systematically with age and gender, valid comparisons of sample data with norms and reference values require suitable adjustment (Hjermstad *et al.* 1998b).

Usually norms are used to interpret group-based differences. For example, a study of 192 Australian women with early stage breast cancer (King *et al.* 2000) showed that the mean physical, emotional and role function scores of young patients were considerably lower (by about 10, 10 and 20 points, respectively) than the means of women of similar age in the Norwegian adult population (Hjermstad *et al.* 1998a). The means of the oldest two age groups in the cancer sample were generally comparable with or slightly higher (up to five points) than those of women of similar age from this population. In the other dimensions of HRQoL, the cancer patients' means were similar to those of the norm. These results suggest that the diagnosis and treatment for early stage breast cancer has the greatest impact on young women, and that it is likely to have a large impact on physical, role and emotional function. It also suggests, somewhat counter-intuitively, that the experience of cancer can actually improve people's perception of their HRQoL. The reasons for this are unknown.

Interpretation of sample scores by comparison with norms can be further facilitated by a calculation (standardization or transformation) that expresses the sample scores as deviations from the norm. This facilitates comparison across domain scales within an instrument, which usually have different means and standard deviations due to different content and coverage. This can be done in one or two steps. The one-step version involves only standardization; the mean of the study sample is subtracted from the mean of the norm and divided by the standard deviation (SD) of the norm (Garratt et al. 1993). This is equivalent to transforming the observed distribution to a Z-score, with a mean of 0 and a SD of 1. (It is also an effect size calculation, although in this case the mean and SD of the normative or reference population are used rather than that of the primary data set.) In the two-step version, the Z-score is further transformed into a T-score. For example, the calculation of the SF-36 Physical and Mental Health Summary multiplication by 10 and addition of 50 to give a distribution with a mean of 50 and a SD of 10 (Ware et al. 1994).

While normative data are useful for interpretation, they are not yet available for many instruments: organizing the appropriate sample surveys is complex and expensive. The issue of systematic differences in HRQoL scores across different language and culture groups needs to be addressed to increase our confidence in norms for valid cross-cultural comparisons. Furthermore, even though apparently significant differences between a study sample and a norm can be demonstrated, the differences are not expressed in terms that allow users to understand whether there are clinically important differences in the study subjects' well-being.

Global ratings of change

In earlier work, the 'minimal clinically important difference' (MID) was defined as 'the smallest difference … which patients perceive as beneficial and which would mandate, in the absence of troublesome side effects and excessive cost, a change in the patient's management' (Jaeschke et al. 1989). Another, somewhat similar term is the 'subjectively significant difference' (SSD) which is the smallest change, either beneficial or deleterious, that is perceptible (discernable) to the subject (Osoba et al. 1998). This definition does not imply that a change in a patient's management is necessarily mandated, or that troublesome side effects or excessive cost be absent. As a result, the definition of the MID has been recently modified, taking these differences in the two definitions into account (Guyatt et al. 2002). More recently, it has been proposed that the term 'minimal difference' be used to denote the difference derived from individual anchor-based (externally-referenced) methods (Norman *et al.* 2003).

While various methods have been proposed for estimating the MID (Guyatt *et al.* 1991), empirical studies to date have generally relied on patients' global ratings of change in their own health. In this approach, the subject is asked to retrospectively judge whether a particular aspect of their health has improved, stayed the same, or worsened, using a single item with several response options across a range from 'much worse' through 'no change' to 'much better'. The degree of change on the global rating scale is then related back to the magnitude of change in the analogous dimension of an HRQoL questionnaire in order to obtain a numerical value denoting the MID (or SSD).

This approach has a number of methodological problems as a gold-standard measure of change. First, because judgements are retrospective, they may be prone to recall bias (Ross 1989). It has been observed that patients' retrospective estimates of change are highly correlated with their present state (Norman *et al.* 1997). Second, they are single items, and so are more prone to measurement error than are multi-item scales. Third, these response items have not been formally evaluated as measures of change. However, small, moderate or large changes in QLQ-C30 scores were found to be similar to small, moderate and large effect sizes (Osoba *et al.* 1998). Wyrwich *et al* (1999, 2002) applied the MID results from (Jaeschke *et al.* 1989) to individual change scores, and found good agreement between the MID value of about 6–7 per cent of the scale breadth and one SEM. Norman *et al.* (2003) reviewed a large number of studies and concluded that effect sizes associated with the MID averaged 0.5. Beaton (2003), however, argues convincingly that to suggest 0.5 SD as a universal answer may be too simple and gives several exceptions to this number. Thus, the global rating approach would appear to have some external validity, but questions still remain and more research is required.

Patients' global change ratings have been used for assessing the significance of HRQoL changes in asthma (Juniper *et al.* 1994), chronic heart and lung disease (Jaeschke *et al.* 1989), osteoarthritis (Ehrich *et al.* 2000), and cancer (Osoba *et al.* 1998). Despite the range of disease groups studied and the variety of HRQoL instruments used, remarkably, these studies generally yielded similar estimates, indicating that patients were able to discern a 6–7 per cent change in the breadth of the relevant instrument scale (approximately one half of a standard deviation of the patients' baseline scores). It has been recommended that a 10 per cent change be used as a cut-off for calculating the proportions of patients whose HRQoL improves, or deteriorates, during or after an intervention (Osoba *et al.* 1998, 2000, 2002) A 10 per cent cut-off is less likely to include false positives than are smaller cut-offs. It is an easy rule of thumb to remember and seems sensible to clinicians. Larger cut-offs of 15 per cent and 20 per cent could also be used in a sensitivity analysis to determine the benefit of treatment, but cut-offs that are too stringent may underestimate the treatment benefit.

It is conceptually appealing to have a single standard, the minimum discernible difference (judged by patients), that would be suitable for all situations, but it may not be the same as the clinically significant difference (judged by health care professionals). The clinically significant difference may differ with context. In adjuvant therapy for cancer, it can be defined as the smallest decrease in HRQoL during therapy that would be tolerated for the increased chance of survival (Coates 1993). For palliative therapy, it may be the smallest improvement in HRQoL, (for example, improvement in physical functioning), that would be worthwhile given the associated toxicity, such as nausea, alopecia and fatigue. In curative therapy, different aspects of HRQoL may be weighed against others. For example, prostatectomy may improve urinary symptoms, but may also cause incontinence and impotence (Fowler *et al.* 1988). In clinical practice, the clinical relevance of HRQoL findings may require a complex judgement which includes the relative importance of different dimensions of HRQoL together with the importance of other clinically meaningful measures derived from physical examination, laboratory and imaging studies. Costs may also need to be considered (O'Brien and Drummond 1994).

Future directions

Several issues need further attention. For example, we have discussed methods for interpretation of HRQoL data that are primarily helpful in understanding group data, but can the same interpretation guidelines be applied to individual patients?

Although there is a remarkable convergence of results from various methods indicating that a half of a standard deviation (or equivalently an effect size of 0.5 or 6–7 per cent of the scale breadth) is a minimum discernable difference (Norman *et al.* 2003), there are some who are skeptical of the arguments and evidence for this conclusion (Beaton 2003; Wright 2003).

Guidelines, where all useful methods and all available data are collated and summarized, are helpful (Cella *et al.* 2002b; Ware *et al.* 1993), but they also need to provide information on what is a clinically useful change.

The potential of cross-instrument calibration using Item Response Theory may help to provide standard health metrics and add evidence for the interpretation of various instruments. In addition, IRT methods have the potential to make individual-level measurement reliable enough for practical use in individual patient management. However, it will still be necessary to examine the IRT data for the minimum discernable difference and for clinical significance (see Chapter 1.5).

An important area that has not yet received sufficient attention is the reporting of results according to the proportion of patients whose HRQoL improves, or deteriorates, after an intervention (Detmar *et al.* 2002, Langendijk *et al.* 2000, Osoba 2002, Osoba *et al.* 2000, Taenzer *et al.* 2000, Velikova *et al.* 2002). The proportion of patients whose scores have improved by at least 0.5 SD, or 1 SEM, or more than 7 per cent (preferably 10 per cent, see above) better than their own baseline scores can be used to calculate the number of patients that need to be treated (NNT) for one patient to benefit (Guyatt *et al.* 2002). This is important information that clinicians can use to make clinical decisions about the value of an intervention. We would highly recommend that results of clinical trials be reported in this fashion, since decision-making based on the proportion of patients whose HRQoL improves or deteriorates makes sense both to clinicians and to policy makers, the ultimate users of HRQoL data.

The approaches to the interpretation that we have summarized are described in general terms and may be applied from the perspectives of most users of HRQoL data. Although each has been described in isolation from the others, it is often helpful to use more than one method in a given study, to provide richness of detail and to allow comparison between methods for further consideration. For example, providing p values, effect sizes and proportions of patients who benefit would help physicians to become familiar with the meaning of effect sizes, a metric with which many are not currently familiar. The provision of information about the 'real world' relevance of HRQoL scores by comparing them with known clinical parameters such as days lost from work, number of days in hospital, and the financial burdens to the individual and society would make changes in HRQoL scores more meaningful to physicians and policy makers. In the end, it is they who need to be most well informed because it is they who make the decisions that most profoundly affect health care.

References

Aaronson, N. K., Cull, A., Kaasa, S., and Sprangers, M. A. G. (1996). The European Organisation for Research and Treatment of Cancer (EORTC) modular approach to quality of life assessment in oncology: An update. In B. Spilker (ed.) *Quality of Life and Pharmacoeconomics in Clinical Trials*, pp. 179–189. Philadelphia: Lippincott-Raven Publishers.

Anastasi, A. and Urbina, S. (1997). *Psychological Testing*. London: Prentice-Hall International.

Beaton, D. E. (2003). Simple as possible? Or too simple? Possible limits to the universality of the one half standard deviation [comment]. *Medical Care*, 41, 593–596.

Cella, D., Bullinger, M., Scott, C., Barofsky, I., and Clinical Significance Consensus Meeting Group. (2002a). Group vs individual approaches to understanding the clinical significance of differences or changes in quality of life. *Mayo Clinic Proceedings*, 77, 384–392.

Cella, D., Eton, D. T., Lai, J. S., Peterman, A. H., and Merkel, D. E. (2002b). Combining anchor and distribution-based methods to derive minimal clinically important differences on the Functional Assessment of Cancer Therapy (FACT) anemia and fatigue scales. *Journal of Pain & Symptom Management*, 24, 547–561.

Coates, A. (1993). Quality-of-life considerations in the adjuvant setting: critical review. *Recent Results in Cancer Research*, 127, 243–245.

Cohen, J. (1988). *Statistical Power Analysis for the Behavioural Sciences*. Hillsdale, NJ: Lawrence Erlbaum Associates.

Cormier, L., Guillemin, F., and Valeri, A., *et al.* (2002). Impact of prostate cancer screening on health-related quality of life in at-risk families. *Urology*, 59, 901–906.

Detmar, S. B., Muller, M. J., Schornagel, J. H., Wever, L. D., and Aaronson, N. K. (2002). Health-related quality-of-life assessments and patient-physician communication: a randomized controlled trial. *Journal of the American Medical Association*, 288, 3027–3034.

Ehrich, E. W., Davies, G. M., Watson, D. J., Bolognese, J. A., Seidenberg, B. C., and Bellamy, N. (2000). Minimal perceptible clinical improvement with the Western Ontario and McMaster Universities osteoarthritis index questionnaire and global assessments in patients with osteoarthritis. [comment]. *Journal of Rheumatology,* **27,** 2635–2641.

Fayers, P. M. and Machin, D. (2000). *Quality of Life: Assessment, Analysis and Interpretation.* Chichester: John Wiley & Sons Ltd.

Fayers, P. M., Weeden, S., and Curran, D. (1998). *EORTC QLQ-C30 Reference Values.* Brussels: EORTC Study Group on Quality of Life.

Fowler, F. J., Wennberg, J. E., Timothy, R. P., Barry, M. J., Mulley, A. G., and Hanley, D. (1988). Symptom status and quality of life following prostatectomy. *Journal of the American Medical Association,* **259,** 3018–3022.

Garratt, A. M., Ruta, D. A., Abdalla, M. I., Buckingham, J. K., and Russell, I. T. (1993). The SF36 health survey questionnaire: an outcome measure suitable for routine use within the NHS? [comment]. *BMJ,* **306,** 1440–1444.

Gonin, R., Lloyd, S., and Cella, D. (1996). Establishing equivalence between scaled measures of quality of life. *Quality of Life Research,* **5,** 20–26.

Guyatt, G. H., Feeny, D. H., and Patrick, D. L. (1991). Issues in quality of life measurement in clinical trials. *Controlled Clinical Trials,* **12,** 81S–90S.

Guyatt, G. H., Osoba, D., Wu, A. W., Wyrwich, K. W., Norman, G. R., and Clinical Significance Consensus Meeting Group. (2002). Methods to explain the clinical significance of health status measures. *Mayo Clinic Proceedings,* **77,** 371–383.

Hays, J., Ockene, J. K., and Brunner, R. L., *et al.* (2003). Effects of estrogen plus progestin on health-related quality of life. *New England Journal of Medicine,* **348,** 1839–1854.

Hjermstad, M. J., Fayers, P. M., Bjordal, K., and Kaasa, S. (1998a). Health-related quality of life in the general Norwegian population assessed by the European Organization for Research and Treatment of Cancer Core Quality-of-Life Questionnaire: the QLQ-C30 (+ 3). *Journal of Clinical Oncology,* **16,** 1188–1196.

Hjermstad, M. J., Fayers, P. M., Bjordal, K., and Kaasa, S. (1998b). Using reference data on quality of life–the importance of adjusting for age and gender, exemplified by the EORTC QLQ-C30 (+3). *European Journal of Cancer,* **34,** 1381–1389.

Jaeschke, R., Singer, J., and Guyatt, G. H. (1989). Measurement of health status: Ascertaining the minimal clinically important difference. *Controlled Clinical Trials,* **10,** 407–415.

Juniper, E. F., Guyatt, G. H., Willan, A., and Griffith, L. E. (1994). Determining a minimal important change in a disease-specific Quality of Life Questionnaire. *Journal of Clinical Epidemiology,* **47,** 81–87.

King, M. T. (1996). The interpretation of scores from the EORTC quality of life questionnaire QLQ-C30. *Quality of Life Research,* **5,** 555–567.

King, M. T. (2001). Cohen confirmed? Empirical effect sizes for the QLQ-C30. *Quality of Life Research,* **10,** 278.

King, M. T., Kenny, P., Shiell, A., Hall, J., and Boyages, J. (2000). Quality of life three months and one year after first treatment for early stage breast cancer: influence of treatment and patient characteristics. *Quality of Life Research,* **9,** 789–800.

Langendijk, J. A., ten Velde, G. P., Aaronson, N. K., de Jong, J. M., Muller, M. J., and Wouters, E. F. (2000). Quality of life after palliative radiotherapy in non-small cell lung cancer: a prospective study. *International Journal of Radiation Oncology, Biology, Physics,* **47,** 149–155.

Lohr, K. N., Aaronson, N. K., and Alonso, J., *et al.* (1996). Evaluating quality-of-life and health status instruments: development of scientific review criteria. *Clinical Therapeutics,* **18,** 979–992.

Lydick, E. and Epstein, R. S. (1993). Interpretation of quality of life changes. *Quality of Life Research,* **2,** 221–226.

McHorney, C. A. and Tarlov, A. R. (1995). Individual-patient monitoring in clinical practice: are available health status surveys adequate? *Quality of Life Research,* **4,** 293–307.

Norman, G. R., Stratford, P., and Regehr, G. (1997). Methodological problems in the retrospective computation of responsiveness to change: the lesson of Cronbach. *Journal of Clinical Epidemiology,* **50,** 869–879.

Norman, G. R., Sloan, J. A., and Wyrwich, K. W. (2003). Interpretation of changes in health-related quality of life: the remarkable universality of half a standard deviation [comment]. *Medical Care,* **41,** 582–592.

O'Brien, B. J. and Drummond, M. F. (1994). Statistical versus quantitative significance in the socioeconomic evaluation of medicines. *PharmacoEconomics,* **5,** 389–398.

Osoba, D. (2002). A taxonomy of the uses of health-related quality-of-life instruments in cancer care and the clinical meaningfulness of the results.[comment]. *Medical Care,* **40** (Suppl III), 31–38.

Osoba, D., Brada, M., Yung, W. K., and Prados, M. (2000). Health-related quality of life in patients treated with temozolomide versus procarbazine for recurrent glioblastoma multiforme. *Journal of Clinical Oncology,* **18,** 1481–1491.

Osoba, D., Slamon, D. J., Burchmore, M., and Murphy, M. (2002). Effects on quality of life of combined trastuzumab and chemotherapy in women with metastatic breast cancer. *Journal of Clinical Oncology,* **20,** 3106–3113.

Osoba, D., Rodrigues, G., Myles, J., Zee, B., and Pater, J. (1998). Interpreting the significance of changes in health-related quality-of-life scores. *Journal of Clinical Oncology,* **16,** 139–144.

Redelmeier, D. A., Guyatt, G. H., and Goldstein, R. S. (1996). Assessing the minimal important difference in symptoms: a comparison of two techniques [see comments]. *Journal of Clinical Epidemiology,* **49,** 1215–1219.

Ross, M. (1989). Relation of implicit theories to the construction of personal histories. *Psychological Review,* **96,** 341–357.

Taenzer, P., Bultz, B. D., and Carlson, L. E., *et al.* (2000). Impact of computerized quality of life screening on physician behaviour and patient satisfaction in lung cancer outpatients. *Psycho-Oncology,* **9,** 203–213.

Velikova, G., Brown, J. M., Smith, A. B., and Selby, P. J. (2002). Computer-based quality of life questionnaires may contribute to doctor-patient interactions in oncology. *British Journal of Cancer,* **86,** 51–59.

Ware, J. E. and Keller, S. D. (1996). Interpreting general health measures. In B. Spilker (ed.) *Quality of Life and Pharmacoeconomics in Clinical Trials,* pp. 445–460. New York: Lippincott-Raven.

Ware, J. E., Kosinski, M., and Keller, S. D. (1994). *SF-36 Physical and Mental Health Summary Scales: a User's Manual.* Boston, MA: Health Assessment Lab, New England Medical Center.

Ware, J. E., Snow, K. K., Kosinski, M., and Gandek, B. (1993). *SF-36 Health Survey Manual and Interpretation Guide.* Boston, MA: The Health Institute, New England Medical Center.

Wilson, I. B. and Cleary, P. D. (1995). Linking clinical variables with health-related quality of life. A conceptual model of patient outcomes. *Journal of the American Medical Association,* **273,** 59–65.

Wright, J. G. (2003). Interpreting health-related quality of life scores: the simple rule of seven may not be so simple [comment]. *Medical Care,* **41,** 597–598.

Wyrwich, K. W., Tierney, W. M., and Wolinsky, F. D. (1999). Further evidence supporting an SEM-based criterion for identifying meaningful intra-individual changes in health-related quality of life. *Journal of Clinical Epidemiology,* **52,** 861–873.

Wyrwich, K. W., Tierney, W. M., and Wolinsky, F. D. (2002). Using the standard error of measurement to identify important changes on the Asthma Quality of Life Questionnaire. *Quality of Life Research,* **11,** 1–7.

Health-related quality of life outcomes in clinical trials

David Osoba

Introduction

Outcomes in clinical trials

Health-related quality of life (HRQoL) outcomes may be measured as either a primary outcome or as secondary outcome in addition to other, more traditional outcomes, e.g. survival, time to progression of disease, duration of remission of disease, days lost from work, and economic impact of illness. A combination of HRQoL measurement with a measurement of these other outcomes can provide a comprehensive assessment of the effects of a disease and/or its treatment. The feature that distinguishes HRQoL assessment from the other assessments is that it is self-assessed by the patient and not by an observer (except in the unusual case of proxy assessments). HRQoL measurement has similarities to health status assessment and symptom assessment, since these are also reported by patients; thus, it has been grouped with them under the term 'patient-reported outcomes' (PROs) (Acquadro *et al.* 2002). It is probably reasonable to view them as being related to each other like the components of a Venn diagram.

Types of clinical trials

Clinical trials may be classified simply as either phase I, II, or III trials. Phase I trials are intended to explore the toxicity of a new treatment and to determine the safe dosage that can be further tested in phase II and III trials. HRQoL assessments are not usually a part of phase I studies because of the small numbers of patients enrolled at each dosage level (often only three or four) and the small number enrolled overall. Thus, conclusions about the effects on HRQoL at each dosage level may not be reliable. Nevertheless, they can provide informative results (e.g. LoRusso *et al.* 2003). In phase II trials, which are intended to explore the possible efficacy of a treatment, HRQoL is often measured at one point in time (cross-sectional), but it is possible to compare a cross-sectional point in time with baseline data to ascertain if there has been either an improvement or deterioration that may be associated with therapy (e.g. Osoba *et al.* 2000a). The most common use of HRQoL assessment is in phase III trials.

Usually, large numbers of patients are enrolled and comparisons are made between two or more treated groups of patients at either one point in time or, longitudinally, over several time points. In addition, comparisons may also be made between defined times on treatment and baseline data within each treated group (e.g. Osoba *et al.* 2002).

Purpose of HRQoL assessment and applications in clinical trials settings

HRQoL assessments are carried out in clinical trials for a variety of reasons that can be classified in different ways (Guyatt *et al.* 1989; Osoba *et al.* 1991; Jaeschke *et al.* 1992; Osoba 2002). The classification presented here is based on the purpose of the assessment and its application in the health care setting in which it is used (Table 4.3.1). Not all of the applications lend themselves to ready testing in randomized controlled clinical trials, e.g. monitoring population health or predicting survival.

A classification based on the purpose of assessment

Most purposes for assessing HRQoL can be grouped under five main headings: screening, prevention, health profile description, health care (clinical) decision-making, predicting outcomes, and preference (utility) assessment (Table 4.3.1). Within each purpose, HRQoL may be assessed in a wide variety of applications and health care settings.

Applications of HRQoL assessment in health care settings

HRQoL assessment in clinical settings may occur at three broad levels of heath care: the macro level of government and health care policy-setting relating to population health, the meso level of institutions and clinical trials pertaining to groups of patients, and the micro level of individual patient care (Sutherland and Till 1996; Osoba 2002).

Most of the HRQoL information at the various levels of health care arises from clinical trials designed to help decide if one intervention is better than another. These studies may be either descriptive (no control arm), or evaluative (to decide whether one treatment approach is preferable to another). The studies have included virtually all the care settings referred to in Table 4.3.1. Because the best decision-making outcomes are derived from randomized, controlled (Phase III) trials, most of the examples below are drawn from those situations. However, only a small number can be cited here and some results are summarized in Table 4.3.2.

Screening

Effect of a screening procedure Screening of large population samples is intended to identify individuals with particular characteristics of interest. An example is the screening of men for elevated levels of prostate-specific antigen (PSA) to narrow down the sample that should be further investigated for possible prostate cancer. One study

Table 4.3.1 Classification based on the purpose and applications of HRQoL assessment

Purpose	Examples of Applications	Amenable to testing in RCTs*?
Screening	Effect of a screening procedure	Yes
Health-profile description	Effect of a disease or its treatment	No
Health-care (clinical) decision-making	Primary and secondary prevention	Yes
	Active treatment to cure a disease	Yes
	Active treatment to prolong life without cure	Yes
	Palliative treatment to control symptoms	Yes
	Supportive care	Yes
	Palliative care	Yes
	Communication in routine patient care	Yes
Prediction of outcomes	Prediction of morbidity	No
	Predicting response to treatment	No
	Prediction of survival	No
Preference (utility) assessment	Monitoring population health	No
	Assessing preferences for health states	Yes

* RCTs = Randomized controlled clinical trial

of the effects of this screening procedure on HRQoL involved 220 men who were related to men who had known prostate cancers and who had PSA levels of 4 mg/mL or less. Forty per cent reported either a minimal or a moderate increase in anxiety during the screening process (Cormier *et al.* 2002). Increased anxiety was associated with age between 50–60 years, having more than two relatives with prostate cancer, having an anxious personality and a high level of education. The identification of such men before they are screened may allow for the provision of appropriate intervention measures, such as counselling, during the screening process.

Health-profile description

Understanding the effects of a disease or therapy HRQoL profiles are available for a variety of diseases using a variety of HRQoL questionnaires. For example, using the Medical Outcomes Study Short Form (MOS SF-36), a generic questionnaire, the functional capacity and the presence of common symptoms such as fatigue and pain have been described for patients with diabetes, rheumatoid arthritis, heart disease, and a variety of cancers, to cite only some of these studies (Ware *et al.* 1994). Similar data has been obtained with the Sickness Impact Profile (Bergner *et al.* 1981). With disease-specific questionnaires, such as the European Organization for Research and Treatment

Table 4.3.2 Summary of examples of studies and results from clinical trials

Reference	Study	Sample Size; Condition	HRQoL Result	Parameter	Proportions Benefiting		Statistical Significance
Day et al. (1999); Day et al. (2001)	RCT of Tamoxifen vs. control	11,064 women	0.74–1.24% more problems with tamoxifen	Aspects of sexual function	Not applicable		$P = 0.031 - 0.016$
Kornblith et al. (2002)	RCT of azacytidine vs. supportive care	191 patients	Azacytidine better than supportive care	Fatigue Dyspnoea Physical function Positive affect	Not determined		$P = 0.0001$ $P = 0.0014$ $P = 0.0002$ $P = 0.0077$
Osoba et al. (2000b)	RCT of temozolomide vs. procarbazine	179; malignant glioma	Better with TMZ	Role function Social function Visual Motor Communication	TMZ 27% 32% 34% 32% 40%	PCB 18% 18% 24% 18% 19%	Not tested
Murray et al. (1999)	RCT of CODE vs. CAV/EP	77; small cell lung cancer	Worse with CODE	Global QoL Physical function Fatigue	Not applicable		$P = 0.018$ $P < 0.001$ $P = 0.001$
Tannock et al. (1996); Osoba et al. (1999)	RCT of Mitoxantrone + prednisone vs. prednisone	161 men; hormone-resistant prostate cancer	Improved with mitoxantrone + prednisone	Pain Physical function Global QoL Fatigue Pain impact	Mitoxantrone 29% 50% 63% 59% 59%	Prednisone 12% 32% 42% 38% 38%	$P = 0.01$ Not calculated

Study	Purpose	Sample	Result	Measure	Values	P value
Littlewood et al. (2001)	RCT of epoietin alfa vs. placebo	349; cancer chemotherapy	Better with epoietin	FACT-G Fatigue subscale Anaemia subscale	Not calculated	$P = 0.004$ $P = 0.004$ $P = 0.007$
Detmar et al. (2002)	RCT of HRQoL – informed consultation vs. control	10 physicians (randomized); 214 patients with cancer	More communication about HRQoL issues	Social function Fatigue Dyspnoea	Informed 22% 54% 23% — Control 11% 37% 13%	Composite $P = 0.01$
Osoba et al. (1997)	Prediction of postchemotherapy emesis	832 patients with various cancers	Additional predictors to previously known ones	Social function (in multivariate analysis)	Not applicable	Prediction of risk for emesis increased; 20 to 76%
Eton et al. (2003)	Prediction of various risk factors	573 patients with non-small cell lung cancer	Improved predictability	Response to treatment Risk of death Risk of disease progression	Not applicable	Odds ratio 1.09, $P = <0.001$ Risk ratio 0.95, $P = <0.001$ Risk ratio 0.98, $P = <0.001$
Coates et al. (1997)	Prediction of survival in cancer	656 patients with various cancers	Independent predictor of survival	Social function Global QoL	Not applicable	Hazard ratio 0.993, $P = 0.001$ Hazard ratio 0.989, $P < 0.001$

of Cancer (EORTC) Quality of Life Questionnaire (QLQ-C30) and the Functional Assessment of Chronic Illness Therapy (FACIT) scales, many studies have assessed patients with various kinds of cancer and a variety of associated conditions such as anaemia, nausea and vomiting, and fatigue.

An example of the value of such profiles in patients with cancer is the study of 433 patients with recurrent glioblastoma multiforme or anaplastic astrocytoma who were assessed by the QLQ-C30 before treatment for the progression of their disease (Osoba *et al.* 2000). The results were compared to similar assessments in patients with a variety of cancers at various stages of disease. Several domains of HRQoL were severely impaired in the brain cancer patients, on a par with patients having late stage lung cancer and with heterogeneous metastatic cancers. Cognitive functioning in those with brain cancer was more severely impaired, but pain was a lesser problem than in other patients. This information should help clinicians to better understand the severity of HRQoL impairment in such patients and, as a result, to plan appropriate interventions.

Health-care (clinical) decision-making

Primary prevention In a study of tamoxifen for the primary prevention of breast cancer, 11,064 women were randomized to receive either 20 mg of tamoxifen or a placebo daily over a planned five years (Day *et al.* 1999). HRQoL was assessed with the Center for Epidemiological Studies Depression Scale (CES-D), the SF-36, the MOS scales for sexual functioning and a checklist of items designed for the study. Women taking tamoxifen reported more vasomotor and gynaecological problems, more difficulties with sexual interest, with becoming sexually aroused and with having an orgasm than did the control group, but these did not have a statistically significant impact on HRQoL (Day *et al.* 1999, 2001). The mean differences in sexual problems between women taking tamoxifen and those not taking tamoxifen were small in absolute terms, varying between 0.74 per cent and 1.24 per cent, but they were statistically significant ($p = 0.031$ to 0.016) due to the large sample size (Table 4.3.2). However, it is unlikely that these differences had clinical significance. Nevertheless, women who are about to be given tamoxifen should be counselled about the potential side effects of this agent.

Active treatment to cure disease or to prolong life The value of azacytidine C (Aza C) was compared to supportive care in 191 patients (median age of 67.5 years, 69 per cent male) with myelodysplastic syndrome (Kornblith *et al.* 2002). Aza C was given for seven days every four weeks and patients on supportive care could be crossed over to Aza C if there was progression of their state into leukaemia. HRQoL was assessed with the EORTC QLQ-C30 and the Mental Health Inventory at baseline, 50, 106 and 182 days. It was found that patients taking Aza C had less fatigue and dyspnoea, had better physical functioning and positive affect than did patients on the supportive care arm (Table 4.3.2). Since there was also a delayed time to disease progression and to death, it was concluded that these benefits were accompanied by HRQoL benefits as well, and that Aza C is an important treatment option for myelodysplastic syndrome.

Active treatment to prolong life without cure The recurrence of Grade 3 and 4 malignant gliomas after initial treatment harbours a poor prognosis. Median survival after the recurrence of glioblastoma multiforme (Grade 3) is from two to three months if it is untreated. In an attempt to find more effective chemotherapy, 225 patients were treated with either temozolomide (the new therapy) or procarbazine (the reference therapy), and of these, 179 completed HRQoL assessment using the QLQ-C30 plus a Brain Cancer Module consisting of 20 items (BN 20) (Yung *et al.* 2000; Osoba *et al.* 2000b). Eighty-nine patients were treated with temozolomide and 90 with procarbazine. Median progression-free survival was 2.89 months and 1.88 months for the two groups, respectively ($P = 0.063$), but overall median survival was not statistically significantly different, being 7.34 and 5.66 months, respectively. Before progression of disease, higher proportions of patients treated with temozolomide than with procarbazine were found to have an improvement (at least 10 per cent over baseline scores lasting for at least eight weeks) in role functioning and social functioning, visual disorder, motor dysfunction and communication deficit (Table 4.3.2). These improvements also lasted longer in the temozolomide-treated group than in the procarbazine-treated group. Thus, despite no statistically significant difference in overall survival, more patients treated with temozolomide experienced improvement in several HRQoL domains before disease progression than did patients treated with procarbazine.

Another example of a clinical trial in which HRQoL data was helpful in decision-making was the comparison of a dose intensive regimen of chemotherapy with standard chemotherapy in patients with extensive-stage small-cell lung cancer (Murray *et al.* 1999). The new treatment, consisting of cyclophosphamide, vincristine, cisplatin and etoposide (CODE) was given weekly to 109 patients, while the standard regimen of cyclophosphamide, doxorubicin and vincristine alternating with etoposide and cisplatin (CAV/EP) was given every three weeks to 110 patients. Radiation therapy was administered to the thorax and to the cranium in patients whose disease responded to CODE, and at the discretion of the treating physicians to patients on the CAV/EP arm. HRQoL was assessed using the QLQ-C30 every three weeks. It was shown that the dose intensity of the CODE therapy was twice that of the four most active drugs in the CAV/EP therapy. The response rate was higher in the CODE arm (87 per cent) than in the CAV/EP arm (70 per cent), but overall survival was not significantly different (median survival time of 0.98 and 0.91 years, respectively). The rates of developing neutropenic fever were similar on both arms but there were 9 deaths on the CODE arm and only one death on the CAV/EP arm. This led to early termination of the study. Furthermore, the HRQoL data showed worse global QOL, physical functioning and more fatigue in patients treated with CODE than with CAV/EP (Table 4.3.2). Thus, in addition to the mortality data, the HRQoL data helped the investigators to conclude that CODE therapy was not suitable for patients with extensive-stage small-cell lung cancer.

These two examples led to entirely different conclusions. In the first example, it was concluded that the new treatment was preferable, while in the second example it was deleterious, compared to a standard treatment. Thus, HRQoL data helped in the decision as to whether or not to adopt a new therapy.

Palliative treatment to control symptoms Symptom control, either for its own sake or with the expectation of only minor prolongation of life, is a common treatment situation in oncology. The control of symptoms that are of major concern to patients, such as pain or fatigue, would be expected to improve HRQoL and the measurement of HRQoL might seem unnecessary. However, it is by no means certain that this would occur, since the control of one symptom may be accompanied either by bothersome side effects or may unmask other symptoms that were secondary so long as the main symptom was dominant (e.g. the control of pain with opioids may be accompanied by somnolence or severe constipation, or may unmask debilitating fatigue). Thus, HRQoL assessment is important in symptom control.

An example of a study that was carried out solely for improving symptom control without an expectation of increased survival was the treatment of men with metastatic, hormone-resistant, prostate cancer (MHRPC) with mitoxantrone and prednisone (Tannock *et al.* 1996; Osoba *et al.* 1999). One hundred and sixty one men were randomized to receive either prednisone alone or prednisone and mitoxantrone. The primary end point was an improvement in pain without an increase in analgesics. Pain was measured using the McGill Present Pain Intensity Index, while HRQoL was measured by a combination of the EORTC QLQ-C30, a quality-of-life module (QLM-P14) developed for MHRPC, and the Prostate Quality of Life Index (PROSQOLI). As expected, there was no difference in overall survival. A primary pain response was achieved in 29 per cent of men receiving mitoxantrone and prednisone vs. 12 per cent in those receiving only prednisone (Table 4.3.2). The median durations of the response were 11 months and 5 months, respectively ($P < 0.0001$). The HRQoL assessment, using the QLQ-C30, showed that several scores, including global QL, physical, role and social functioning, as well as fatigue, insomnia, drowsiness and constipation, were significantly better in the mitoxantrone and prednisone group than in the prednisone alone group. Hair loss was the only deleterious side effect in those receiving the chemotherapy. More men benefited from mitoxantrone and prednisone than from prednisone alone in several HRQoL domains. These improvements lasted significantly longer in the combined therapy group than in the prednisone alone group ($0.004 < P < 0.05$).

Recently, a review of the evaluation of HRQoL in advanced prostate cancer, using a checklist for determining the robustness of the HRQoL assessment, showed that the HRQoL data in eight of 24 studies were informative for clinically decision-making (Efficace *et al.* 2003). An interesting finding in this review was that seven of the eight studies were published since 1998, indicating that recent studies tend to exhibit better HRQoL design and study execution than do earlier ones.

Supportive care The use of medroxyprogesterone acetate in the treatment of anorexia and weight loss in patients with advanced cancer has shown that appetite and weight loss can be improved, but the HRQoL benefits are uncertain. One study claimed benefits (Bruera *et al.* 1998) but others have shown deterioration in HRQoL scores in both the treated and control groups (Simons *et al.* 1996; Rowland *et al.* 1996). The use of hydrazine sulfate has been found to have deleterious effects on HRQoL (Loprinzi *et al.* 1994).

Several studies have shown that erythropoietin products are effective in increasing haemoglobin levels in patients undergoing chemotherapy for cancer or who are anaemic as a result of the cancer or its treatment (Littlewood *et al.* 2001; Gabrilove *et al.* 2001; Crawford *et al.* 2002). A substantial gain in haemoglobin is associated with an improvement in fatigue, activity level and energy. For example, in one randomized study of 349 patients with cancer, the mean change scores on the Functional Assessment of Cancer Therapy-General (FACT-G) and the fatigue and anaemia subscales of the FACT-Anaemia scale were statistically significantly better in patients who received epoetin alfa vs. placebo, regardless of change in haemoglobin (Littlewood *et al.* 2001) (Table 4.3.2). However, there was no calculation of the proportions of treated patients who benefited.

A study of the effects of chemotherapy-induced emesis (post-chemotherapy nausea and vomiting) found that nausea and even one or two episodes of vomiting were associated with significant deterioration in HRQoL from baseline scores on the EORTC QLQ-C30 (Osoba *et al.* 1997a). This was part of the evidence leading to the recommendation that the goal of antiemetic therapy should be the complete control of nausea and vomiting (Gralla *et al.* 1999).

Palliative care Palliative care is often directed towards the control of symptoms that tend to occur near the end of life (e.g. pain, shortness of breath, dehydration, constipation, etc.) and it would seem to be an ideal setting for trials in symptom control. Yet the individual-focused care that is a tenet of palliative care seems to mitigate against randomized, controlled trials. Thus relatively few trials have included HRQoL assessment. In part, this is because questionnaires designed for ambulatory patients seem unsuitable for those who are less mobile and near the end of life, when existential and spiritual concerns seem more important than earlier in the illness trajectory (Cohen *et al.* 2000; Steinhauser *et al.* 2002). Also, long-term studies are difficult in this setting because of high attrition rates (McMillan and Weitzner 2003). Thus, most of the studies are descriptive in nature, but are still providing important information (Goodwin *et al.* 2003; Lo *et al.* 2002; Klepstad *et al.* 2002; Weisbord *et al.* 2002; Trail *et al.* 2003). Nevertheless, randomized controlled studies of a shorter-term nature should be possible.

Communication in routine patient care Since the ultimate goal of health care is to restore or preserve HRQoL, HRQoL should be monitored in individual patient care as a means of following the progress of the patient's illness. Does the provision of HRQoL data at each clinic visit facilitate physician-patient communication and allow the recognition of problems uncovered by the HRQoL assessment? To answer this question, 10 physicians were randomized, in a cross-over design, to receive HRQoL information on 214 patients being seen in the clinic (Detmar *et al.* 2002). Communication was assessed with audiotapes of the patient–physician interviews and awareness of problems by comparing patients' ratings on an independent measure of HRQoL. At the time of the fourth clinic visit, consultations discussing HRQoL issues were statistically significantly higher in the intervention group than in the control group with respect to social functioning, fatigue and dyspnoea (Table 4.3.2). All of the physicians and 87 per cent of the patients thought that the HRQoL information facilitated communication. In addition, physicians identified a larger proportion of patients with moderate-to-severe health problems in the intervention group than in the control group.

Although other studies (Taenzer *et al.* 2000; Velikova *et al.* 2002) did not randomize physicians, they showed, nevertheless, that communication between physicians and patients was improved by presenting the individual patient's HRQoL data to the physicians during the clinic visit.

Prediction of outcomes

Predicting morbidity In a study of 412 men, aged 50–72 years, with treated hypertension and high risk factors for stroke and myocardial infarction, the patients completed the Minor Symptoms Evaluation Profile at baseline and were then followed for a median of 6.6 years (Agewall *et al.* 1998). During follow-up, statistically significant predictors of stroke but not of myocardial infarction, even after adjustment for potential cardiovascular risk factors, were low contentment and vitality. Thus these domains provided additional predictive value to the usual risk factors.

Predicting response to treatment Scores on the physical well-being (PWB) scale and the trial outcome index (TOI) of the FACT-Lung questionnaire predicted response to treatment, risk of disease progression and risk of death in 573 patients with advanced non-small cell lung cancer (Eton *et al.* 2003). A higher baseline PWB score was associated with a better response to treatment (odds ratio 1.09; $P < 0.001$) and lower risk of death (risk ratio 0.95; $P < 0.001$), whereas a higher baseline TOI score was associated with a lower risk of disease progression (risk ratio 0.98; $P < 0.001$).

Predicting survival The ability of HRQoL data to predict overall survival in cancer to a greater extent than more conventional predictive factors, such as performance status, has now been demonstrated in several advanced/metastatic cancers, e.g. bladder cancer (Roychowdhury *et al.* 2003), breast cancer (Coates *et al.* 1987, 1992), melanoma (Coates *et al.* 1993), colorectal cancer (Earlam *et al.* 1996), lung cancer (Ganz *et al.* 1991), and heterogeneous groups of patients comprising several cancers (Dancey *et al.* 1997; Coates *et al.* 1997). For example, in a multi-institutional study of 656 patients from 10 countries, it was found that social functioning and global QOL remained predictive, in addition to age and Eastern Cooperative Group Performance Status (hazard ratios 0.993 and 0.989; confidence intervals 0.988 to 0.997 and 0.984 to 0.995;

$P = 0.001$ and <0.001, respectively) (Coates *et al.* 1997). It seems that patients are able to convey information, through the responses to HRQoL questionnaires, about their survival that is not captured in other ways, such as by laboratory tests or by assessing performance status (Coates *et al.* 1993).

Preference (utility) assessment

Monitoring population health Preference-based, rather than psychometrically derived, measures have been applied to studying population health. The main reason is that utility measures are designed to provide an outcome that can be expressed in a single number. This can then be combined with length of survival to produce a single number that is useful for economic applications. These single numbers, in turn, are preferred by policy decision-makers at the macro level (see Chapter 6.2). The study of population health is not often the subject of randomized controlled studies, since these are usually observational studies.

Assessing patients' preferences for health states Clinical trials have used utility assessment as a method of determining the efficacy of treatment in phase III studies (e.g. Schunnemann *et al.* 2003; Moskowitz *et al.* 2003; Raynauld *et al.* 2002) and for evaluating the cost of therapy (e.g. van Dieten *et al.* 2003). Preference assessment has been used as a means of determining stated patient preferences within a choice of treatments (Lubeck *et al.* 2002; Coyle *et al.* 2001; Brundage *et al.* 1998; Sullivan *et al.* 2002; Siderowf *et al.* 2002,) and decision-making in patient care (Bruera *et al.* 2001).

Unexpected outcomes

There are several examples of how HRQoL assessment has either produced counterintuitive results or led to findings that were serendipitous. A counterintuitive result was obtained in a study of women who were randomized to receive either continuous or intermittent chemotherapy for metastatic breast cancer (Coates *et al.* 1987). It was expected that interrupted chemotherapy would have fewer deleterious side effects and, therefore, that HRQoL would be better in this group. However, the outcome was to the contrary, with women who received continuous chemotherapy reporting higher HRQoL in several domains. This was suspected to be attributable to more effective disease remission and was eventually confirmed by slightly longer duration of survival. Another unexpected finding is the predictive value of HRQoL status for survival as demonstrated in several cancers (see the section Predicting response to treatment above).

Caveats, recommendations, and summary

The use of HRQoL assessment is growing (Sanders *et al.* 1998). Over the 17 years prior to 1998, there was an increase in HRQoL reporting from 0.63 per cent to 4.2 per cent of all trials. This increase was greatest in oncology trials, rising from 1.5 per cent to

8.2 per cent. Since then the increase has accelerated and the quality of reporting is improving (Efficace *et al.* 2003). However, only a few studies have used HRQoL outcomes as the primary outcomes and more such studies are needed.

There is still inadequate/incomplete reporting in many clinical trials of important information including patient characteristics, reasons for missing data, how the missing data was dealt with in the analysis, and how the results were interpreted for clinical meaningfulness or significance (Bernhard *et al.* 1998; Fairclough 2002; Fayers and Machin 2000; Lee and Chi 2000; Guyatt *et al.* 2002; Efficace *et al.* 2003).

Most clinical trials have concentrated on reporting differences between groups of patients and, thus, statistical methods appropriate for analysing differences between group data (tests of the null hypothesis and effect sizes) have been commonly used. Unfortunately, the clinical importance of such differences often remains unclear and very few studies have addressed the meaning of differences in terms of the numbers, or proportion, of patients who benefit (e.g. Langendijk *et al.* 2000; Osoba *et al.* 2000, 2002) (see Chapter 4.2).

The use of computer adaptive testing, based on item response theory, may help to make measurements more precise (see Chapter 2.3). However, work is still required to improve the reliability of assessment tools for individual subjects above that which is acceptable for groups of individuals. The clinical significance of differences in scores obtained by this method will need to be determined.

Not all clinical trials that have assessed HRQoL could be documented here. Only a few examples of clinical trials can be given for each of the purposes and applications of HRQoL assessment, but they should serve to illustrate the diversity of the settings and the richness of the information that has been achieved by HRQoL studies. Since the ultimate goal of all health care is to improve, restore, and preserve HRQoL, there is a role for HRQoL assessment at every level of health care and in every setting.

References

Acquadro, C., Berzon, R., and Dubois, D., *et al.* (2003). Incorporating the patient's perspective into drug development and communication: An ad hoc task force report of the Patient-reported Outcomes (PRO) Harmonization Group meeting at the Food and Drug Administration, February 16, 2001. *Value in Health*, **6**, 522–531.

Agewall, S., Wikstrand, J., and Fagerberg, B. (1998). Stroke was predicted by dimensions of quality of life in treated hypertensive men. *Stroke*, **29**, 2329–2333.

Bergner, M., Bobbitt, R. A., Carter, W. B., and Gilson, B. S. (1981). The Sickness Impact Profile: development and final revision of a health status measure. *Medical Care*, **19**, 787–805.

Bernhard, J., Cella, D., and Coates, A. S., *et al.* (1998). Missing quality of life data in cancer clinical trials: serious problems and challenges. *Statistics in Medicine*, **17**, 517–532.

Bruera, E., Ernst, S., and Hagen, N., *et al.* (1998). Effectiveness of megestrol acetate in patients with advanced cancer: a randomized, double-blind, crossover study. *Cancer Prevention and Control*, **2**, 74–78.

Bruera, E., Sweeney, C., Calder, K., Palmer, L., and Benisch-Tolley, S. (2001). Patient preferences versus physician perceptions of treatment decisions in cancer care. *Journal of Clinical Oncology*, **19**, 2883–2885.

Brundage, M. D., Davidson, J. R., Mackillop, W. J., Feldman-Stewart, D., and Groome, P. (1998). Using a treatment-trade-off method to elicit preferences for the treatment of locally advanced non-small-cell lung cancer. *Medical Decision Making*, **18**, 256–267.

Coates, A., Gebski, V., and Bishop, J. F., *et al.* (1987). Improving the quality of life during chemotherapy for advanced breast cancer. A comparison of intermittent and continuous treatment strategies. *New England Journal of Medicine*, **317**, 1490–1495.

Coates, A., Gebski, V., and Signorini, D., *et al.* (1992). Prognostic value of quality-of-life scores during chemotherapy for advanced breast cancer. Australian New Zealand Breast Cancer Trials Group. *Journal of Clinical Oncology*, **10**, 1833–1838.

Coates, A., Porzsolt, F., and Osoba, D. (1997). Quality of life in oncology practice: prognostic value of EORTC QLQ-C30 scores in patients with advanced malignancy. *European Journal of Cancer*, **33**, 1025–1030.

Coates, A. S., Thomson, D., and McLeod, G. R. M., *et al.* (1993). Prognostic value of quality of life scores in a trial of chemotherapy with or without interferon in patients with metastatic malignant melanoma. *European Journal of Cancer*, **29A**, 1731–1734.

Cohen, S. R. and Mount, B. M. (2000). Living with cancer: 'Good Days' and 'Bad Days' – what produces them? Can the McGill Quality of Life Questionnaire distinguish between them? *Cancer*, **89**, 1854–1865.

Cormier. L., Guillemin. F., and Valeri, A., *et al.* (2002). Impact of prostate cancer screening on health-related quality of life in at-risk families. *Urology*, **59**, 901–906.

Coyle, D., Wells, G., Graham, I., and Lee, K. M., *et al.* (2001). The impact of risk on preference values: implications for evaluations of postmenopausal osteoporosis therapy. *Value Health* **4**, 385–391.

Crawford, J., Cella, D., and Cleel, C. S., *et al.* (2002). Relationship between changes in hemoglobin level and quality of life during chemotherapy in anemic cancer patients receiving epoetin alfa therapy. *Cancer*, **95**, 888–895.

Dancey, J., Zee, B., and Osoba, D., *et al.* (1997). Quality of life score: an independent prognostic variable in a general population of cancer patients receiving chemotherapy. *Quality of Life Research*, **6**, 151–158.

Day, R., Ganz, P. A., and Costantino, J. P. (2001). Tamoxifen and depression: more evidence from the National Surgical Adjuvant Breast and Bowel Project's Breast Cancer Prevention (P-1) randomized study. *Journal of the National Cancer Institute*, **93**, 1615–1623.

Day, R., Ganz, P., Costantino, J. P., Cronin, W. M., Wickerham, D. L., and Fisher, B. (1999). Health-related quality of life and tamoxifen in breast cancer prevention: A report from the National Surgical Adjuvant Breast and Bowel P-1 study. *Journal of Clinical Oncology*, **17**, 2659–2669.

Detmar, S. B., Muller, M. J., Schornagel, J. H., Wever, L. D., and Aaronson, N. K. (2002). Health-related quality-of-life assessments and patient-physician communication: a randomized controlled trial. *Journal of the American Medical Association*, **288**, 3027–3034.

Earlam, S., Glover, C., Fordy, C., Burke, D., and Allen-Mersh, T. G. (1996). Relation between tumour size, quality of life, and survival in patients with colorectal liver metastases. *Journal of Clinical Oncology*, **14**, 171–175.

Eton, D. T., Fairclough, D. L., Cella, D., Yount, S. E., Bonomi, P., Johnson, D. H., and Eastern Cooperative Oncology Group (2003). Early change in patient-reported health during lung cancer chemotherapy predicts clinical outcomes beyond those predicted by baseline report: results from Eastern Cooperative Oncology Group Study 5592. *Journal of Clinical Oncology*, **21**, 1536–1543.

Efficace, F., Bottomley, A., and Osoba, D., *et al.* (2003). Beyond the development of health-related quality-of-life (HRQoL) measures: a checklist for evaluating HRQoL outcomes in cancer clinical trials – does evaluating HRQoL in prostate cancer research inform clinical decision-making? *Journal of Clinical Oncology,* **21,** 3502–3511.

Fairclough, D. L. (2002). *Design and Analysis of Quality of Life Studies in Clinical Trials.* Boca Raton: Chapman & Hall/CRC.

Fayers, P. and Machin, D. (2000). *Quality of Life: Assessment, Analysis and Interpretation.* Chichester: J Wiley & Sons.

Gabrilove, J. L., Cleeland, C. S., Livingston, R. B., Sarakhan, B., Winer, E., and Einhorn, L. H. (2001). Clinical evaluation of once-weekly dosing of epoeitin alfa in chemotherapy patients: improvements in hemoglobin and quality of life are similar to three-times-weekly dosing. *Journal of Clinical Oncology,* **19,** 2875–2882.

Ganz, P. A., Lee, J. J., and Siau, J. (1991). Quality of life assessment. An independent prognostic variable for survival in lung cancer. *Cancer,* **67,** 3131–3135.

Guyatt, G., Osoba, D., and Wu, A., *et al.* (2002). Methods to explain the clinical significance of health status measures. *Mayo Clinic Proceedings,* **77:** 371–383.

Goodwin, D. M., Higginson, I. J., Myers, K., Douglas, H. R., and Normand, C. E. (2003). Effectiveness of palliative day care in improving pain, symptom control, and quality of life. *Journal of Pain and Symptom Management,* **25,** 202–212.

Gralla, R. J., Osoba, D., and Kris, M. G., *et al.* (1999). Recommendations for the use of antiemetics: evidence-based, clinical practice guidelines. American Society of Clinical Oncology. *Journal of Clinical Oncology,* **17,** 2971–2994.

Guyatt, G. H., Veldhuzen Van Zanten, S. J. O., and Feeny, D. H., *et al.* (1989). Measuring quality of life in clinical trials: a taxonomy and review. *Canadian Medical Association Journal,* **140,** 1441–1448.

Jaeschke, R., Guyatt, G. D., and Cook, D. (1992). Quality of life instruments in the evaluation of new drugs. *PharmacoEconomics,* **1,** 84–94.

Klepstad, P., Hilton, P., Moen, H., Fougner, B., Borchgrevink, P. C., and Kaasa, S. (2002). Self-reports are not related to objective assessment of cognitive function and sedation in patients with cancer pain admitted to a palliative care unit. *Palliative Medicine,* **16,** 513–519.

Kornblith, A. B., Herndon, J. E., 2nd, and Silverman, L. R., *et al.* (2002). Impact of azacytidine on the quality of life of patients with myelodysplastic syndrome treated in a randomized phase III trial: a Cancer and Leukemia Group B study. *Journal of Clinical Oncology,* **20,** 2441–2452.

Langendijk, J. A., Ten Velde, G. P. M., and Aaronson, N. K., *et al.* (2000). Quality of life after palliative radiotherapy in non-small-cell lung cancer: A prospective study. *International Journal of Radiation Oncology Biology and Physics,* **47,** 149–155.

Littlewood, T. J., Bajetta, E., and Nortier, J. W. R., *et al.* (2001). Effects of epoeitin alfa on hematologic parameters and quality of life in cancer patients receiving non-platinum chemotherapy: results of a randomized, double-blind, placebo-controlled trial. *Journal of Clinical Oncology,* **19,** 2865–2874.

Lee, C. W. and Chi, K. N. (2000). The standard of reporting of health-related quality of life in clinical cancer trials. *Journal of Clinical Epidemiology,* **53,** 451–458.

Lo, R. S., Woo, J., and Zhoc, K. C., *et al.* (2002). Quality of life of palliative care patients in the last two weeks of life. *Journal of Pain and Symptom Management,* **24,** 388–397.

Loprinzi, C. L., Kuross, S. A., and O'Fallon, J. R., *et al.* (1994). Randomized placebo-controlled evaluation of hydrazine sulfate in patients with advanced colorectal cancer. *Journal of Clinical Oncology,* **12,** 1121–1125.

LoRusso, P. M., Herbst, R. S., and Rischin, D., *et al.* (2003). Improvements in quality life and disease-related symptoms in phase I trials of the selective oral epidermal growth factor receptor tyrosine kinase inhibitor ZD1839 in non-small lung cancer and other solid tumors. *Clinical Cancer Research*, **9**, 2040–2048.

Lubeck, D. P., Grossfeld, G. D., and Carroll, P. R. (2002). A review of measurement of patient preferences for treatment outcomes after prostate cancer. *Urology*, **60**, 72–7 (3 suppl 1); discussion 77–78.

McMillan, S. C. and Weitzner, M. A. (2003). Methodologic issues in collecting data from debilitated patients with cancer near the end of life. *Oncology Nursing Forum*, **30**, 123–129.

Moskowitz, R. W., Sunshine, A., Brugger, A., Lefkowith, J. B., Zhao, W. W., and Geis, G. S. (2003). American Pain Society pain questionnaire and other pain measures in the assessment of osteoarthritis pain: a pooled analysis of three celecoxib pivotal studies. *American Journal of Therapeutics*, **10**, 12–20.

Murray, N., Livingston, R. B., and Shepherd, F. A., *et al.* (1999). Randomized study of CODE versus alternating CAV/EP for extensive-stage small-cell lung cancer: An intergroup study of the National Cancer Institute of Canada Clinical Trials Group and the Southwest Oncology Group. *Journal of Clinical Oncology*, **17**, 2300–2308.

Osoba, D. (2002). A taxonomy of the uses of health-related quality of life (HRQoL) instruments in cancer care and the clinical meaningfulness of the results. *Medical Care, 2002*, (40), 31–8 (suppl III).

Osoba, D., Aaronson, N., and Till, J. E. (1991). A practical guide for selecting quality-of-life measures in clinical trials and practice. In D. Osoba (ed.) *Effect of Cancer on Quality of Life*, pp 89–104. Boca Raton: CRC Press.

Osoba, D., Brada, M., Prados, M. D., and Yung, W. K. A. (2000). Effect of disease burden on health-related quality of life in patients with malignant gliomas. *Neuro-Oncology*, **2**, 221–228.

Osoba, D., Brada, M., Yung, W. K. A., and Prados, M. (2000a). Health-related quality of life in patients with anaplastic astrocytoma during treatment with temozolomide. *European Journal of Cancer*, **36**, 1788–1795.

Osoba, D., Brada, M., Yung, W. K. A., and Prados, M. (2000b). Health-related quality of life in patients treated with temozolomide versus procarbazine for recurrent glioblastoma multiforme. *Journal of Clinical Oncology*, **18**, 1481–1491.

Osoba, D., Slamon, D. J., Burchmore, M., and Murphy, M. (2002). Effects on quality of life of combined trastuzumab and chemotherapy in women with metastatic breast cancer. *Journal of Clinical Oncology*, **20**, 3106–3113.

Osoba, D., Tannock, I. F., Ernst, D. S., and Neville, A. J. (1999). Health-related quality of life in men with metastatic prostate cancer treated with prednisone alone or mitoxantrone and prednisone. *Journal of Clinical Oncology*, **17**, 1654–1663.

Osoba, D., Zee, B., Warr, D., Latreille, J., Kaizer, L., and Pater, J. (1997a). Effect of postchemotherapy nausea and vomiting on health-related quality of life. *Supportive Care in Cancer*, **5**, 307–313.

Raynauld, J. P., Torrance, G. W., and Band, P. A. *et al.* (2002). A prospective, randomized, pragmatic, health outcomes trial evaluating the incorporation of hylan G-F 20 into the treatment paradigm for patients with knee osteoarthritis (Part 1 of 2): clinical results. *Osteoarthritis Cartilage*, **10**, 506–517.

Rowland, K. M. Jr. Loprinzi, C. L., and Shaw, E. G., *et al.* (1996). Randomized double-blind placebo-controlled trial of cisplatin and etoposide plus megestrol acetate in extensive-stage small-cell lung cancer: A North Central Cancer Treatment Group Study. *Journal of Clinical Oncology*, **14**, 135–141.

Roychowdhury, D. F., Hayden, A., and Liepa, A. M. (2003). Health-related quality-of-life parameters as independent prognostic factors in advanced or metastatic bladder cancer. *Journal of Clinical Oncology*, **21**, 673–678.

Sanders, C., Egger, M., and Donovan, J., *et al.* (1998). Reporting on quality of life in randomised controlled trials: bibliographic study. *British Medical Journal*, **317**, 1191–1194.

Schunnemann, H. J., Griffith, L., Stubbing, D., Goldstein, R., and Guyatt, G. H. (2003). A clinical trial to evaluate the measurement properties of 2 direct preference instruments administered with and without hypothetical marker states. *Medical Decision Making*, **23**, 140–149.

Siderowf, A., Ravina, B., and Glick, H. A. (2002). Preference-based quality-of-life in patients with Parkinson's disease. *Neurology*, **59**, 103–108.

Simons, J. P. F. H. A., Aaronson, N. K., and Vansteenkiste, J. F., *et al.* (1996) Effects of medroxyprogesterone acetate on appetite, weight, and quality of life in advanced-stage non-hormone-sensitive cancer: a placebo-controlled multicentre study. *Journal of Clinical Oncology*, **14**, 1077–1084.

Steinhauser, K. E., Bosworth, H. B., and Clipp, E. C., *et al.* (2002). Initial assessment of a new instrument to measure quality of life at the end of life. *Journal of Palliative Medicine*, **5**, 829–841.

Sullivan, S. D., Lew, D. P., Devine, E. B., Hakim, Z., Reiber, G. E., and Veenstra, D. L. (2002). Health state preference assessment in diabetic peripheral neuropathy. *PharmacoEconomics*, **20**, 1079–1089.

Sutherland, H. J. and Till, J. E. (1993). Quality of life assessments and levels of decision making: differentiating objectives. *Quality of Life Research*, **2**, 221–226.

Taenzer, P., Bultz, B. D., and Carlson, L. E., *et al.* (2000). Impact of computerized quality of life screening on physician behaviour and patient satisfaction in lung cancer patients. *Psycho-Oncology*, **9**: 203–213.

Tannock, I. F., Osoba, D., and Stockler, M. R., *et al.* (1996). Chemotherapy with mitoxantrone plus prednisone or prednisone alone for symptomatic hormone-resistant prostate cancer; A Canadian randomized trial with palliative end points. *Journal of Clinical Oncology*, **14**, 1756–1764.

Trail, M., Nelson, N. D., Van, J. N., Appel, S. H., and Lai, E. C. (2003). A study comparing patients with amyotrophic lateral sclerosis and their caregivers on measures of quality of life, depression, and their attitudes toward treatment options. *Journal of Neurological Science*, **209**, 79–85.

Van Dieten, H. E., Perez, R. S., and van Tulder, M. W., *et al.* (2003). Cost effectiveness and cost utility of acetylcysteine versus dimethyl sulfoxide for reflex sympathetic dystrophy. *Pharmacoeconomics*, **21**, 139–148.

Velikova, G., Brown, J. M., Smith, A. B., and Selby, P. J. (2002). Computer-based quality of life questionnaires may contribute to doctor-patient interactions in oncology. *British Journal of Cancer*, **86**, 51–59.

Ware, J. E., Kosinski, M., and Keller, S. D. (1994). *SF-36 Physical and Mental Health Summary Scales: A User's Manual*. Boston, MA: The Health Institute, New England Medical Center.

Weisbord, S. D., Carmody, S. S., and Bruns, F. J., *et al.* (2003). Symptom burden, quality of life, advance care planning and the potential value of palliative care in severely ill haemodialysis patients. *Nephrology Dialysis Transplantation*, **18**, 1345–1352.

Yung, W. K., Albright, R. E., and Olson, J., *et al.* (2000). A phase II study of temozolomide vs. procarbazine in patients with glioblastoma multiforme at first relapse. *British Journal of Cancer*, **83**, 588–593.

Response shift: you know it's there but how do you capture it? Challenges for the next phase of research

Carolyn Schwartz, Mirjam Sprangers and Peter Fayers

Introduction

Health is not a given. Whether confronted with sudden or gradual changes in health, individuals must accommodate and adapt to these changed conditions. There is an increasing recognition that when people experience changes in health, they may change their internal standards, their values, and/or their conceptualization of health-related quality of life (HRQoL).

These 'response shifts' make comparisons over time difficult to interpret. For example, in the context of treatment evaluations, response shifts may attenuate estimates of treatment effects if patients adapt to treatment toxicities or disease progression over time. Consequently, patient adaptation to treatment toxicities or to improvements in health may result in an inaccurate assessment of quality of life over time. Although toxicity to which patients accommodate is arguably of less concern than toxicity to which they cannot adapt, differences in quality of life across treatment arms may also be obscured when response shift affects the treatment groups differentially despite randomization (Bernhard *et al.* 1999; Sprangers and Schwartz 1999a).

While response shift is not new from a clinical (Wilson 1999) or intuitive (Breetvelt and Van Dam 1991) perspective, its recent application to QoL research has led to new methodological and theoretical developments. The study of response shift alerts the researcher to the underlying and unmeasured forces that can influence the HRQoL findings, and emphasizes the need to look beyond the surface of measurement in longitudinal research. The purpose of this chapter is to review briefly the extant literature and why it is important to measure response shift, to examine the magnitude and clinical significance of response shift, and to explore the competing explanations and current areas of confusion related to the construct. A more comprehensive discussion of the role and importance of response shift is presented by chapters in Schwartz and Sprangers (2000).

Background on response shift

The concept of response shift has its foundation in research on educational training interventions (Howard and Dailey 1979) and management science (Golembiewski *et al.* 1976). Howard and Dailey defined response shift in terms of changes in internal standards of measurement. Refining the definition of response shift, Golembiewski and colleagues delineated a typology of change that distinguished actual change (alpha change) from changes in internal standards (beta change) and meaning (gamma change). Changes in values were inherent to Golembiewski's description of reconceptualization, but were not explicitly seen as a separate component. These concepts led to the working definition proposed by Sprangers and Schwartz (1999a): Response shift refers to a change in the meaning of one's self-evaluation of a target construct as a result of (a) a change in the respondent's internal standards of measurement (scale recalibration); (b) a change in the respondent's values (reprioritization); or (c) a redefinition of the target construct (reconceptualization). Reprioritization is thus an added explicit component of this definition.

Why measure response shift?

Assessment of response shift is important in HRQoL research when evaluating change over time, examining cross-sectional differences between groups, or exploring psychological processes. Special cases of each of these contexts are described briefly below.

Change over time

A major reason for studying response shift is that it could lead to inaccurate estimates of treatment effects when analysing *clinical trials*. Response shift might lead to an underestimation of the true effect if there were different patterns of response shifts between treatment groups, possibly leading to false negative conclusions (Oort *et al.* in press). It might also lead to differential recalibration by treatment arm (Bernhard *et al.* 1999). There is clearly a need to clarify the impact of recalibration response shift in clinical trials research. Additionally, response shifts may compromise *cost utility evaluations* if they have a substantial impact on utility scores; response shift may distort the reported changes in HRQoL (in either or both treatment arms of a trial), and any attempt to combine HRQoL with cost will be flawed.

Cross-sectional differences

Many attempts at determining the '*minimally clinical significant change*' of HRQoL outcomes are based on asking patients whether they have noted any change in their condition, and how important any such change is to them. Their answers are then compared to the past and present assessments. The tacit assumption is that no response shift has occurred between past and present assessment times.

Response shift may also explain the differences commonly observed between patients' *self-assessments* and *proxy assessments*. Although a proxy may be sensitive to a patient's response shift, and may consciously or subconsciously attempt to make a corresponding allowance, response shift could account for part of the substantial discrepancies between patient and proxy. Further, it is possible that proxies themselves undergo response shift in their judgements, and recalibrate or reprioritize the importance of issues.

Insight into psychological processes

When a nurse or clinician talks about 'coping' or '*adaptation to illness*', they are referring to cognitive, affective or behavioural mechanisms that may lead to response shifts. Many patient management interventions are thus attempting to induce response shifts, either as their main objective or as an adjunct to active therapy. However, multiple forms of response shift may in fact be occurring, and should be distinguished and evaluated. In addition, a better understanding of the response-shift processes may lead to more effective ways of helping patients to adapt to illness.

Response shift has also been described as one type of *placebo effect*, in which specific psychological mechanisms lead to changes in a patient's self-assessed health in the absence of known biological and physiological effects (Wilson 1999). Conversely self-assessed health can remain stable in the presence of changes in biological and physiological health. There are several reasons for using placebos in clinical trials, but one aim might be to minimize the impact of different expectations between the patient groups that could have an independent effect on QoL. Use of placebos cannot remove response shift, but it makes it more plausible that the expectations would be similar in the two groups. It would not, however, mitigate the differential response shifts due to different effects or side effects of the treatment arms.

Current methods for assessing response shift

A range of response shift detection procedures have been used, some of which originated from management or educational sciences, others from the area of HRQoL. Recent empirical work in HRQoL has investigated response shift using design approaches (Sprangers *et al.* 1999), preference-based techniques (Lenert *et al.* 1999; Schwartz *et al.* 2002), individualized approaches (O'Boyle *et al.* in Schwartz and Sprangers 2000), qualitative methods (Rapkin, in Schwartz and Sprangers 2000), and statistical approaches (Oort *et al.* in press). A brief review of the most widely used or promising methods will follow; Schwartz and Sprangers (2000) provide a more comprehensive account of some of these methods.

The most widely used design approach for assessing response shift in HRQoL research is the retrospective pretest–post-test ('then-test') design to assess changes in internal standards (Howard *et al.* 1979). This method asks respondents at follow-up to re-evaluate their baseline level of functioning. The comparison of baseline and retrospective-pretest (then-test) measures changes in the respondent's internal standards. Since the follow-up assessment and the then-test are completed at the same time, it is assumed that respondents use the same internal standards when answering items. The comparison between then-test and follow-up indicates actual change. This approach has been used to investigate response shifts among people with cancer, people with hearing impairment and people with multiple sclerosis (Sprangers *et al.* 1999; Joore *et al.* 2002; Schwartz *et al.* 2004a). Despite its wide use, the scientific study of its psychometric characteristics in HRQoL applications is relatively undeveloped. For example, the validity of its assumption (i.e. similar standards at follow-up and then-test) has not been established, although current efforts are underway to investigate this assumption (Oort *et al.* in press). Further, recent research has suggested that then-test scores reflect both recall bias (i.e. memory distortion) and recalibration (Schwartz *et al.* 2004a). Oort *et al.* found convergence between results of the then-test and structural equation modelling approaches to assessing response shift. These findings suggest that recall bias does not invalidate the then-test, although it is likely to lead to measurement with a substantial amount of noise.

Preference-based approaches are another family of methods that can be used to assess response shift, with a focus on reprioritization and reconceptualization. Lenert *et al.* (1999) used utility measures and demonstrated that people in poor health valued intermediate health states almost as much as near-normal states, whereas patients in good health valued intermediate states nearly as little as poor health states. This cross-sectional study inferred response shift, but did not assess it directly since it did not follow patients over time. Schwartz *et al.* (2002) conducted a randomized clinical trial of an advance care planning intervention for ambulatory geriatric patients. Using a standard treatment preference measure to look at preference change, they reported that participants of the advance care planning intervention reprioritized their values regarding the desirability of life-sustaining treatments, as compared to the control group. Additionally, the participants and not the controls were found to reconceptualize HRQoL in terms of how tolerable they would find poor health states, as measured by a Beliefs and Values questionnaire (Pearlman *et al.* 1999). These preference-based methods can be relatively straightforward to include and interpret in longitudinal research, but further research is needed to document their psychometric robustness.

For those researchers who seek to understand more of the meaning beneath the numbers, individualized and qualitative methods hold the most promise. The most popular individualized measure appears to be the Schedule for the Evaluation of Individual Quality of Life (SEIQoL), as described in Chapter 4.1. Respondents nominate the five most relevant domains to their HRQoL. They then assess their current status within each domain using a visual analogue scale with anchors ranging from 'best possible' to 'worst possible'. The SEIQoL generates an overall index that summarizes satisfaction with and relative importance of each domain. Although not the original intent of this measure, Schwartz and Sprangers (1999) proposed adapting it as follows to measure response shift. One can repeat the described exercises at subsequent assessment points and compare the described domains. A change in values (reprioritization) would be suggested by changes in the weight/order of the domains, whereas a change in conceptualization would be suggested by changes in the content of the domains (O'Boyle *et al.* in Schwartz and Sprangers, 2000). Although the SEIQOL has the advantage of being able to assess these aspects of response shift, it can be challenging to compare intra- or inter-individual data because the domain content changes between assessments within and across individuals.

Qualitative approaches involve open-ended interviews, in contrast to the semi-structured interviews that often characterize individualized approaches. An example of a qualitative measure is the Idiographic Assessment of Personal Goals (Rapkin and Fischer 1992). This semi-structured interview investigates respondents' goals and self-evaluation of the goals according to a series of dimensions, such as level of effort needed to pursue the goal. Reconceptualization response shift would be evident in the change in goal content from one interview to the next, whereas reprioritization would be reflected by a reordering of goals over time (Rapkin, in Schwartz and Sprangers, 2000). This qualitative measure proved amenable to multivariate quantitative analysis in examining the impact of illness in personal goal content among persons with AIDS.

Finally, there are promising statistical methods for response shift research. These methods build on covariance analytic techniques originally developed for response shift research in education and management science, taking advantage of the substantial technological advances of the past two decades. Recently Oort *et al.* (in press) applied item response theory (IRT) and factor analysis (FA), using a detection procedure based on structural equation modelling (SEM). They interpreted reconceptualization response shift as variation in factor loading *patterns*; reprioritization response shift as significant changes in factor loading *values*; and recalibration response shift as significant changes in the specific factor *means*. These three changes are among 11 types of change that can theoretically be identified; depending on circumstances, the detectable number is smaller. This approach has been found to be useful in detecting all three types of response shifts in longitudinal data on cancer patients undergoing invasive surgery. Recalibration response shift was found to lead to an underestimation of the true deterioration in physical health. Similar results were obtained from both the IRT and then-test approaches. While this technique requires further testing, it has the advantage that collection of additional HRQoL data is not required.

Clinical significance of response shift

To date, the published research evaluating response shift has sought to document whether the phenomenon exists at all, rather than focusing on the magnitude of the effect.

Table 4.4.1 Clinical significance of response shift effects in published studies with n >100

Response Shift Method(s) Used	Type of Study	Patient Population	Reference	Outcome Assessed	Effect Size
Then test	Longitudinal observational study	Cancer patients receiving radiotherapy (n = 199)	Visser et al. (2000)	Recalibration response shift in fatigue.	+0.18[a] (P <0.01)
Then test	Randomized controlled trial	Colon cancer undergoing adjuvant chemotherapy (n = 132)	Bernhard et al. (2001)	Recalibration response shift in subjective health in all treatment arms.	−0.25[a] (P <0.001)
Then test	Longitudinal observational study	Stroke patients (n = 144) and caregiver controls (n = 50)	Ahmed et al. (in press)	Response shift in VAS of the EQ-5D. 10% lower retrospective rating in stroke patients as compared to controls.	Not given.
Then-test Ideographic assessment of personal goals	Longitudinal observation study	Prostate cancer patients (n = 166)	Lepore and Eton (in Schwartz and Sprangers 2000)	Recalibration response shift in social-emotional QoL and buffering effect of reprioritization response shift.	ES not given but significant effects reported for recalibration (P <0.001) and reprioritization (P <0.05)

Ideographic assessment of personal goals	Longitudinal observation study	AIDS patients (n = 140)	Rapkin (2000)	Reprioritization response shift explained variance in global well-being, mental functioning, and pain.	ES not given but significant effects reported for reprioritization (P <0.001, 0.01, and 0.05).
Preference change	Psychometric study with retest	Seriously ill patients (n = 168)	Schwartz et al. (2004a)	Reprioritization of preference for life-sustaining treatments.	+0.25[b]
Statistical: structural equation modelling	Longitudinal observational study	Cancer patients undergoing invasive surgery (n = 170)	Oort et al. (in press)	Reconceptualization of physical and mental functional status.	0.16 and − 0.48 ES; Accounting for RS changed size of true change in physical health from medium to large.
Statistical: General Linear Model[e]	Longitudinal case-control study	Low-risk breast cancer patients (n = 462); matched controls (n = 604)	Groenvold et al. (1999)	Differences in the prevalence of anxiety and depression.	+0.17[c] (P <.021) +0.21[c] (P <.001)

[a] Standardized response mean was not given by authors, but was estimated from their published data.

[b] Effect size = (Then-test − Pre-test) divided by average SD of Then-test and Pre-test.

[c] Effect size = Difference between patients and general population, divided by SD of population.

[d] Based on Oort's typology of change (Oort, in press).

[e] Mean scores were compared using ANCOVA (age as covariate) as well as using a non-parametric partial gamma with age grouped in 10-year intervals, to compare the proportion of cases defined as clinically anxious or depressed.

Although there is already ample recognition of the importance of response shift, its clinical significance is only beginning to be investigated rigorously. As a preliminary step to address the clinical significance of response shift phenomena, we reviewed published QoL literature on response shift. This included 22 empirical papers, of which only three were randomized trials. In the interest of space, we present summaries of the longitudinal studies with samples larger than 100 (Table 4.4.1). Effect size refers (ES) to the mean difference divided by the standard deviation. Not all authors provided the ES, in which case it was estimated; the exact form of ES used is defined in the footnote to the table, and varied according to what data were available in each publication. The median ES for all studies was 0.25, and 0.18 for studies with n>100. Additionally, observational studies had a slightly larger ES, with a median of 0.39 for all studies and 0.20 for studies with n>100. The ES for randomized controlled trials was 0.25 for all studies, but −0.25 for the one study with n>100. The direction of the ES is not consistent across studies (i.e. some find a positive ES and others find a contradictory negative value).

The limitations of this review should be noted. These estimates are based on a small number of studies using varying outcomes tools and response shift methods. We could not correct for multiple comparisons made in the original papers, from which only statistically significant results were reported. The item characteristics of the various tools used and of the then-test are not known, although we have standardized the metric of the comparisons so that higher scores indicate better functioning. Thus this informal review only provides an indication of the possible effect sizes. It does suggest, however, that response shift may play a significant role in QoL research, and that the direction of this shift may be different across studies. Future research should adopt a standard of reporting ES, so that there is a standardized metric for assessing the clinical significance of the phenomenon.

Theoretical developments

Proposed models

Sprangers and Schwartz (1999a) proposed a theoretical model where response shift is the result of a catalyst and the interaction of 'antecedents' and 'mechanisms'. Whereas antecedents refer to stable characteristics of the individual, mechanisms represent the behavioural, cognitive and affective processes that adjust to the change in health state. The interaction of antecedents and mechanisms leads to response shift, and affects perceived HRQoL. Lepore and Eton (in Schwartz and Sprangers 2000) tested this model in prostate cancer patients, and found that response shift moderated (buffered) rather than suppressed the impact of changes in health and HRQoL. Other work testing this model is in progress. Although useful for hypothesizing relationships among key constructs relevant to QoL assessment, the model presents some problems of logical circularity.

Rapkin and Schwartz (2004) extend the above model by adding appraisal variables and clinical indicators of change (e.g. clinician judgment, performance tests, or family caregiver ratings). They define the following four appraisal parameters: (1) induction of a frame of reference; (2) recall and sampling of salient experiences; (3) application of standards of comparison used to appraise experiences; and (4) combination of appraisals using a subjective algorithm to arrive at an HRQoL rating. They propose that changes in appraisal reflect response shifts. Response shift is inferred when the discrepancy between expected and observed changes in perceived HRQoL is explained by changes in appraisal. By measuring appraisal and inferring response shift, this model avoids the circularity of defining mechanisms and response shift similarly. It also yields testable hypotheses about partitioning variance in HRQoL change scores, and is a promising avenue for empirical research.

These theories provide but a starting point for response shift research, and lead to more questions than they can answer. For example, the idea that health state changes are catalysts of response shift does not indicate when and how often one should search for response shift. Is response shift likely immediately after diagnosis of threatening illness? One week later? One year later? If response shifts lead to a successive series of new thresholds of internal standards, new prioritizations of values, and modified conceptualizations of HRQoL, then we need to know what signals the next 'window' for a given meaning of HRQoL, and how long it will last. Since these windows are likely to be specific to the individual, we need to know which methods and designs are most effective at capturing these patterns. A further question is how big the health state change needs to be to lead to response shifts. Would episodic illness patterns lead to different thresholds at different times, depending on whether the patient is in remission or having an exacerbation? Finally, health state changes and response shifts do not always go together: one may occur without the other. What are the necessary conditions or person characteristics for response shifts with and without health state changes? These questions are challenges for the next phase of research. At present, not detecting response shift may be due to not recognizing this successive series of 'windows' and thus not measuring at the right time(s). A better understanding of what constitutes sufficient health state change to be a catalyst of response shift will facilitate the design and interpretation of longitudinal studies.

Is it the 'emperor's new clothes' or not?

Response shift is a phenomenon recognized by many clinicians in their daily practice, leading some social scientists to wonder whether response shift is merely a new umbrella-term for familiar phenomena that can better be studied in their own right (e.g. coping, adaptation). Others, however, wonder whether response shift is one of the most important new concepts helping us to understand HRQoL assessment, especially as it influences the measurement characteristics of standard tools. While a decade ago response shift was a rare term in HRQoL research, it now seems to have evolved into a buzz word that is often used in circumstances where contradictory 'findings we do not understand' are described. If we allow response shift to encompass 'everything', it has lost its meaning, and loses its potential to further HRQoL science. Therefore alternative hypotheses for unexplained shifts should be considered prior to labelling them as 'response shifts'.

Implicit theories of stability and change propose that when people are asked to recall past events, their judgement is based on an '*implicit theory*' in which an evaluation of their current state is modified according to their perception of the change that has taken place (Ross 1989). Thus patients may in effect say to themselves, 'I have pain now, but it was much worse before and so my previous pain must have been xxx.' Accordingly, implicit theories can guide or misguide any response to a retrospective question when a subject has an imperfect knowledge of the prior state (Norman 2003). We suggest that the same implicit-theory processes described by Ross could also determine the response to prospective questions, and could account for the same pattern of HRQoL scores as response shift but without affecting changes in internal standards, values, or meaning of HRQoL (see Figure 4.4.1). If, however, these implicit theories

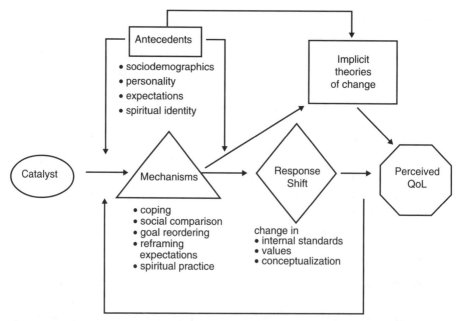

Fig. 4.4.1 Implicit theories as alternative explanations for HRQoL. If implicit theories have an independent effect on HRQoL, then they would not influence response shift. In contrast, if they influence one's internal standards, values or conceptualization of QoL, then they might act as antecedents or mechanisms in the Sprangers and Schwartz (1999a) model of response shift and QoL.

cause response shifts, they are not alternative explanations but rather antecedents or mechanisms of response shift. Furthermore, it is possible that perception of change may itself also be subject to response shift – for example, reprioritization might result in altered perception of the magnitude of change. Future research should test competing hypotheses regarding implicit theories.

Table 4.4.2 shows how examples of response shift methods could be confounded by implicit theories. Implicit theories can play a role in any prospective or retrospective self-report tool, and also in response shift measures. Prospective methods are particularly susceptible to implicit theories affecting processes such as *expectations* (e.g. about the course of one's disease), *denial* (e.g. about health state deterioration), and *impression management* (e.g. playing the 'good patient'). Impression management may be particularly prevalent in measures that require an interviewer (e.g. SEIQoL and Idiographic Assessment of Personal Goals), and may also play some role in treatment preference assessment if patients endorse the treatments advocated by their health care provider. Filtering information about oneself to try to consciously or unconsciously impress others can influence self-reports. *Effort justification* may also affect prospective measurement when respondents choose a response at follow-up that reinforces the effort invested during the interim (e.g. enduring a toxic treatment). Similarly, *cognitive dissonance* may affect a follow-up response when patients choose an answer that is consonant with their behaviour or cognition in an effort to appear consistent.

Retrospective measures such as the then-test are prone to all of the implicit theories that affect prospective measures, as well as *recall bias*. In QoL research, recall bias refers to memory distortion (in contrast with epidemiological research, in which it can be a bias in recall because of the respondents' increased awareness of the research object). If memory distortion is random, it only increases the error variance in measurement and would reduce statistical power but not result in bias, because there is no reason why it should be in a certain direction. Bias would, however, result if respondents cannot accurately recall what was answered previously, but use a rule to reconstruct or fill in memory gaps as proposed by implicit theories of change. There is ample evidence that memory is susceptible to distortion (e.g. Herrmann 1995), and thus methods founded on recall are suspect and may fail to evaluate the target construct. Schwartz *et al.* (2004a) examined then-test responses over extended follow-up (i.e. five years) and found that the then-test captured recall bias along with recalibration response shift. Ahmed *et al.* (in press) found similar effects of recall bias among stroke patients over a shorter follow-up (i.e. 6 and 24 weeks). Both effort justification and cognitive dissonance responding are likely to affect then-test responses, but their effect on other measures of response shift is less clear.

The phenomena in Table 4.4.2 are not all mutually exclusive, and may not be universally considered to be 'implicit theories'. In the older psychological literature there are many more labels ('self-fulfilling prophecy', 'demand characteristics', 'social desirability', 'response sets' and 'response styles', etc.) to describe phenomena that interfere with the

Table 4.4.2 Implicit theories possibly affecting response shift methods

Response Shift Method Example	Response Shift Type Assessed	Implicit Theories				Impression Management	Effort Justification	Cognitive Dissonance Responding
		Recall Bias	Expectations	Denial				
Prospective								
Preference change	Reprioritization		✓	✓		✓✓		
SEIQoL	Reprioritization and Reconceptualization		✓	✓		✓✓		
Idiographic assessment of personal goals	Reprioritization and Reconceptualization		✓	✓		✓✓		
IRT on data collected prospectively	Recalibration Reprioritization Reconceptualization		✓	✓		✓		
Retrospective								
Then-test	Recalibration	✓	✓	✓		✓	✓	✓

validity of self-report measures. Highlighting these phenomena might make one think that it is impossible to measure anything through self-report – a conclusion that we do not endorse. Rather, we propose that a rigorous consideration of all explanations is necessary for the growth of the field. Future research would benefit from the systematic investigation of the relative importance of these implicit theory explanations as compared to response shift theory explanations.

Definitional confusion: different understandings of response shift

When talking with colleagues about response shift, we are always struck by the diverse meanings associated with the term. Although the conceptual definitions proposed by Golembiewski *et al.* (1976) and Howard and Dailey (1979) are subsumed under the Sprangers and Schwartz model, the operational definitions and detection procedures vary widely. This diversity is appropriate in the exploratory phases of response shift research, and triangulation of different methods may help the field mature. Referring to different ideas with the same name can, however, lead to miscommunication and confusion.

Table 4.4.3 summarizes the principal interpretations of the term 'response shift'. First, some people consider response shift to be a *bias* that needs to be corrected for, whereas to others it is a *meaningful change* worth investigating in its own right. Second, some consider it a *measurement characteristic* whereas to others it is a *subject characteristic*. Third, response shift is considered by some to be an ad hoc *explanation* of counterintuitive empirical findings, whereas others conceive it as a *phenomenon* that can be scientifically studied. Fourth, some label *temporary* changes in internal standards, values, and conceptualization as response shift, whereas others reserve the term for *long lasting* and relatively permanent changes. Fifth, some consider response shift to be only catalysed by an *event* whereas others see response shift resulting from the mere *passage of time*. Finally, according to some the events *unrelated to health* changes may lead to response shifts, whereas others only acknowledge *health-related* events as inducing response shifts. These dimensions, which are not mutually exclusive or exhaustive, are proposed to stimulate thought about the conceptual and operational definitions of response shift.

Epilogue

Response shift is a phenomenon that appeals to many people, but there is little consensus on if and how it can be made 'visible'. An analogy that comes to mind is a dolphin swimming in the open ocean, and every once in a while jumping up out of the water to breathe. One can know that the dolphin is there, and witness when it jumps out of the water, but knowing when and where to look exceeds our current understanding. We suggest that current priorities for research are to determine what constitutes a response

Table 4.4.3 Definitional clarifications of response shift exemplified in the context of clinical trials

Dimension of cross-talk

Dimension of cross-talk		
Bias vs. meaningful change	If one is only interested in the 'pure' effects of a treatment, then response shift confounds treatment effect estimates, and thus needs to be adjusted to yield distilled treatment effects.	If one believes it is worthwhile to understand which treatments or toxicities are most amenable to adaptation, then response shift is informative and thus worth assessing for its own merit.
Measurement vs. subject characteristics	Response shift may occur as a result of measures that are invalid (e.g. undefined standard of comparison) and unreliable (e.g. item too global to elicit same construct at retest).	Patients may change their internal standards, values, or conceptualizations of HRQoL as a result of treatment-related benefits or toxicities.
Explanation vs. phenomenon	Response shift is one of the *ad hoc* explanations (along with implicit theories) that can account for paradoxical trial results (e.g. stable reported HRQoL despite substantial disease progression).	Response shift can be measured and therefore scientifically studied in a clinical trial.
Temporary vs. long-lasting	Short-lived changes in internal standards, values or conceptualization can be induced by the clinical research context (e.g. modifying the order of questionnaires or administering the questionnaire along with different questionnaires at different time points).	Only relatively permanent changes constitute 'response shifts,' and any short-term changes in internal standards, values, or conceptualization are considered to be noise. How long is 'permanent' and how short is 'short-term' are yet to be defined.
Event vs. passage of time	Response shift is catalysed by treatment and other real events that occur during the clinical trial (e.g. disease progression).	The mere passage of time without apparent salient events is sufficient for stimulating response shift, even among no-treatment control group participants.
Unrelated to health vs. related to health	Other events (e.g. losing one's job) that took place during but were unrelated to the clinical trial might have led to response shifts that affect HRQoL answers.	Only health-related events occurring during the clinical trial are relevant to response shift in HRQoL.

shift catalyst (i.e. when and where to look), and to explore how often and how long one should measure. Validating existing and new measures of response shift will depend upon this characterization. The field would also benefit from the systematic investigation of the circumstances under which implicit theories are operating, rather than response shift phenomena. It is our hope that further examination of the definitional distinctions provided herein will help to create a common language and a clearer research agenda for advancing this line of investigation.

Acknowledgements

We gratefully acknowledge helpful comments from Frans Oort Ph.D., Mechteld Visser Ph.D. and Geoff Norman Ph.D. on earlier drafts of this manuscript.

References

Ahmed, S., Mayo, N. E., Wood-Dauphinee, S., and Hanley, J. (in press). Response shift influences estimates of change in health-related quality of life (HRQL) post-stroke. *Journal of Clinical Epidemiology*.

Bernhard, J., Hürny, C., Maibach, R., Herrmann, R., and Laffer, U. (1999). For the Swiss Group for Clinical Cancer Research (SAKK) . Quality of life as subjective experience: reframing of perception in patients with colon cancer undergoing radical resection with or without adjuvant chemotherapy. Swiss Group for Clinical Cancer Research (SAKK) *Annals of Oncology*, **10**, 775–782.

Bernhard, J., Lowy, A. Maibach, R., and Hürny, C. (2001). Response shift in the perception of health for utility evaluation: an explorative investigation. *European Journal of Cancer*, **37**, 1729–1735.

Breetvelt, I. S. and Van Dam, F. S. A. M. (1991). Underreporting by cancer patients: The case of response shift. *Social Science and Medicine*, **32**, 981–987.

Golembiewski, R. T., Billingsley, K., and Yeager, S. (1976). Measuring change and persistence in human affairs: Types of change generated by OD designs. *Journal of Applied Behavioral Science*, **12**, 133–157.

Groenvold, M., Fayers, P. M., Sprangers, M. A., Bjorner, J. B., Klee, M. C., Aaronson, N. K., Bech, P., and Mouridsen, H. T. (1999). Anxiety and depression in breast cancer patients at low risk of recurrence compared with the general population: a valid comparison? *Journal of Clinical Epidemiology*, **52**(6), 523–530.

Herrmann, D. (1995). Reporting current, past, and changed health status: what we know about distortion. *Medical Care*, **33**, (4), AS89–AS94.

Howard, G. S. and Dailey, P. R. (1979). Response shift bias: a source of contamination of self-report measures. *Journal of Applied Psychology*, **64**, 144–150.

Howard, G. S. Dailey, P. R., and Gulanick, N. A. (1979). The feasibility of informed pretests in attenuating response-shift bias. *Applied Psychology Measurement*, **3**, 481–494.

Joore, M. A., Potjewijd, J., Timmerman, A. A., and Anteunis, L. J. C. (2002). Response shift in measurement of quality of life in hearing impaired adults after hearing aid fitting. *Quality of Life Research*, **11**, 299–307.

Lenert, L. A., Treadwell, J. R., and Schwartz, C. E. (1999). Associations between health status and utilities: implications for policy. *Medical Care*, **37**, 479–489.

Norman, G. (2003). Hi! How are you? Response shift, implicit theories and differing epistemologies. *Quality of Life Research*, **12**, (3), 239–249.

Oort, F. J. (in press). Types of change: Using structural equation modelling to detect response shifts. *Quality of Life Research*.

Oort, F. J., Visser, M. R. M., and Sprangersm M. A. G. (under review). Detecting response shifts in quality of life data from cancer patients undergoing invasive surgery: A structural equation modelling approach. *Quality of Life Research*.

Pearlman, R., Starks, H., Cain, K., Cole, W., Rosengren, D., and Patrick, D. (1999). *Your life, your choices: Planning for future medical decisions: How to prepare a personalized living will.* Washington, DC: Department of Veterans Affairs, Veterans Health Administration.

Rapkin, B. D. and Fischer, K. (1992). Personal goals of older adults: issues in assessment and prediction. *Psychology and Aging*, **7**, 127–137.

Rapkin, B. D. and Schwartz, C. E. (2004). Toward a theoretical model of quality-of-life appraisal: Implications of findings from studies of response shift. *Health and Quality of Life Outcomes*, **2**, 14.

Ross, M. (1989). Relation of implicit theories to the construction of personal histories. *Psychological Review*, **96**, (2), 341–357.

Schwartz, C. E., Sprangers, M. A. G., Carey, A., and Reed, G. (2004a). Exploring response shift in longitudinal data. *Psychology and Health*, **19**, 51–69.

Schwartz, C. E., Merriman, M., Reed, G., and Hammes, B. (2004b). Measuring patient treatment preferences in end-of-life care research: Applications for advance care planning interventions and response shift research. *Journal of Palliative Medicine*, **7**, 233–245.

Schwartz, C. E. and Sprangers, M. A. G. (1999). Methodological approaches for assessing response shift in longitudinal quality of life research. *Social Science and Medicine*, **48**, 1531–1548.

Schwartz, C. E. and Sprangers, M. A. G. (eds) (2000). *Adaptation to Changing Health: Response Shift in Quality-of-Life Research.* Washington, DC: American Psychological Association.

Schwartz, C. E., Wheeler, H. B., Hammes, B., Basque, N., Edmunds, J., Reed, G., Ma, Y., Li, L., Tabloski, P., Yanko, Y., and the UMass End-of-Life Working Group. (2002). Early intervention in planning end-of-life care with ambulatory geriatric patients: results of a pilot trial. *Archives of Internal Medicine*, **162**, 1611–1618.

Sprangers, M. A. G. and Schwartz, C. E. (1999b). Integrating response shift into health-related quality-of-life research: A theoretical model. *Social Science and Medicine*, **48**, 1507–1515.

Sprangers, M. A. G. and Schwartz, C. E. (1999a). The challenge of response shift for quality-of-life-based clinical oncology research. *Annals of Oncology*, **10**, 747–749.

Sprangers, M. A. G., Van Dam, F. S. A. M., Broersen, J., Lodder, L., Wever, L., Visser, M. R. M., Oosterveld, P., and Smets, E. M. A. (1999). Revealing response shift in longitudinal research on fatigue: The use of the then-test approach. *Acta Oncologica*, **38**, 709–718.

Visser, M. R., Smets, E. M., Sprangers, M. A., and de Haes, H. J. (2000). How response shift may affect the measurement of change in fatigue. *Journal of Pain & Symptom Management*, **20**, (1), 12–18.

Wilson, I. B. (1999). Clinical understanding and clinical implications of response shift. *Social Science and Medicine* **45**, 1577–1588.

Individual patient monitoring

Galina Velikova and Penny Wright

During the twentieth century a change in the pattern of diseases in the developed countries occurred, with a predominance of chronic conditions. This led to a shift in the understanding of health as a satisfactory physical and psychosocial functioning of the individual, not merely an absence of disease (WHO 1952). There was a movement away from the limited biomedical model of health and illness to a bio-psychosocial model (Engel 1977). This fundamental shift in the health-related thinking led to an increasing interest in the measurement of health status, functioning and well-being and in the use of these measures in health care research and practice (Greenfield and Nelson 1992). Many reliable and valid instruments for measurement of health status were developed, which were widely applied in the research setting. Since the 1990s there has been a steady interest in the use of HRQoL instruments in clinical practice in the care of individual patients.

The use of health status and health-related HRQoL measures in clinical practice was the main focus of two conferences on Advances in Health Status Assessment held in 1989 and 1992 (Lohr 1989; Lohr 1992). Potential uses of health status measures in clinical settings were identified as:

- screening for psychological and functional problems;
- monitoring disease symptoms or therapeutic response;
- facilitating doctor–patient communication;
- assessing quality of care;
- providing case-mix adjustment for comparing other outcomes between patient groups (Deyo and Patrick 1989).

The potential suggested by these possible applications had not yet been realized. Several barriers to the use of HRQoL measurement in clinical practice were identified:

- *Practical barrier* – if HRQoL measurements are to be used in clinical practice the data has to be collected and processed rapidly and results presented to physicians in 'real time', in an understandable format, allowing quick identification of problems. The costs of data collection and analysis should be considered, and special attention should be paid to how the measurement process is integrated into the usually busy clinical routine.

- *Methodological and conceptual barriers* – concerns whether HRQoL instruments developed for group comparisons can be used in individual patients; clinical meaning of HRQoL scores; determining the smallest clinically significant difference in HRQoL scores; clinicians' uncertainty as to how to interpret the results and how to use the information.

- *Relative lack of research data* on the possible benefits of HRQoL information for the patients and for the process of care.

- *Attitudinal barrier* – scepticism among physicians and researchers about the validity and importance of self-rated measures of health. Physicians continue to prefer physiologic outcomes, and most of them are not sufficiently familiar with health status questionnaires.

In this chapter recent research data will be reviewed, addressing each of the above barriers separately. Examples from the authors' own work in applying regular HRQoL measurement in cancer patients will be given.

Practical issues of collection and processing of HRQoL data

Data collection

Traditionally, HRQoL data have been collected by patient self-report questionnaires administered on a paper, with responses then manually entered onto a database. This method is unsuitable for busy clinical practices. Optical mark recognition systems can be used to transfer data from paper forms to a database, allowing the processing of large amounts of data. This method is very useful for postal surveys, but has some shortcomings for use in clinical practice, such as the requirement of special forms, recognition of multiple answers, missing data, need for verification and examination of the database for errors. A computer processing system (RT-2000) was developed for SF-36 which was based on optical mark-recognition technology, computer analysis of responses and print-out of patients results in graphic form, together with 95 per cent CI, normative data for comparison, and information on the quality of the data (Ware *et al.* 1994).

Electronic data collection and computer information technology allows HRQoL data to be collected, stored and scored automatically, allowing physicians to have immediate information about their patients' present HRQoL as well as cumulative HRQoL information from previous clinic visits. Individual patient's HRQoL profiles can be presented in a meaningful graphic or numeric format, similar to that of other widely used laboratory and instrumental tests. The results can be used in individual patient care and can become part of larger clinical databases containing information on patients medical history, investigations, treatment plans etc. The electronic questionnaires can be administered with a variety of devices. Increasingly, computers with touch-screen monitors are used due to ease of administration, but also standard desktop computers

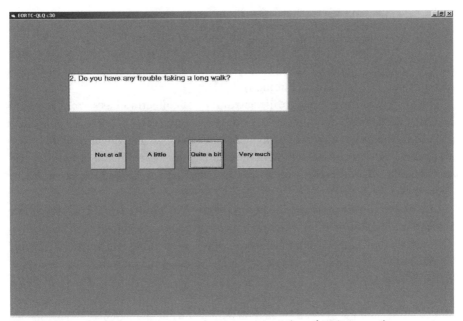

Fig. 4.5.1 Examples of the computer touch screen presentation of HRQoL questions.

with a mouse or portable tablet computers can be applied (Figure 4.5.1). A number of surveys in patients with diabetes, gastrointestinal diseases, in psychiatry and in oncology have shown that interactive computer programmes were well accepted by the patients and provided reliable information (Buxton *et al.* 1998; Lewis *et al.* 1996; Pouwer *et al.* 1998; Roizen *et al.* 1992; Taenzer *et al.* 1997). In a randomized cross-over trial of 149 cancer patients completing the EORTC QLQ-C30 and the Hospital Anxiety and Depression Scale (HADS) on paper and by touch-screen, we found that 52 per cent of the patients preferred the touch-screen to paper, irrespective of age, sex and presentation order, and 24 per cent had no preference. The quality of the data collected with the touch-screen system was very good, without missing responses. At group level the differences between scores from the two modes of administration of the instruments were small, suggesting equivalence for most of the HRQoL scales. At the level of individual patient the agreement between the HRQoL scores on the two versions was good, with Kappa coefficients from 0.57 to 0.77 and percentage global agreement from 69 per cent to 97 per cent. In a test–retest study of 81 patients the electronic questionnaires showed good test–retest reliability, with correlation coefficients from 0.78 to 0.95 and Kappa coefficients of agreement between 0.60 and 0.90 (Velikova *et al.* 1999).

A potential disadvantage of touch-screen systems is the requirement for patients to attend the clinic or hospital in order to complete the questionnaires. With the wider use of the Internet, the administration of electronic HRQoL questionnaires can also be extended to patients' homes. In addition, systems for telephone data collection are in development and pilot testing, which would allow patients to answer clinically relevant questions from their homes at frequent intervals, with the data automatically scored and entered on a database with facilities to alert physicians of potential problems (Susan Yount, personal communication).

The described experience with electronic data collection has so far been with standard fixed length questionnaires. Computer administration systems would allow the use of Computer Adaptive Testing (CAT) to administer individually tailored questionnaires, with precise measurement of specific domains, reduction of test time and comparability of scores across studies and diseases. CAT is described in Chapter 2.2, by Bjorner and Ware.

Interactive computer systems can also be used in a more simple way to collect patient-specific information with branching questionnaires. Patients can be asked to choose their most important problems from a list of symptoms and functional impairments, and further questions can be then asked to assess the frequency and severity of the problems.

Integration of HRQoL measurement into clinical routine

Routine HRQoL assessment in outpatient clinics will only be achieved if patients are willing and able to be involved with the process. We performed two studies field-testing the feasibility and patient compliance of routine HRQoL assessment that can be achieved using computer touch-screen systems in oncology practice (Wright *et al.* 2003). First, compliance was assessed in a cohort of 272 patients who gave informed consent to enter the study. The patients were asked to complete the EORTC QLQ-C30 and HADS every time they attended the oncology outpatient clinic over a period of six months. They were shown how to use the computer touch-screens at baseline, but after that the onus was on them to complete the assessment with no prompting from staff. At the end of the study, compliance with HRQoL assessment was calculated by dividing the number of assessments completed by the number of visits attended. Thirty-six per cent of patients did not complete any HRQoL assessments after the baseline visit, 22 per cent completed the HRQoL assessment at every visit. Forty-two percent of patients were 'partial compliers', that is, they completed the HRQoL assessment at some appointments but not at others. The median compliance for this group was 50 per cent with a range from 10 per cent to 93 per cent.

The results of this study led to a second strategy in which all patients attending selected clinics in a practice were asked to complete the touch-screen systems at each visit over a set three month period (n = 1,291), an 'all-comers' approach. The touch-screen system was integrated into clinic practice, with patients being asked to complete the assessment as part of the clerking-in process. For this latter approach, permission was given by the institutional ethics committees to offer patients the HRQoL assessments without prior individual informed consent in order to mimic as closely as possible routine clinical practice. A substantial proportion of patients complied completely (67 per cent); a significant minority did not complete the touch-screen questionnaires at all (24 per cent) and there were few 'partial compliers' (9 per cent). In the last group of patients the median compliance was 50 per cent with range from 25 per cent to 87 per cent. Those who did not complete the assessment included people who would have not been eligible due to not speaking English or being unwell to physically use the touch-screen. However, there remained a significant minority who chose to 'opt out' of the assessment.

It is feasible to use the computer touch-screen systems to generate data on a high proportion of large numbers of patients attending oncology clinics. An approach which incorporates data collection into routine clinical practice generates better compliance overall and, in particular, better data to describe changes over time than an approach which identifies a separate cohort prospectively. For HRQoL assessment to become a routine part of clinical practice, a system that is fully integrated into standard procedures is the most likely to prove successful.

Methodological and conceptual barriers

An important concern over the use of standard HRQoL instruments for individual patients, including EORTC QLQ-C30, is the fact that these instruments have been developed for comparing groups of patients in clinical research. Therefore the reliability coefficients of the subscales usually meet the 0.70 reliability criterion commonly accepted for group comparisons, but not the 0.90 criterion recommended for interpretation of scores at the level of individual patients (Nunnally and Bernstein 1994). Some researchers hold the view that the available health status instruments are not suitable for monitoring individual patients in clinical practice due to lack of precision, low reliability and wide 95 per cent confidence intervals (McHorney and Tarlov 1995). Others accept that in situations where the tests results will be used to highlight areas of concerns and will be followed by further standard clinical assessment, more liberal reliability criteria might be acceptable (Hays *et al.* 1993).

It makes sense to use similar questionnaires, if possible, both in clinical research and practice so that clinicians can become familiar with their content and interpretation. Furthermore clinical usefulness may be demonstrated as clinical experience broadens (McHorney and Tarlov 1995). The developers of the general health survey SF-36 provide guidelines on the use of individual patient profiles (Meyer *et al.* 1994; Ware, *et al.* 1994). They recommended the use of 95 per cent CI around individual patient scores and use of normative data for interpretation, and discussed the potential use of SF-36 for monitoring patients in clinical practice and its mental health scale as screening tool for psychological morbidity.

Kazis *et al.* (1988) developed and tested patient profiles based on Arthritis Impact Measurement Scales. The profiles were computer-generated, single page summary reports of patient scores, together with population scores and descriptive information.

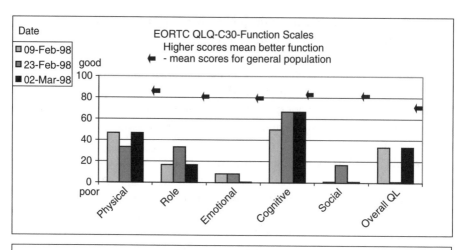

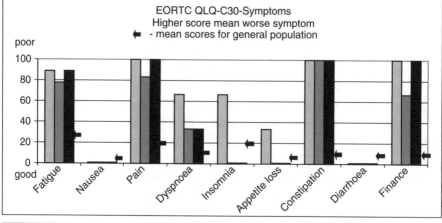

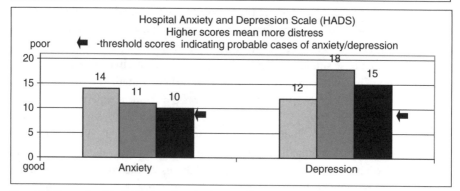

Fig. 4.5.2 Example of individual patient HRQoL profile.

Interpretation of the profile: The EORTC QLQ-C30 results during three clinic visits in February and March 1998 showed rather low scores on all functional scales. The most significant limitations were in role (possibly work) and social functioning. Very low score on emotional

continued

The authors assessed professionals' understanding of the information by a health status ranking exercise involving 123 rheumatologists and arthritis health professionals. They found that the professionals were able to understand the health information and could use it to produce consistent estimates of patient health status.

The EORTC QLQ-C30 has been used in individual oncology patients either as a graphic summary of the results (Detmar and Aaronson 1998), or as a computer-generated written report listing the items for which the patient indicated a deficit in performance or a presence of a symptom (Taenzer *et al.* 1997). Both methods were considered acceptable by clinicians.

With the aim of investigating the applicability of a standard HRQoL questionnaire to individual cancer patients, we compared the HRQoL results of 114 cancer patients with the corresponding medical records at both individual and group level (Velikova *et al.* 2001). When individual scores were presented in a clear graphic format including assessments at multiple points of time, it was possible to recognize patterns in individual patient responses. The HRQoL scores and their change over time corresponded to the severity of disease and treatment course in individual patients. Figure 4.5.2 presents an example of an individual patient profile from the study with explanation of the clinical background and brief interpretation of the HRQoL results. The example illustrates the direct correspondence between HRQoL scores and recorded symptoms. However, the HRQoL questionnaires had more information on emotional distress and other functional limitations, which was not present in the medical records. At group

....

Fig. 4.5.2 (Continued) function and high levels of anxiety and depression on Hospital Anxiety and Depression Scale (HADS) suggested clinically significant psychological distress. The scores on the functional scales showed very little change over time. HADS scale suggested possibly some reduction of anxiety, but still remaining around the cut-off point. However scores on depression became worse and clinical assessment for depression should be recommended. The patient reported multiple symptoms – fatigue, pain, dyspnoea, insomnia, appetite loss and constipation as well as financial problems related to her disease. Fatigue, pain, constipation and financial problems remained the same over time with possibly some temporary minor improvement in pain. Dyspnoea, insomnia and appetite loss improved.
Summary of the medical records: This profile is from a 54-year-old woman with recurrent ovarian cancer with pelvic mass who was unable to work since diagnosis. The main problems described in the initial annotation were low back pain radiating to posterior aspect of thigh, accompanied by abnormal sensation and affecting walking; also constipation, shortness of breath and low energy levels. The tiredness and the shortness of breath were noted, but not the insomnia. Pain had been identified as the major problem together with constipation. Symptomatic drugs including morphine, amitriptyline and dexamethasone were adjusted. However, pain control was difficult to achieve, although some initial response to dexamethasone was noted in the second annotation. This resulted in good night sleep. Later the pain returned and following a review of the CT scan the patient received radiotherapy to the pelvis. The emotional distress was not identified in the medical records.

level, a higher proportion of patients reported problems on the HRQoL questionnaire than were mentioned in the medical records. Most often clinicians mentioned pain (22–39 per cent), and at the initial visit role (66 per cent) and social issues (77 per cent). For the rest of the symptoms and functions, the problems were recorded in between 1 and 25 per cent of the notes, but 20 to 76 per cent of the patients reported HRQoL impairment. Problems not recorded in the medical notes tended to be of low severity with a significant trend observed for pain, fatigue, nausea/vomiting, dyspnoea, loss of appetite and physical function. These observations, although descriptive, support the validity of standard HRQoL measures in individuals, and suggest that despite some reliability limitations the questionnaires can be useful for monitoring symptoms and functional problems of patients in daily clinical practice.

It is believed that longitudinal assessment at multiple time points should establish a personal norm for each individual patient. Then changes over time for that individual may be best judged in relation to what is 'normal' for that patient. It can also be expected that as HRQoL assessment becomes more common in clinical settings, intuitive familiarity will develop both through individual and collective experience, as has occurred for more established measures of disease activity and severity.

Research data on the possible benefits for the patients and for the process of care

The use of HRQoL instruments for individual patients in practice has been studied in both observational studies and randomized controlled studies. In a longitudinal practice-based project, Meyer *et al.* (1994) and Kurtin *et al.* (1992) reported three years of experience with quarterly assessment of self-reported health of dialysis outpatients using SF-36. The longitudinal results were presented to the clinicians in a graphic format with 95 per cent CI around individual scores. Two case reports were discussed, comparing information from SF-36 with the dialysis team's assessment of the patient according to the medical records. The serial measurement of health status allowed recognition of clear patterns in patient responses. The SF-36 was found to reveal new information, rather than merely restate the clinicians' intuition about their patients' functioning and well-being, despite the fact that the dialysis clinicians had regular and frequent contacts with their patients.

Several earlier randomized studies in general medicine suggested that health status reports provided useful information, facilitated communication between patients and doctors, but had smaller impact on patients' functional status (Kazis *et al.* 1990; Rubenstein *et al.* 1989, 1995; Wagner *et al.* 1997). Several possible explanations for these results were suggested. The health status information was collected some time prior to the clinic visit and might have become irrelevant by the time of the consultation. The clinicians were usually given health status information from one assessment without further longitudinal data. Physicians were not offered specific management suggestions for improving the functional status of their patients. Indeed the only trial with positive results had incorporated specific management recommendations together with the HRQoL report (Rubenstein *et al.* 1995).

Two recent systematic reviews of the randomized trials in general medicine recommended further evaluation of this type of intervention. Greenhalgh and Meadows (1999) reviewed 13 randomized studies from 1987–97 for evidence of effectiveness of patient-based measures of health in routine practice in terms of improving process and outcome of patient care. The detection of psychological and to a lesser extent functional problems was improved, but less impact was found on patient management. The review found little evidence to suggest improvement in outcomes of patient care. Espallargues *et al.* (2000) reviewed 21 randomized studies assessing the impact of health status measures (including mental health measures) in clinical practice and reached similar conclusions – feeding back information to health professionals about patients' self-reported health status had an effect on at least one indicator of the process of care, but not on the outcomes of care. The meta-analysis of 11 studies feeding back mental health status information showed higher rates of diagnosis (odds ration 1.91, 95 per cent CI 1.28–2.83) and notations in the medical charts in the intervention group. No significant effect on treatment or patient outcomes was observed. The authors concluded that screening for mental health problems may have a role in routine clinical practice, but a need remains for a more thorough evaluation of this type of intervention.

There is a growing interest in using HRQoL measurement in cancer medicine and significant evidence has been accumulated from several randomized studies. Detmar *et al.* (2002a) investigated the impact of HRQoL information (results from EORTC QLQ-C30 in a graphic format) on patient–doctor communication regarding HRQoL issues and on physicians' awareness of patients' physical and psychosocial problems. This was done in a randomized cross-over study of 214 patients treated with palliative chemotherapy, who completed the HRQoL questionnaire on 4 consecutive clinic visits. At the forth visit a positive effect on patient-doctor communication was found (effect size 0.38). Ten of the 12 HRQoL issues were discussed more frequently: social functioning (22 per cent in intervention visits vs. 11 per cent in control visits), fatigue (56 per cent vs. 35 per cent respectively and dyspnoea (24 per cent vs. 12 per cent respectively). Within the intervention group an increase over time of at least 10 per cent of physician recognition of moderate to severe problems was observed for daily activities, feelings, social activities, pain and fatigue. In the control group this was observed only for pain and daily activities. However, the identification of more problems did not play a role in the treatment decisions regarding palliative chemotherapy (Detmar *et al.* 2002b). The intervention had no effect on patients' well-being, as measured by a general health survey SF-36.

In a randomized study McLachlan *et al.* (2001) collected and made available to the health care team information on patient-reported cancer needs, HRQoL and psychological screening. The intervention was administered at a single point in time to 450 cancer patients at various stages of their disease and treatment. All patients completed the questionnaires on touch-screen computers, but information was fed back to the health care team only for the intervention group. Patients were assessed at two and six months after randomisation. No difference between the two groups was found in respect to HRQoL, cancer needs, psychological functioning or satisfaction with care. Subgroup analysis of patients who were depressed at baseline, suggested significant reduction in depression at two and six months in the intervention group. In the control group 73 per cent and 90 per cent of the patients who were moderately to severely depressed at baseline, remained depressed at two and six months. In the intervention arm these percentages were reduced to 58 per cent and 45 per cent respectively.

Taenzer *et al.* (2000) studied the impact of computerized HRQoL screening on physician behaviour and patient satisfaction in a cross-sectional study of 53 lung cancer patients. The study employed a sequential recruitment design and a single completion of EORTC QLQ-C30. The authors found that the HRQoL screening was effective in increasing detection of HRQoL problems during the clinic appointment. Patients in the experimental arm indicated that on average 50 per cent of HRQoL items they identified were addressed during the clinic appointment, compared with 24 per cent for patients in the control group. A small increase in the actions being taken in relation to HRQoL problems was noted. Actions were taken on 73 per cent of HRQoL categories in the experimental group compared with 65 per cent in the control group.

In a randomized study including 286 patients and 28 oncologists, we tested the hypothesis that regular collection and transfer of HRQoL data to practicing oncologists may have positive impact on the process of medical care and may result in benefits for the patients. The study employed a prospective randomized design with three groups – an intervention group (regular completion of HRQoL questionnaire on touch-screen computer over six months and feeding back results to clinicians); an attention-control group (regular completion of HRQoL questionnaires without feedback of information to clinicians); and a control group (no completion of HRQoL questionnaires in clinics). Primary outcomes were patient well-being, measured by Functional Assessment of Cancer Therapy-General questionnaire (FACT-G), and doctor–patient communication and clinical management, measured by content analysis of tape-recorded consultations. Secondary outcomes were other process measures (tests, drugs, medical records), continuity of care and patient satisfaction. The results of the study suggested an impact of the intervention on the content of patient–doctor communication with more frequent enquiry about non-specific symptoms, including fatigue (60 per cent of intervention consultations vs. 42 per cent of attention-control vs. 48 per cent of control consultations), insomnia (31 per cent vs. 8 per cent vs. 18 per cent respectively), lack of appetite (48 per cent vs. 35 per cent vs. 25 per cent) and a trend for more frequent discussion of emotional issues (54 per cent vs. 46 per cent vs. 41 per cent). No significant effect on patient management was found. Using mixed-effects modelling to analyse the longitudinal HRQoL outcomes data, a significant improvement in patient well-being over

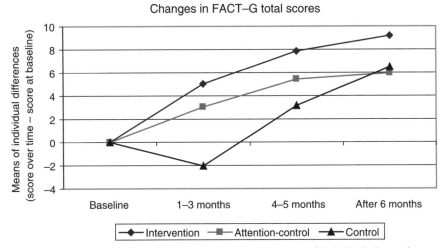

Fig. 4.5.3 Changes in patient well-being overtime (mean values of individual changes).

(a) FACT-G total scores.*

*Intervention vs. Control groups, $P = 0.006$; Intervention vs. Attention-control $P = 0.80$; Attention-control vs. Control group $P = 0.01$.

time was observed for patients in both intervention and attention-control group (who completed the HRQoL questionnaires on a regular basis) in comparison with the control group (Figure 4.5.3a). No significant difference was found between the intervention and the attention-control group. The HRQoL differences between intervention and control group were also clinically significant. Forty percent of the patients in the intervention group showed clinically meaningful improvement in HRQoL (FACT-G change > 7 points), in comparison with 32 per cent in the attention-control and 24 per cent in the control group. The number needed to 'treat' for one patient to benefit was 4.2. The effect of the intervention diminished over time. Similar results, with main differences between the intervention and control, but not between intervention and attention-control, were observed separately for Physical well-being and Functional well-being. However, for patient Emotional well-being an effect was observed only for in the intervention group, but not in attention-control group (Figure 4.5.3b). An improvement was found in patient perceptions of the continuity of their care. All patients were highly satisfied with the quality of medical care and no between-group differences were observed (Velikova *et al.* 2004).

Data from physicians' self-reported use of HRQoL information showed significant variability between clinicians. The audiotapes from a cross-sectional sample of clinic encounters demonstrated that the HRQoL results were explicitly used in 64 per cent of the visits. Doctors' attention was focused mainly on symptoms, to some extent on

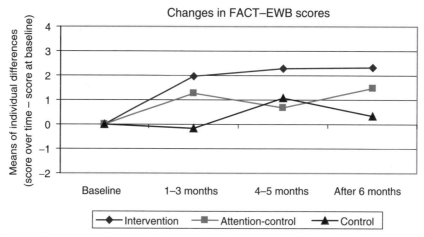

Fig. 4.5.3 Changes in patient well-being overtime (mean values of individual changes). (b) FACT-E Emotional well-being (EWB).*

* Intervention vs. control groups, $P = 0.008$; Intervention vs. Attention-control $P = 0.43$; Attention-control vs. control group $P = 0.12$.

emotional issues, but the data on functional limitations was largely ignored. In a multiple regression model improvements in patient well-being were associated with explicit use of HRQoL data during the encounters ($P = 0.016$), discussion of pain ($P = 0.046$) and role function ($P = 0.046$). Therefore, it could be speculated that the relatively small patient benefits from the intervention may be due to the fact that despite training in interpretation of the questionnaires, physicians were unsure how to use the HRQoL data and how to respond to it. These observations are in concordance with the conclusions of the systematic review on the use of patient-based health measures in routine practice (Greenhalgh and Meadows 1999). These issues naturally lead to the discussion of the role of physicians' and health professionals' attitudes to HRQoL assessments in clinical practice.

Attitudinal barrier

Physicians participating in surveys or clinical studies using regular HRQoL measurement have in general expressed very positive views of the clinical usefulness of the data (Bezjak *et al.* 2001; Detmar *et al.* 2002a; Meyer *et al.* 1994; Wagner *et al.* 1997). The health status information was found to identify additional problems for discussion and to be useful to patient management. In our work oncologists found HRQoL data useful in approximately two-thirds of the consultations. As stated above, individual physicians' attitude and use of data was variable. Physicians were concerned that using the HRQoL data will open a Pandora's box by identifying multiple problems, leading to prolongation of the encounters. In practice, none of the studies detected any lengthening of the consultations as a result of using HRQoL data.

Despite expressed positive attitude towards HRQoL data and willingness to use the data, in practice oncologists rarely based their decisions on HRQoL information, even in the palliative setting (Detmar *et al.* 2002b). The preference for physiological outcomes is still very strong, and physicians are not confident in using more 'subjective' outcomes like HRQoL. Wider application would be promoted by training health care providers about the methods of health status assessment, comparing newer functional measures with older scales with which clinicians are familiar and with clinical and laboratory measures. For individual health status scores to be useful to clinicians, attention should be given to clear graphic presentations of the data, comparison of results with previous scores from the same patients, trends over time, and comparison with norms for a general population or for relevant patient subgroups. It may be helpful to provide clinicians with the functional scores and with interpretations of the absolute score, as well as changes in the score and recommendations about management (Deyo and Carter 1992).

Additional information can be added to the HRQoL instruments to make the data more medically relevant, for example information on symptoms severity, frequency, duration, and effectiveness of particular drugs. It is likely that for individual patient monitoring disease-specific questionnaires will be more clinically relevant than generic instruments.

The physicians in our study indicated that it would be very useful if HRQoL data were plotted against significant clinical data like chemotherapy cycles, tests results, and major treatment decisions.

Conclusions and future directions

Monitoring HRQoL of individual patients in clinical practice is possible and feasible using electronic data collection. Results can be processed immediately and fed back to the physicians for use in patient care. The procedure for data collection can be incorporated into busy clinics. The serial measurement of HRQoL allowed recognition of patterns over time corresponding to disease course, thus providing evidence for the validity of these measures in the assessment of the individual. The HRQoL profiles had more information than the medical records on symptoms, and particularly on functional issues, such as emotional distress and physical performance.

Patients found the measurement acceptable and felt it was helping them to tell the doctors about their problems. Evidence from several randomized studies confirmed that using HRQoL screening in clinical practice can lead to an increased discussion of quality of life issues, and can facilitate patient–doctor communication without increasing consultation time. Most of the studies found no significant effect on patient management or patient well-being. However, positive effect on identification of depression was suggested. In one study routine assessment of cancer patients' HRQoL not only had a positive impact on doctor–patient communication, but also resulted in benefits for some patients, who had better HRQoL and emotional functioning.

Clearly, further research using randomized controlled studies is necessary before monitoring of individual patients HRQoL is recommended for routine use in clinical practice, but the findings are encouraging and suggest that such a simple intervention has the potential for improving patient care. These results justify further work in several directions:

- evaluating the approach in more diverse clinical settings;

- investigating ways of increasing the positive effects of HRQoL information.

Increased impact of HRQoL measurements can be expected if better instruments are used to assess psychological distress, symptoms and functioning. Physicians indicated that sometimes the standardized questionnaires provided rather general information and more patient-specific data would be clinically beneficial. Individualized HRQoL measures exist, as described in Chapter 4.1 by O'Boyle *et al.*, but the experience with them is relatively limited and their suitability for regular longitudinal monitoring of patients in clinical practice needs further investigation. The development of precise and flexible measures of HRQoL, based on item response theory analysis and computer adaptive testing as described in Chapters 2.2 (Bjorner and Ware) and 2.3 (Cella *et al.*), is expected to revolutionize the measurement of individual patient HRQoL and to be particularly suitable for clinical practice.

The methods by which HRQoL results are implemented and fed back to clinicians are very important. Education alone might not be sufficient for changing clinical practice and formal implementation strategies should be employed, guided by theories of individual and organizational change (Deyo and Carter 1992; Greenhalgh and Meadows 1999).

In the not so distant future, the principle of collection of patient-based data, including HRQoL information using touch-screen, Internet or telephone-based computer technology, will no doubt be further developed to form an important part of the electronic patient records.

References

Bezjak, A., Ng, P., Skeel, R. T., DePetrillo, A. D., Comis, R., and Taylor, K. M. (2001). Oncologists' use of quality of life information: Results of a survey of Eastern Cooperative Oncology Group physicians, *Quality of Life Research*, **10**, 1–13.

Buxton, J., White, M., and Osoba, D. (1998). Patients' experiences using a computerized program with a touch-sensitive video monitor for the assessment of health-related quality of life. *Quality of Life Research*, **7**, 513–517.

Detmar, S. B. and Aaronson, N. K. (1998). Quality of life assessment in daily clinical oncology practice: a feasibility study. *European Journal of Cancer*, **34**, 1181–1186.

Detmar, S. B., Muller, M. J., Schornagel, J. H., Wever, L. D., and Aaronson, N. K. (2002a). Health-related quality-of-life assessments and patient-physician communication: a randomized controlled trial. *JAMA*, **288**, 3027–3034.

Detmar, S. B., Muller, M. J., Schornagel, J. H., Wever, L. D., and Aaronson, N. K. (2002b). Role of health-related quality of life in palliative chemotherapy treatment decisions. *Journal of Clinical Oncology*, **20**, 1056–1062.

Deyo, R. A. and Patrick, D. L. (1989). Barriers to the use of health status measures in clinical investigation, patient care, and policy research. *Medical Care*, **27**, S254–S268.

Deyo, R. A. and Carter, W. B. (1992). Strategies for improving and expanding the application of health status measures in clinical settings. A researcher-developer viewpoint. *Medical Care*, **30**, (Suppl.) MS176–186 .

Engel, G. L. (1977). The need for a new medical model: a challenge for biomedicine. *Science,* **196**, 129–136.

Espallargues, M., Valderas, J. M., and Alonso, J. (2000). Provision of feedback on perceived health status to health care professionals: a systematic review of its impact, *Medical Care*, **38**, 175–186.

Greenfield, S. and Nelson, E. C. (1992). Recent developments and future issues in the use of health status assessment measures in clinical settings. *Medical Care*, **30**, (Suppl) MS23–41.

Greenhalgh, J. and Meadows, K. (1999). The effectiveness of the use of patient-based measures of health in routine practice in improving the process and outcomes of patient care: a literature review, *Journal of Evaluation in Clinical Practice*, **5**, 401–416.

Hays, R. D., Anderson, R., and Revicki, D. (1993). Psychometric considerations in evaluating health-related quality of life measures. *Quality of Life Research*, **2**, 441–449.

Kazis, L. E., Anderson, J. J., and Meenan, R. F. (1988). Health status information in clinical practice: the development and testing of patient profile reports, *Journal of Rheumatology*, **15**, 338–344.

Kazis, L. E., Callahan, L. F., Meenan, R. F., and Pincus, T. (1990). Health status reports in the care of patients with rheumatoid arthritis, *Journal of Clinical Epidemiology*, **43**, 1243–1253.

Kurtin, P. S., Davies, A. R., Meyer, K. B., DeGiacomo, J. M., and Kantz, M. E. (1992). Patient-based health status measures in outpatient dialysis. Early experiences in developing an outcomes assessment program, *Medical Care*, **30**, (Suppl.) MS136–149.

Lewis, G., Sharp, D., Bartholomew, J., and Pelosi, A. J. (1996). Computerized assessment of common mental disorders in primary care: effect on clinical outcome, *Family Practice*, **13**, 120–126.

Lohr, K. N. (1989). Advances in health status assessment. Overview of the conference, *Medical Care*, **27**, S1–11.

Lohr, K. N. (1992). Applications of health status assessment measures in clinical practice. Overview of the third conference on advances in health status assessment, *Medical Care*, **30**, MS1–14.

McHorney, C. A. and Tarlov, A. R. (1995). Individual-patient monitoring in clinical practice: are available health status surveys adequate? *Quality of Life Research*, **4**, 293–307.

McLachlan, S. A., Allenby, A., and Matthews, J., *et al.* (2001). Randomized trial of coordinated psychosocial interventions based on patient self-assessments versus standard care to improve the psychosocial functioning of patients with cancer, *Journal of Clinical Oncology*, **19**, 4117–4125.

Meyer, K. B., Espindle, D. M., DeGiacomo, J. M., Jenuleson, C. S., Kurtin, P. S., and Davies, A. R. (1994). Monitoring dialysis patients' health status, *American Journal of Kidney Diseases*, **24**, 267–279.

Nunnally, J. C. and Bernstein, I. H. (1994). *Psychometric Theory*, 3rd edn. New York, St Louis, San Francisco, Auckland, Bogota: McGraw-Hill, Inc.

Pouwer, F., Snoek, F. J., van der Ploeg, H. M., Heine, R. J., and Brand, A. N. (1998). A comparison of the standard and the computerized versions of the Well-being Questionnaire (WBQ) and the Diabetes Treatment Satisfaction Questionnaire (DTSQ). *Quality of Life Research*, **7**, 33–38.

Roizen, M. F., Coalson, D., and Hayward, R. S., *et al.* (1992). Can patients use an automated questionnaire to define their current health status? *Medical Care*, **30**, (Suppl.) MS74–84.

Rubenstein, L. V., Calkins, D. R., and Young, R. T., *et al.* (1989). Improving patient function: a randomized trial of functional disability screening, *Annals of Internal Medicine*, **111**, 836–842.

Rubenstein, L. V., McCoy, J. M., and Cope, D. W., *et al.* (1995). Improving patient quality of life with feedback to physicians about functional status, *Journal of General Internal Medicine*, **10**, 607–614.

Taenzer, P., Bultz, B. D., and Carlson, L. E., *et al.* (2000). Impact of computerized quality of life screening on physician behaviour and patient satisfaction in lung cancer outpatients, *PsychoOncology*, **9**, 203–213.

Taenzer, P. A., Speca, M., and Atkinson, M. J., *et al.* (1997). Computerized quality-of-life screening in an oncology clinic, *Cancer Practice*, **5**, 168–175.

Velikova, G., Wright, E. P., and Smith, A. B., *et al.* (1999). Automated collection of quality of life data: a comparison of paper and computer-touchscreen questionnaires. *Journal of Clinical Oncology*, **17**, 998–1007.

Velikova, G., Wright, P., and Smith, A. B., *et al.* (2001). Self-reported quality of life of individual cancer patients: concordance of results with disease course and medical records, *Journal of Clinical Oncology*, **19**, 2064–2073.

Velikova, G., Booth, L., and Smith, A. B., *et al.* (2004). Measuring quality of life in routine oncology practice improves communication and patient well-being – a randomized controlled trial. *Journal of Clinical Oncology*, **22**, 714–724.

Wagner, A. K., Ehrenberg, B. L., Tran, T. A., Bungay, K. M., Cynn, D. J., and Rogers, W. H. (1997). Patient-based health status measurement in clinical practice: a study of its impact on epilepsy patients' care. *Quality of Life Research*, **6**, 329–341.

Ware, J. E., Jr, Kosinski, M., and Keller, S. D. (1994). *SF-36 Physical and Mental Health Summary Scales: a user's manual*. Boston, MA: The Health Institute, New England Medical Center.

WHO (1952). *Constitution of the WHO*, 5th edn. Geneva: World Health Organization.

Wright, E. P., Selby, P. J., and Crawford, M., *et al.* (2003). Feasibility and compliance of automated measurement of quality of life in oncology practice. *Journal of Clinical Oncology*, **21**, 374–382.

Section 5

Measures for clinical trials

5.1

Self-rated health

Jakob B. Bjorner, Peter Fayers and Ellen Idler

Many health-related quality of life questionnaires and health surveys contain questions of the type: 'In general, would you say your health is: excellent, very good, good, poor or fair?' or 'What do you think of your own health condition compared to that of other men of your age?' Such global questions concerning the general perception of a respondent's own health have been focus of increasing interest in public health research during the past decades – for four reasons:

1. Answers to such questions have been shown to be surprisingly strong predictors of subsequent mortality, morbidity, discharge from the labour force, and use of medical services. The associations generally persist even after controlling for numerous other risk factors.

2. The questions maximize sensitivity to respondent views of health because they allow respondents to weight together different aspects of health status, putting most emphasis on those aspects of health that they consider relevant. In this aspect they differ from the multi-item health components and health utility indexes often used in quality of life research.

3. These questions provide researcher with a simple and convenient way of including information on health in a survey. Thus, numerous surveys have included a single global question on self-rated health, permitting a flurry of secondary analyses once the research community took interest in the ability of self-rated health to predict other health outcomes.

4. The questions on self-rated health are fairly abstract, prompting an interest in studying the meaning respondents assign to such questions – using qualitative methods – as a laboratory for understanding respondents' cognitive processing of health-related information.

The purpose of this chapter is to provide an introduction to the research on self-rated health by reviewing the research concerning the four topics mentioned above. Further, we will discuss the measurement of self-rated health, and how and to what extent self-rated health should be included in clinical studies.

Various names have been used to describe the concept discussed here: general health perceptions (Ware 1976), self-perceived health (Wannamethee and Shaper 1991;

Marmot *et al.* 1991), self-assessed health (Idler 1993), self-evaluated health (Idler *et al.* 1990), and self-rated health (Liang *et al.* 1991). This chapter will use the name self-rated health.

Part of the fascination with self-rated health can be formulated as: 'how come a global subjective rating of health performs so well?' We know that people differ in their frame of reference. Some respondents will probably – consciously or subconsciously – compare themselves with others of the same age, whilst others may consider how they were before they became ill. The phenomenon of response shift (see Chapter 4.4) might occur for self-rated health. This would imply that people change their response criteria over time. Those with a chronic illness or a severe disability may learn to cope, or may change their expectations and claim improved overall health, even though their illness seems stable to an observer. If such processes occur, differences in self-rated health between two groups would be smaller than their difference in medically-defined health. On the other hand, self-ratings may be influenced by personality factors such as hypochondria, so that self-ratings reflected personality more than health per se (Barsky *et al.* 1992). Throughout the chapter we will examine whether empirical data points to such problems in the interpretation of data on self-rated health.

Measurement of self-rated health

A diverse set of questions and response options have been used to measure self-rated health (Table 5.1.1). In the majority of health surveys self-rated health is measured by a single item, although some use multi-item scales. The time frame may be unspecified or, for example, stated as at present, within the last year, or 'since your illness'. In most cases the question is posed without any comparison group, but alternatively the respondents can be asked to rate themselves relative to a peer group, such as those of similar age or those with similar illness. Another option is to use an earlier time as the reference value, for example 'Compared to one year ago, how would you rate your health now?' with options from 'much better' to 'much worse'. Most instruments have used ordered categorical response options, most commonly with four or five states. Numerical rating scales with more than five response categories have also been used, as have visual analogue scales, typically anchored at the extremes by 'Best' or 'Worst' imaginable health state.

In predictive studies, no systematic differences between different wordings have been found, suggesting that they all tap into the same concept (Idler and Benyamini 1997). The few head-to-head comparisons of self-rated health questions show good overall agreement between questions with and without an explicit same-aged peers comparison group (Baron-Epel and Kaplan 2001). In one small study the question using the same-age comparison group predicted mortality better for men but not for women (Manderbacka *et al.* 2003). In summary, there is scarce direct evidence of superiority for any particular wording. However, there are advantages in using standard items that

Table 5.1.1 Examples of questions on self-rated health

Question	Response choices				
Do you consider yourself a healthy, fairly healthy, sick or very sick person?[1]	Healthy	Fairly healthy	Sick	Very sick	No answer
How would you rate your own health within the last year?[2]	Excellent	Good	Fair	Poor	Miserable
How would you describe your health status at present?[3]	Excellent	Good	Fair	Poor	
Do you feel healthy, rather healthy, moderately healthy or not healthy?[4]	Healthy	Rather healthy	Moderately healthy	Not healthy	
Do you consider yourself a healthy, fairly healthy, sick or very sick person?[5]	Healthy	Fairly healthy	Sick	Very sick	
All in all, would you say your health is excellent, good, fair or poor?[6]	Excellent	Good	Fair	Poor	
What do you think of your own health condition compared to that of other men of your age?[7]	Better	Same	Worse		
How would you assess your own health condition?[8]	Excellent	Good	Fairly healthy	Not very healthy	Not healthy at all
In general would you say your health is:[9]	Excellent	Very good	Good	Fair	Poor
We would like you to indicate on this scale how good or bad your own health state is today[10]	Visual analogue scale: Best imaginable health state = 100		Worst imaginable health state = 0		
How would you rate your overall health during the past week?[11]	7-point numerical rating scale: Excellent = 7			Very poor = 1	

[1] (Kaplan et al. 1988), [2] (Møller et al. 1996), [3] (Wannamethee and Shaper 1991), [4] (Pijls et al. 1993), [5] (Kaplan et al. 1988) [6] (Kaplan and Camacho 1983), [7,8] (Appels et al. 1996), [9] (Ware et al. 1993), [10] (Brooks 1996), [11] (Fayers et al. 2001).

permit comparison across studies and which are available in a wide range of rigorously tested translations. It is also important to avoid items that have skew distributions with floor or ceiling effects. Ceiling effects is the more frequent problem because many items do not adequately discriminate positive states of health. The question with the most widespread use is: *'In general, would you say your health is:'* with the response options: *'Excellent; Very Good; Good; Fair; Poor'*. This item also provides good discrimination between positive states of health (Bjorner *et al.* 1996). It is included in the SF-36 Health Outcomes Survey (Ware *et al.* 1993) as well as in many other health surveys.

Multi-item scales with 5 to 32 item have also been proposed (Ware 1976; Davies and Ware Jr. 1981; Stewart *et al.* 1992; Ware *et al.* 1993). These scales cover subdimensions such as current health, prior health, resistance/susceptibility, health outlook, health worry/concern, sickness orientation, rejection of sick role, and attitude toward going to the doctor. Although the original long forms were scored as multiple scales, subsequent psychometric analysis has reduced the number of subconcepts involved, for example to current health, health outlook, and resistance to illness (Ware *et al.* 1993) and found that they can be considered belonging to one overall dimension (Bjorner and Kristensen 1999).

Self-rated health as a summary measure of health

Self-rated health is often a convenient approach to assess health – because it is brief (often one item will do) and because the assessment results in only one score. Single global assessments of overall health or overall quality of life have long been used by health economists and policy makers, who require a single summary score for each patient. However, most health-related quality of life questionnaires are multidimensional profile instruments, measuring many aspects of quality of life, symptoms of disease and side effects of treatments. If provided, a summary score for overall health or quality of life is often based on either simple or weighted summation over the individual items. Such scores have the advantage that the investigator knows exactly what items have contributed to the score, but the disadvantage that the items included may not at all be relevant for the particular patient. In contrast, when subjects respond to a global question they can base their response on the information they deem relevant, but we cannot be sure what they have in mind – for example, some may be focusing on mental health, others on physical health; some may be using implicit theories about their expectations, or comparisons with a peer group.

Self-rated health as a predictor of outcome

An impressive number of epidemiological studies have found that self-rated health is a strong independent predictor of subsequent mortality; for reviews see (Idler 1992; Idler and Benyamini 1997; Benyamini and Idler 1999; Bjorner *et al.* 1996), and in this

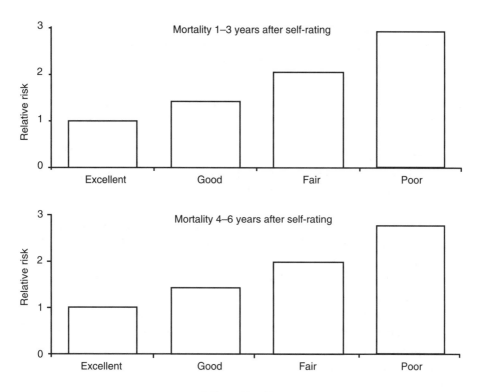

Fig. 5.1.1 Self-rated health as predictor of mortality (Mossey and Shapiro 1982).

Multivariate analyses controlled for 'objective health' (doctors' visits, hospitalizations, and self-reported diseases), gender, age, income, life satisfaction and living area (n = 3,128).

book Chapter 4.3. Figure 5.1.1 shows results from one of the important early studies (Mossey and Shapiro 1982); results that are characteristic of most of these studies:

1. A strong increase in relative risk of mortality for poorer self-rated health, with a clear trend for each category. Thus, even a rating of '*good*' has increased risk compared to '*excellent*'.

2. Multivariate analyses has controlled for potential confounders – most notably 'medical health'. In some studies, 'medical health' has been operationalized crudely as self-reported diagnoses, in other studies a clinical examination has been performed and several other covariates (often cardiovascular risk factors) have been included. In most studies, the predictive power of self-rated health is robust and not explained by other covariates. In the few studies where the effect disappears in multivariate analyses, the analyses often include very similar variables (e.g. Bath 2003).

3. The effect is not only short term. Some studies have followed respondents up to 16 years. Although a few studies do not find a long term predictive effect of self-rated health (Benyamini *et al.* 2003), most studies do.

Most studies have been performed in general population samples, often – but not always – focused on elderly populations. In the studies that have examined disease-specific causes of death, self-rated health is predictive of survival through a broad range of fatal diseases (Bjorner *et al.* 1996). Studies in specific disease groups, like coronary heart disease (Bosworth *et al.* 1999) and cancer (Coates *et al.* 1997; Osoba 1999; Shadbolt *et al.* 2002), also find self-rated health to be a powerful predictor of subsequent mortality, and better than clinical assessments including stage of disease and performance status.

Fewer studies have been carried out for other outcomes than mortality, but the results consistently support self-rated health as an important risk indicator. Thus it has been found to predict future decline in physical functioning (Idler and Kasl 1995; Lee, 2000), discharge from the labour force (Lund and Borg 1999), and future use of medical services (Kravitz *et al.* 1992).

These results provide strong evidence of criterion validity of self-rated health as a measure of health. Further, the ability to predict mortality, even when multiple other health covariates are included in the model, has led to speculations about exactly what is measured by these questions that can explain the strong relation with mortality. Explanations are of two broad types:

1. That self-rated health is an effective health indicator because it integrates many different health-related factors – more than would be included as covariates in a standard study. Such factors could include pre-clinical stages of disease, family disposition for high mortality, a general susceptibility, personality traits such as pessimism, anger or hostility, health behaviours, medically diagnosed disease, life events, social network and socio-economic status (Bjorner *et al.* 1996). Also, self-rated health may capture the person's evaluation of the trajectory of his/her health (Idler and Benyamini 1997).

2. Self-evaluation of health may also affect subsequent health. For example, health optimists may be more likely to engage in healthy lifestyles or to be motivated to undertake efforts at recovery from adverse health events such as stroke or heart attack (Idler and Benyamini 1997; Bjorner *et al.* 1996).

Diehr and colleagues performed an elegant study exploring the relation between self-rated health and mortality (Diehr *et al.* 2001b). They followed 5888 elderly people at six-month intervals for eight years. For the 1464 persons who died during the study, Figure 5.1.2 shows self-ratings of health organized by time to death. It is clear that the self-ratings steadily decline till the time of death, with accelerated decline in the last nine months. For the survivor group, self-rated health only declined slightly (Diehr *et al.* 2002). Thus the trajectory of self-rating of health seems to reflect disease processes

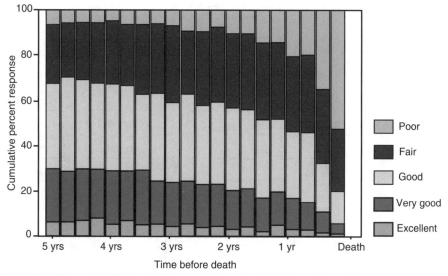

Fig. 5.1.2 Self-rated health in the five years before death (Diehr *et al.* 2001b).

leading to death. Diehr and colleagues also examined the trajectory before and after other sentinel health events. Cancer diagnosis, first incidence of coronary heath disease, myocardial infarction, and hip fractures all showed a clearly declining trajectory of self-ratings before the event, while for stroke the self-ratings do not decline prior to the event, suggesting absence of precursor symptoms (Diehr *et al.* 2001b). In conclusion, these results provide further support for the interpretation of self-rated health as a measure of health and do not suggest that response-shift has occurred (although it cannot be ruled out). Further, the predictive validity of self-rated health does not support the hypothesis that self-ratings of health mostly reflect personality.

Diehr and colleagues (2001a) have developed a coding for self-rated health that includes death as an outcome; a code is assigned to each of the response choices, reflecting the probability of being in good health two years later. The codes (excellent: 95, very good: 90, good: 80, fair: 30, poor: 15, dead: 0) were stable over several data sets, and offer a coherent approach to combining self-ratings with mortality information. However, there are general statistical and conceptual arguments against aggregation of quality of life data and mortality (Cox *et al.* 1992).

Factors associated with self-ratings of health

Since self-ratings of health allow the respondent to weight together different aspects of health status, it becomes an empirical and theoretical question to understand what factors influence the global ratings. Figure 5.1.3 presents a model proposed by Wilson and Cleary that has been very influential in shaping the understanding of the relationship

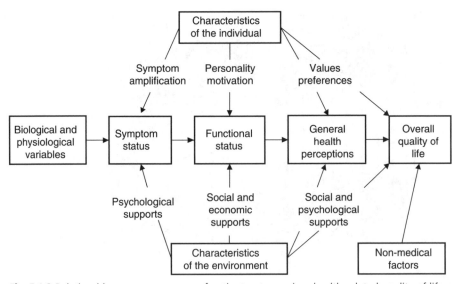

Fig. 5.1.3 Relationship among measures of patient outcome in a health-related quality of life conceptual model (Wilson and Cleary 1995).

between specific and generic outcome measures (Wilson and Cleary 1995). The model hypothesizes a causal chain from very specific physiological processes over disease-specific symptoms and functional status to self-rated health (general health perceptions). This causal chain is hypothesized to be influenced by characteristics of the individual (symptom amplification, personality, motivation, values, and preferences) and of the environment (psychological, social, and economic supports).

Bjorner and colleagues (1996) performed a systematic literature review of explanatory variables for self-ratings of health. Most studies were cross-sectional, a few were longitudinal. The studies differed markedly in population, explanatory variables included, and success in explaining self-rated health (R^2 ranged from 5 to 75 per cent). Four types of explanatory variables were consistently and strongly associated with self-rated health (Figure 5.1.4): medical diagnoses, physical symptoms, physical function, and mental symptoms. Gender, marital status, and social network were not significantly associated with self-ratings, when controlling for other measures of health. Age seemed to have a slightly U-shaped relation with age, the youngest and the oldest age groups having the best self-ratings. Weak associations with self-rated health were seen for ethnicity (Caucasians having better self-ratings) and employment (people employed having better self-ratings). Longer education was consistently associated with better self-ratings of health, even for people of equal health status according to other health indicators. Further, some studies suggest that education or income group modifies the association between self-rated health and other health indicators (Johnston and Ware 1976). For high income groups, self-rated health was highly associated with both physical

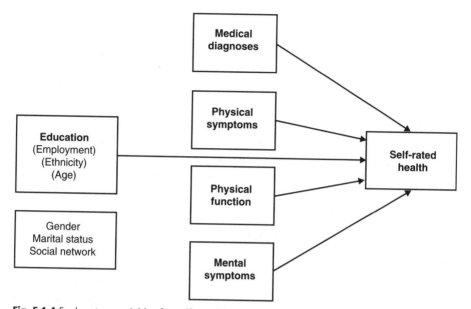

Fig. 5.1.4 Explanatory variables for self-rated health (Bjorner *et al.* 1996).

and mental health variables. For low income groups, self-rated health was strongly associated with physical health variables and only weakly with mental health variables.

Recent research on the relationship of clinical risk factors to self-ratings of health shows associations across a wide set of biomarkers (Goldman *et al.* 2004). Body mass index, waist to hip ratio, total to HDL cholesterol ratio, cortisol to DHEA-S ratio, and norepinephrine are all significantly associated with self-rated health, even when number of medical diagnoses, physical functioning, mental health, behavioural risk factors, stress, and SES are accounted for. In a small longitudinal study decrease in self-rated health was associated with an increase in s-prolactin and these changes predicted a high score on a measure of vital exhaustion at follow-up (Halford *et al.* 2003). The association between self-rated health and biomarkers that appear to lack a perceptual basis may partly be explained by the biomarkers being part of disease processes that the respondents can perceive but are not adequately captured by the other health measures included in the studies. However, this remains a promising area for future research.

Questionnaires such as the SF-36 place the self-rated health item at the beginning of the questionnaire, so that the respondents are uninfluenced by other health-related items; others, such as the EORTC 30-item quality of life questionnaire (QLQ-C30), deliberately place the self-rated health items at the end so that the earlier items serve as a frame, indicating to patients that the investigator is interested in physical, emotional, role, social, and cognitive functioning, as well as the effects of disease-specific symptoms (Fayers *et al.* 2001). However, a randomized study, where a question on self-rated health was placed either before or after questions on chronic diseases, found that the position of the global question in relation to specific questions did not matter (Bjorner *et al.* 2003). Some questionnaires place several global self-rating questions together (e.g. the QLQ-C30 has global self-rating question on quality of life next to a global self-rating question on health). The correlation between such items is generally very high and they are often equally good a predicting survival (Coates *et al.* 1997). This may be due to a framing effect (that respondents tend to provide similar answers to two global items placed next to each other). In separate analyses of factors associated with self-rated quality of life (Fayers and Hand 2002), the association with mental health factors is stronger than generally seen for self-rated health, thus supporting the assumption that respondents indeed distinguish between the two concepts.

Qualitative analyses of self-ratings

When answering questions on self-rated health, some respondents may think in terms of specific health problems associated with their particular illness, others in terms of behaviour or physical restrictions and functioning. An approach to understanding respondents' interpretations and their processes in rating their health is to use qualitative methods developed in the field of cognitive aspects of survey methodology (CASM), see e.g. (Tourangeau *et al.* 2000). Global questions on self-rated health have been proposed as a useful focus area for using CASM with quality of life measures, since these questions require the respondent to summarize and integrate various aspects of health (Fayers and Sprangers 2002; Barofsky, 2003). Jylhä (1994) analysed recordings of interviews with 40 elderly respondents. While many respondents followed the logic of the interview and gave unambiguous answers to the questions on self-rated health, a large proportion provided narratives of their health situation that did not fit easily onto the preset questionnaire categories. Jylhä concluded that in the interview situation 'health' is a multidimensional, context-bound phenomenon that can be constructed out of different, even contradictory elements.

A couple of studies have used a debriefing technique in which the self-rated health question was followed by a question like: 'Tell me why you say that.' or 'What goes through your mind when you say that?' and analysed the data by qualitative techniques. Many similarities are seen between the descriptive categories identified in such studies: e.g. presence/absence of illness, health behaviours, and physical ability/performance (Groves *et al.* 1992; Krause and Jay 1994), but the number and labels of categories differ. Borawski and colleagues (1996) classified the health attributions of 885 elderly respondents into five categories (developed by a qualitative study of 50 persons): physical health focused, attitudinal/behavioural, health transcendence, externally focused, and non-reflective. Health attributions were then investigated together with self-rated health as predictors of three-year mortality. Health attributions were significant predictors with respondents using externally focussed health attributions having the lowest mortality, followed by respondents basing their self-ratings on health transcendence. Highest mortality was seen for the non-reflective group (Borawski *et al.* 1996).

Contradictory elements in the narratives (as the ones described by Jylhä) represent a difficulty for classifying respondents into a single category. The above studies tackled this problem by focusing on the first reason mentioned by the respondent, discharging other information. Idler and colleagues (1999) recognized this problem and aimed at solving it by hypothesizing a hierarchy of six categories from the most restrictive and biomedical health definitions to the most holistic and inclusive ones: (1) physical health, diagnoses, symptoms; (2) physical functioning; (3) health risk behaviours; (4) social role activities; (5) social relationships; and (6) psychological, spiritual, emotional. Respondents were categorized after the highest category they used. Respondents using the more inclusive categories had more positive self-ratings judged in comparison with their medical history (Idler *et al.* 1999).

The processing of symptoms and higher order disease concepts might involve perceptual processes similar to those involved in other sensory modalities (Leventhal 1986). The basic process is pattern recognition, in which input from perceptual organs interacts with pre-existent knowledge to form mental representations (e.g. symptoms or health assessments). This pre-existing knowledge (referred to as illness theories or illness *schemata*) enables the individual to organize the sensory information into meaningful categories (Bishop 1991; Leventhal *et al.* 1992). Bjorner *et al* (1996) hypothesized that global health evaluations could be understood as health schemata. This hypothesis implies that people have general beliefs about their health, and that these beliefs affect whether health-related sensory inputs are noticed and whether they are interpreted as disease symptoms or some thing else. Thus, while general health perceptions are influenced by knowledge of medical diagnoses, functioning and symptoms, the health perceptions may also affect how symptoms and functioning are perceived and interpreted.

Conclusion

While self-rated health is included in some popular questionnaires, not all standard generic or disease-specific instruments include items assessing the concept. However, arguably *all* HRQoL instruments should contain at least one simple global question about overall health and/or overall quality of life, allowing respondents to weight together different aspects of their health status, emphasizing those aspects of health that they consider most relevant (Gill and Feinstein 1994). Also, self-rated health is an important risk indicator and can provide predictive information additional to, and better than, traditional clinical assessments of disease and physical performance status. For some clinical trials, overall self-rated health or overall quality of life would seem the most appropriate indicator of outcome, to be included alongside other patient-reported outcomes and clinical measures of treatment efficacy. Based on the conceptual framework that places self-rated health as one of the most generic health concepts, one might anticipate that self-rated health would be less responsive than disease-specific health measures. However, experience from trials shows that significant treatment effects on self-rated health are not infrequent. This may occur if the treatment affects a broad range of outcomes (in which case self-rated health may capture the total treatment effect more efficiently than any specific health outcomes measure) or if the treatment itself may affect the patients' assessment of his/her health, for example coronary angioplasty (Pocock *et al.* 2000).

In light of the demanding cognitive tasks and the inherent subjectivity in self-ratings of health, it is also fair to ask whether such ratings are too fuzzy to provide reliable information. Evaluations of reliability by test–retest and internal consistency methodology show that self-rated health is as reliable as other health status measures (Ware *et al.* 1993). And the effectiveness of self-rated health as a risk indicator also implies that the measure is reliable. While we do not completely understand the cognitive processes used to interpret and answer questions on self-rated health, the results from quantitative and qualitative studies seem to converge on some general conclusions: self-ratings of health do to a large extend reflect health states; for most respondents, self-ratings reflect mainly physical health, but a sizeable minority has a broader definition of health, including social, mental, and even spiritual components. In conclusion, if we were allowed only one question to measure health status, the rating of health as *excellent, very good, good, poor,* or *fair* would be a good candidate.

References

Appels, A., Bosma, H., Grabauskas, V., Gostautas, A., and Sturmans, F. (1996). Self-rated health and mortality in a Lithuanian and a Dutch population. *Social Science and Medicine,* 42, 681–690.

Barofsky, I. (2003). Cognitive approaches to summary measurement: its application to the measurement of diversity in health-related quality of life assessments. *Quality of Life Research,* 12, 251–260.

Baron-Epel, O. and Kaplan, G. (2001). General subjective health status or age-related subjective health status: does it make a difference? *Social Science and Medicine,* 53, 1373–1381.

Barsky, A. J., Cleary, P. D., and Klerman, G. L. (1992). Determinants of perceived health status of medical outpatients. *Social Science and Medicine,* 34, 1147–1154.

Bath, P. A. (2003). Differences between older men and women in the self-rated health-mortality relationship. *Gerontologist,* 43, 387–395.

Benyamini, Y., Blumstein, T., Lusky, A., and Modan, B. (2003). Gender differences in the self-rated health-mortality association: is it poor self-rated health that predicts mortality or excellent self-rated health that predicts survival? *Gerontologist,* 43, 396–405.

Benyamini, Y. and Idler, E. L. (1999). Community studies reporting association between self-rated health and mortality. *Research on Aging,* 21, 392–401.

Bishop, G. D. (1991). Understanding the understanding of illness: lay disease representations. In J. A. Skelton and R. T. Croyle (eds), *Mental Representations in Health and Illness,* pp. 32–59. New York: Springer-Verlag.

Bjorner, J. B. and Kristensen, T. S. (1999). Multi-item scales for measuring global self-rated health. Investigation of construct validity using structural equations models. *Research on Aging*, **21**, 417–439.

Bjorner, J. B., Kristensen, T. S., Orth-Gomér, K., Tibblin, G., Sullivan, M., and Westerholm, P. (1996). *Self-rated Health: A useful concept in research, prevention and clinical medicine*. Stockholm: Swedish Council for Planning and Coordination of Research.

Bjorner, J. B., Ware, J. E., Jr., and Kosinski, M. (2003). The potential synergy between cognitive models and modern psychometric models. *Quality of Life Research*, **12**, 261–274.

Borawski, E. A., Kinney, J. M., and Kahana, E. (1996). The meaning of older adults' health appraisals: congruence with health status and determinant of mortality. *J Gerontol. B. Psychol. Sci Soc Sci*, **51**, S157–70.

Bosworth, H. B., Siegler, I. C., Brummett, B. H., Barefoot, J. C., Williams, R. B., and Clapp-Channing, N. E., *et al.* (1999). The association between self-rated health and mortality in a well-characterized sample of coronary artery disease patients. *Medical Care*, **37**, 1226–1236.

Brooks, R. (1996). EuroQol: the current state of play. *Health Policy*, **37**, 53–72.

Coates, A., Porzsolt, F., and Osoba, D. (1997). Quality of life in oncology practice: prognostic value of EORTC QLQ-C30 scores in patients with advanced malignancy. *European Journal of Cancer*, **33**, 1025–1030.

Cox, D. R., Fitzpatrick, R., Fletcher, A. E., Gore, S. M., Spiegelhalter, D. J., and Jones, D. R. (1992). Quality-of-life assessment: Can we keep it simple? *Journal of the Royal Statistical Society*, **155**, 353–393.

Davies, A. R. and Ware, J. E., Jr. (1981). *Measuring Health Perceptions in the Health Insurance Experiment* (Rep. No. R-2711-HHS). Santa Monica, CA: The RAND Corporation.

Diehr, P., Patrick, D. L. ,Spertus, J., Kiefe, C. I., McDonell, M., and Fihn, S. D. (2001a). Transforming self-rated health and the SF-36 scales to include death and improve interpretability. *Medical Care*, **39**, 670–680.

Diehr, P., Williamson, J., Patrick, D. L., Bild, D. E., and Burke, G. L. (2001b). Patterns of self-rated health in older adults before and after sentinel health events. *J Amer Geriatr. Soc*, **49**, 36–44.

Diehr, P., Williamson, J., Burke, G. L., and Psaty, B. M. (2002). The aging and dying processes and the health of older adults. *Journal of Clinical Epidemiology*, **55**, 269–278.

Fayers, P. M. and Hand, D. J. (2002). Causal variables, indicator variables and measurement scales: an example for quality of life. *Journal of the Royal Statistical Society*, **165**, Part 2, 1–21.

Fayers, P. M. and Sprangers, M. A. (2002). Understanding self-rated health. *Lancet*, **359**, 187–188.

Fayers, P. M., Aaronson, N. K., Boreal, K., Groenvold, M., Curran, D., and Bottomley, A. (2001). *The EORTC QLQ-C30 Scoring Manual*, 3rd edn. Brussels: European Organization for Research and Treatment of Cancer.

Gill, T. M. and Feinstein, A. R. (1994). A critical appraisal of the quality of quality-of-life measurements. *JAMA*, **272**, 619–626.

Goldman, N., Glei, D. A., and Chang, M. C. (2004). The role of clinical risk factors in understanding self-rated health. *Ann. Epidemiol*, **14**, 49–57.

Groves, R. M., Fultz, N. H., and Martin, E. (1992). Direct questioning about comprehension in a survey setting. In J.M. Tanur (ed.) *Questions about Questions. Inquiries into the cognitive bases of surveys*, pp. 49–61. New York: Russell Sage Foundation.

Halford, C., Anderzen, I., and Arnetz, B. (2003). Endocrine measures of stress and self-rated health. A longitudinal study. *J Psychosomatic Research*, **55**, 317–320.

Idler, E. (1992). Self-assessed health and mortality: a review of studies. *Int.Rev.Health Psychol.* **1**, 33–54.

Idler, E. L. (1993). Age differences in self-assessments of health: age changes, cohort differences, or survivorship? *Journal of Gerontology*, **48**, S289–300.

Idler, E. L. and Kasl, S. V. (1995). Self-ratings of health: do they also predict change in functional ability? *J Gerontol B.Psychol Sci Soc Sci*, **50**, S344–53.

Idler, E. L. and Benyamini, Y. (1997). Self-rated health and mortality: a review of twenty-seven community studies. *Journal of Health and Social Behavior*, **38**, 21–37.

Idler, E., Kasl, S., and Lemke, J. (1990). Self-evaluated health and mortality among the elderly in New Haven, Connecticut, and Iowa and Washington counties, Iowa, 1982–1986. *American Journal of Epidemiology*, **131**, 91–103.

Idler, E. L., Hudson, S. V., and Leventhal, H. (1999). The meanings of self-ratings of health. *Research on Aging*, **21**, 458–476.

Johnston, S. A. and Ware, J. E., Jr. (1976). Income group differences in relationships among survey measures of physical and mental health. *Health Serv. Res*, **11**, 416–429.

Jylhä, M. (1994). Self-rated health revisited: exploring survey interview episodes with elderly respondents. *Social Science and Medicine*, **39**, 983–990.

Kaplan, G. A. and Camacho, T. (1983). Perceived health and mortality: a nine-year follow-up of the human population laboratory cohort. *American Journal of Epidemiology*, **117**, 292–304.

Kaplan, G., Barell, V., and Lusky, A. (1988). Subjective state of health and survival in elderly adults. *Journal of Gerontology*, **43**, S114–S120.

Krause, N. M. and Jay, G. M. (1994). What do global self-rated health items measure? *Medical Care*, **32**, 930–942.

Kravitz, R. L., Greenfield, S., Rogers, W., Manning, W. G., Jr., Zubkoff, M., and Nelson, *et al.* (1992). Differences in the mix of patients among medical specialties and systems of care. Results from the medical outcomes study [see comments]. *JAMA*, **267**, 1617–1623.

Lee, Y. (2000). The predictive value of self assessed general, physical, and mental health on functional decline and mortality in older adults. *J Epidemiol. Community Health*, **54**, 123–129.

Leventhal, H. (1986). Symptom reporting: a focus on process. In S. McHugh and T. M. Vallis (eds) *Illness Behavior – A multidisciplinary model*, pp. 219–237. New York: Plenum Press.

Leventhal, H., Diefenbach, M., and Leventhal, E. A. (1992). Illness cognition: Using common sense to understand treatment adherence and affect cognition interactions. *Cognitive Therapy and Research*, **16**, 143–163.

Liang, J., Bennett, J., Whitelaw, N., and Maeda, D. (1991). The structure of self-reported physical health among the aged in the United States and Japan. *Medical Care*, **29**, 1161–1180.

Lund, T. and Borg, V. (1999). Work environment and self-rated health as predictors of remaining in work 5 years later among Danish employees 35–59 years of age. *Exp. Aging. Res.* **25**, 429–434.

Manderbacka, K., Kareholt, I., Martikainen, P., and Lundberg, O. (2003). The effect of point of reference on the association between self-rated health and mortality. *Social Science and Medicine*, **56**, 1447–1452.

Marmot, M. G., Smith, G. D., Stansfeld, S., Patel, C., North, F., and Head, J., *et al.* (1991). Health inequalities among British civil servants: the Whitehall II study. *Lancet*, **337**, 1387–1393.

Møller, L. Kristensen, T. S., and Hollnagel, H. (1996). Self-rated health as a predictor of coronary heart disease. *Journal of Epidemiology and Community Health*, **50**, 423–428.

Mossey, J. M. and Shapiro, E. (1982). Self-rated health: a predictor of mortality among the elderly. *Am. J. Public Health*, **72**, 800–808.

Osoba, D. (1999). What has been learned from measuring health-related quality of life in clinical oncology. *Eur. J Cancer*, **35**, 1565–1570.

Pijls, L. T., Feskens, E. J., and Kromhout, D. (1993). Self-rated health, mortality and chronic diseases in elderly men (The Zutphen Study 1985–1990). *American Journal of Epidemiology,* **138,** 840–848.

Pocock, S. J., Henderson, R. A., Clayton, T., Lyman, G. H., and Chamberlain, D. A. (2000). Quality of life after coronary angioplasty or continued medical treatment for angina: three-year follow-up in the RITA-2 trial. Randomized Intervention Treatment of Angina. *J Am. Coll. Cardiol.* **35,** 907–914.

Shadbolt, B., Barresi, J., and Craft, P. (2002). Self-rated health as a predictor of survival among patients with advanced cancer. *J Clin Oncol,* **20,** 2514–2519.

Stewart, A. L., Hays, R. D., and Ware, J. E., Jr. (1992). Health perceptions, energy/fatigue, and health distress measures. In A.L. Stewart and J. E. Ware, Jr. (eds) *Measuring Functionning and Well-Being: The Medical Outcomes Study Approach,* pp. 143–172. London: Duke University Press.

Tourangeau, R., Rips, L. J., and Rasinski, K. (2000). *The Psychology of Survey Response.* Cambridge: Cambridge University Press.

Wannamethee, G. and Shaper, A. G. (1991). Self-assessment of health status and mortality in middle-aged British men. *Int. J Epidemiol,* **20,** 239–245.

Ware, J. E., Jr. (1976). Scales for measuring general health perceptions. *Health Serv. Res,* **11,** 396–415.

Ware, J. E., Jr., Snow, K. K., Kosinski, M., and Gandek, B. (1993). *SF-36 Health Survey. Manual and interpretation guide.* Boston, MA: The Health institute, New England Medical Center.

Wilson, I. B. and Cleary, P. D. (1995). Linking clinical variables with health-related quality of life. A conceptual model of patient outcomes. *JAMA,* **273,** 59–65.

Generic adult health status measures

Stephen Joel Coons and James W. Shaw

Introduction

As discussed in Chapter 1.1, health status measures can be generic or disease-targeted. Generic health status measures are intended to be applicable across all diseases or conditions, across different medical interventions, and across a wide range of populations (Patrick and Deyo 1989). In clinical trials, a targeted measure may provide more detailed outcome information regarding changes in the particular patient population. In addition, targeted measures may be perceived as being more relevant to patients, clinicians, and researchers (Guyatt *et al.* 1993). However, use of both targeted and generic measures may be optimal in most clinical trials. By using only a targeted measure, the general or overall impact on functioning and well-being may be missed.

The two broad types of generic measures are health profiles and preference-based measures. Health profiles provide an array of scores representing individual domains of health or quality of life. In clinical trials, an advantage of a health profile is that it provides multiple outcome scores that may be useful in measuring differential effects of an intervention. In contrast, preference-based measures provide a single health index score on a continuum from dead (0.0) to perfect health (1.0). The score represents the respondent's subjective health status adjusted by a population-based preference weight for that health state. Preference-based measures are discussed in much greater detail in Chapter 6.2.

Many generic health status measures are available; however, it was necessary to select a manageable number for this chapter. The primary selection criteria were that the measure must (1) address physical, psychological, and social functioning and well-being and (2) appear with sufficient frequency in papers presented at recent relevant scientific meetings. A comprehensive evaluation of the measures selected is not within the scope of this chapter. Except for two of them, the measures have had years of use and testing. Only representative evidence regarding their measurement properties will be provided.

Health profiles

The health profiles selected were the SF-36 and the WHOQOL-BREF. Two profile measures conspicuous in their absence are the Sickness Impact Profile (SIP) and the

Nottingham Health Profile (NHP). Although the contribution and historical significance of the SIP and NHP should not be overlooked, their current level of use did not warrant inclusion. For more extensive reviews of these and other measures, readers are referred to additional sources (e.g., McDowell and Newell 1996; Bowling 1997).

SF-36 – background and description

By far, the SF-36 dominates the field of generic health status measurement. The SF-36 is comprised of 36 items selected from a larger pool of items used by RAND in the Medical Outcomes Study (MOS) (Stewart *et al.* 1992). The 36 items in the SF-36 are distributed by QualityMetric as the SF-36, by RAND as the RAND 36-Item Health Survey 1.0, and by the Psychological Corporation as the RAND-36 HSI. There are minor differences among the three versions in scoring for the pain and general health scales, but more significant differences in the derivation of the physical and mental health summary scores.

An extensive questionnaire battery was administered to the MOS longitudinal panel. The SF-36 items were selected to maximize their associations with the long-form MOS scales from which they were derived. The SF-36 produces eight multi-item scales: physical functioning, role limitations due to physical problems, bodily pain, general health perceptions, vitality, social functioning, role limitations due to emotional problems, and mental health. It also includes a single item that addresses perceived health change. The SF-36 scales are scored on a 0 to 100 possible range, with higher scores representing better functioning and well-being.

Factor analyses of the SF-36 provide strong support for a two-factor model of health. Ware *et al.* (1994) derived physical (PCS) and mental component summary (MCS) measures for the SF-36 using an orthogonal rotation method that forced the two factors to be uncorrelated. Orthogonal factor rotations can lead to counterintuitive results (Hays and Morales 2001; Taft *et al.* 2001). Hays *et al.* (1993) also derived summary measures for the SF-36; however, they used an oblique rotation method that allowed for correlation between the factors.

The SF-36 takes about 7–10 minutes to self-administer. Shorter versions of the instrument have been developed, including the SF-12 (Ware *et al.* 1996) and SF-8 (Ware *et al.* 2001). Individual scale scores and component summary scores may be computed for the SF-8 and the SF-12 Version 2.0 (SF-12v2) (Ware *et al.* 2000). Although there is little difference in reliability between the summary scores for the SF-36, SF-12, and SF-8, individual scale scores for the abbreviated versions tend to be less reliable than the SF-36. This loss of precision can be a problem in small samples or with small anticipated effect sizes.

Measurement properties

There is extensive evidence supporting the internal consistency and test-retest reliability of the SF-36 scales in a variety of populations (Coons *et al.* 2000). The same is true for various forms of validity. To test construct validity, Essink-Bot *et al.* (1997) reported that the SF-36 scales demonstrated the best ability to discriminate between migraine sufferers and their matched controls when compared to the NHP, EQ-5D, and COOP/WONCA. They also tested the ability of the four measures to distinguish between subjects based on absence from work due to illness, and found that the SF-36 performed best. Of five measures compared in a study of individuals with acute or chronic musculoskeletal problems, the SF-36 proved to be the measure most responsive to clinical change (Beaton *et al.* 1997).

Alternate forms and translations

The SF-36 can be self-administered or administered by a trained interviewer in person or by telephone. Several technology-based administration approaches have also been developed (e.g., computer-adaptive dynamic health assessment (DYNHA®), voice recognition, telephone keypad). Alternate forms are available with one- or four-week recall periods.

The SF-36 has been translated into more than 50 languages as part of the most coordinated and systematic testing and adaptation effort undertaken for any health status measure (Ware and Gandek 1998). Also available are the SF-36 Version 2.0 (SF-36v2) and SF-12v2. These newer versions incorporate improvements in instructions, item wording, and response options (Mullen *et al.* 2000). For further information visit http://www.SF-36.org.

WHOQOL-BREF – background and description

Under the auspices of the World Health Organization (WHO), the WHOQOL was developed collaboratively and simultaneously by researchers from 15 countries (The WHOQOL Group 1995). Their purpose was to create an internationally applicable and cross-culturally comparable quality-of-life measure. The pilot instrument included 236 items that addressed 29 facets of quality of life. Following extensive field testing, 100 items were selected for inclusion in the WHOQOL-100.

The WHOQOL-100 taps six domains – physical, psychological, independence, social, environment, spiritual – that encompass 24 facets of quality of life (e.g., pain and discomfort, positive affect, mobility, social support). Each facet is measured using four items, making 96 items in total. An additional four items are used to measure global quality of life and general health. Thus, 25 facet scores and six domain scores are produced.

Although the WHOQOL-100 has been shown to be conceptually and psychometrically sound (Bonami *et al.* 2000), its length makes it impractical for use in large epidemiological studies, clinical trials, or routine clinical practice. To fill this role, an abbreviated 26-item version, the WHOQOL-BREF, was developed. The WHOQOL-BREF contains one item from each of the 24 facets in the WHOQOL-100 and one item each for overall quality of life and general health. In designing the WHOQOL-BREF, the independence and physical domains were merged, as were the psychological and spiritual domains. This resulted in a four-domain (physical, psychological, social, and environment) structure. Table 5.2.1 shows the domains and facets included in the WHOQOL-BREF.

The WHOQOL-BREF produces domain scores but, unlike the WHOQOL-100, does not produce individual facet scores. All items are rated on a five-point response scale. The mean score of items within a domain is used to calculate the domain score. Mean scores are then multiplied by four in order to make them comparable with scores for the WHOQOL-100. Alternatively, scores may be converted to a 0–100 scale using a

Table 5.2.1 Domains and facets included in the WHOQOL-BREF

Domains	Facets addressed by single items
Physical health	Pain and discomfort
	Sleep and rest
	Energy and fatigue
	Mobility
	Activities of daily living
	Dependence on medicinal substances and medical aids
	Work capacity
Psychological	Positive feelings
	Thinking, learning, memory and concentration
	Self-esteem
	Bodily image and appearance
	Negative feelings
	Spirituality/religion/personal beliefs
Social relationships	Personal relationships
	Social support
	Sexual activity
Environment	Freedom, physical safety and security
	Home environment
	Financial resources
	Health and social care: accessibility and quality
	Opportunities for acquiring new information and skills
	Participation in and opportunities for recreation/leisure activity
	Physical environment (pollution/noise/traffic/climate)
	Transport

second transformation method. The domain scores are scaled in a positive direction such that higher scores denote better quality of life.

Measurement properties

Domain scores of the WHOQOL-BREF correlate highly ($r \approx 0.9$) with scores for the corresponding WHOQOL-100 domains. The WHOQOL-BREF's domains also demonstrate good reliability and validity (The WHOQOL Group 1998). Because it is so new, evidence regarding the WHOQOL-BREF's responsiveness is sparse. O'Carroll *et al.* (2000) administered the WHOQOL-100, which encompasses the WHOQOL-BREF, to 50 liver transplant patients both before and three months after transplantation. With the exception of the social domain, similar improvements were noted in the domain scores for both versions of the WHOQOL.

Alternate forms and translations

The WHOQOL-BREF was developed as a self-administered form. In addition, interviewer-assisted and interviewer-administered forms are available. The standard recall period is 'the last two weeks'. The WHOQOL-BREF is available in over 20 different languages. For further information visit http://www.who.int/evidence/assessment-instruments/qol/index.htm.

Preference-based measures

The preference-based measures discussed are the EQ-5D, Quality of Well-Being (QWB) Scale, Health Utilities Index (HUI), and SF-6D. Each measure has a descriptive system to assess health status and a scoring function that is applied to assign preference weights to observed health states. Although the four instruments seek to measure a similar construct, there are important differences among them in how this is accomplished. Kopec and Willison (2003) compared the scoring functions of the four measures discussed here. They reported that preference weights assigned by the four instruments to equivalent health states vary considerably. Conner-Spady and Suarez-Almozor (2003) investigated the implications of estimating quality-adjusted life years (QALYs) gained based on the use of the HUI3, EQ-5D, and SF-6D. They concluded that observed health improvement (e.g., QALYs gained) varied substantially among the measures, and that this necessitates caution when comparing the results of studies using different preference-based measures. O'Brien *et al.* (2003) expressed similar concerns.

Quality of Well-Being (QWB) Scale – background and description

The QWB was one of the first entries in the field of quality-of-life measurement systems (Patrick *et al.* 1973). It was developed as a part of a general health-policy model and was viewed as an alternative to economic cost-benefit analysis for resource allocation (Kaplan and Anderson 1996). The QWB assesses health status using three scales representing related but distinct aspects of daily functioning (Table 5.2.2).

Table 5.2.2 Domains included in the preference-based measures

Measure	
QWB	
Mobility	
Physical activity	
Social activity	
Symptoms/problems	
HUI2	**HUI3**
Sensation	Vision
Mobility	Hearing
Emotion	Speech
Cognition	Ambulation
Self-care	Dexterity
Pain	Emotion
Fertility	Cognition
	Pain
EQ-5D	
Mobility	
Self-care	
Usual activity	
Pain/discomfort	
Anxiety/depression	
SF-6D	
Physical functioning	
Role limitation	
Social functioning	
Mental health	
Bodily pain	
Vitality	

In addition, symptom/problem complexes representing health problems or symptomatic complaints that may hinder functioning and well-being are assessed. The interview-administered version of the QWB includes 26 symptom/problem complexes, whereas the self-administered version, the QWB-SA, includes 58 symptoms (Kaplan *et al.* 1997).

Preference weights for the health states represented by the QWB have been derived, based on category rating scale exercises, through general population studies conducted in San Diego (Kaplan and Anderson 1996). The scoring function integrates the levels of functioning with the most undesirable of the reported symptoms/problems to produce a single score that represents an individual's point-in-time well-being. As with the other preference-based measures, the QWB score ranges from 0.0 to 1.0, representing death and perfect health, respectively.

The QWB has been criticized for being too long and complex. For the first 20 years of its existence, the instrument required a trained interviewer to administer it, because it involves branching and probe questions. Completion time for the interview has been reported to range from 10 to 30 minutes. Unlike the interview-based QWB, the QWB-SA can be self-administered in about 12 minutes (Sieber *et al.* 2000). The self-administered version reduces both respondent and administrative burden and is a more practical measure for clinical trials.

Measurement properties

Estimates of internal consistency reliability are not relevant for preference-based measures. A study of test–retest reliability of both the QWB and QWB-SA demonstrated their scores to be stable over a one-month period (Kaplan *et al.* 1997). A significant amount of data is available to support the QWB's construct validity. For example, Orenstein *et al.* (1989) examined relationships among the QWB score, exercise performance, and three pulmonary function tests in patients with cystic fibrosis. The authors reported that the QWB score was significantly correlated with each variable in the predicted direction. Evidence for the QWB-SA's construct validity was demonstrated by its sensitivity to migraine severity (Sieber *et al.* 2000). A number of studies (e.g., Bombardier *et al.* 1986) have found the QWB to be responsive to important clinical changes following treatment interventions. Data supporting the responsiveness of the QWB-SA is limited, but beginning to emerge (Pyne *et al.* 2003).

Alternate forms and translations

The QWB is administered by trained interviewers, either face-to-face or over the telephone. Initial testing suggested that the QWB-SA scores were essentially equivalent to those of the interviewer-administered QWB (Kaplan *et al.* 1997); however, subsequent work shows significant systematic differences between the scores obtained (Pyne *et al.* 2003).

The QWB was developed in US English. Spanish-, German-, and Indochinese-language versions of the QWB are available. For the QWB-SA, there are French and French-Canadian versions, and Spanish and German versions are nearing completion. For further information visit http://medicine.ucsd.edu/fpm/hoap/qwb.htm.

Health Utilities Index (HUI) – background and description

Torrance and colleagues (1982) based the HUI's conceptual framework on the innovative work of Fanshel and Bush (1970). The HUI was designed to measure health status and describe health-related quality of life (Horsman *et al.* 2003). The first version of the HUI, HUI1, was developed to evaluate outcomes for low birthweight infants. The HUI1 consisted of four attributes and a formula to calculate utility scores (Torrance *et al.* 1982). The HUI1 has evolved into two currently available systems: the HUI2 and HUI3 (Table 5.2.2). The HUI2 consists of seven attributes (with three to five levels per attribute) that describe 24,000 unique health states. Formulas have been developed to allow for the calculation of value and utility scores using HUI2 data.

The most recent and conceptually advanced version, the HUI3, has eight attributes (with five or six levels per attribute) that describe 972,000 unique health states. A multi-attribute utility function was developed for the HUI3 using visual analog scale (VAS) and standard gamble measurements from a random sample of the general population of Hamilton, Ontario (Feeny *et al.* 2002). In addition, unlike the scoring systems for the other preference-based measures, the scoring function is multiplicative (rather than additive) and single attribute utility functions were estimated. As with the EQ-5D, the HUI2 and HUI3 allow for negative scores, which reflect health states considered worse than dead (i.e., < 0.0)

For most studies, the 15-item self-administered HUI2/3 questionnaire (i.e., '15Q') is appropriate. It typically takes 5–10 minutes to complete. Interviewer administration is usually conducted with the '40Q', which typically takes 3–5 minutes.

Measurement properties

Test-retest reliability of the HUI3 was evaluated in the 1991 Statistics Canada General Social Survey (GSS) (Boyle *et al.* 1995). Six of the eight attributes had moderate or better kappa coefficients. According to the authors, the results also indicated that the individual questions, algorithms for determining attribute levels, and a provisional HUI3 index formula provided reliable information about the health status of subjects in the GSS.

Extensive evidence supporting the construct validity of the HUI2 and HUI3 has been published (Horsman *et al.* 2003). Barr *et al.* (1997) provided data demonstrating that the HUI2 and HUI3 were sensitive to the changing adverse event profile in children with acute lymphoblastic leukemia who were in remission and receiving maintenance chemotherapy. Specifically, the HUI attributes (i.e., pain, emotion, and mobility/ambulation) were found to be responsive to toxicity associated with steroid use during the chemotherapy cycle. Blanchard *et al.* (2003) reported that the SF-36, HUI2, and HUI3 were all responsive to clinical change in patients undergoing total hip arthroplasty, with the HUI3 being the most responsive of the generic measures tested.

Alternate forms and translations

The combined HUI2/3 questionnaire is available for interviewer administration (in person or via telephone) and self-completion (Horsman *et al.* 2003). Both have been developed in self-assessment and proxy-assessment forms.

Questionnaires for each of four standard recall periods (one week, two weeks, four weeks, and usual) are available. The 'usual' recall period is often used in long-term follow-up or for population health surveys. All of the alternative forms mentioned above are available in Canadian English. In addition, numerous other language versions exist. For further information visit http://www.healthutilities.com.

EQ-5D – background and description

A multidisciplinary team of European researchers (the EuroQol Group) designed the EQ-5D to be a brief, self-completed instrument for describing and valuing health-related quality of life (Brooks et al. 1996). A multidimensional structure was a goal, although simplicity was considered essential to make it practical for use in population health surveys or in conjunction with condition-targeted instruments for the assessment of outcomes related to specific conditions and/or treatments (EuroQol Group 1990).

The EQ-5D has two parts. The first is a descriptive system that classifies respondents into one of 243 distinct health states. The current descriptive system consists of five dimensions shown in Table 5.2.2. Each dimension has three levels, reflecting 'no problems', 'some problems' and 'extreme problems'. A scoring function assigns a value to self-reported health states from a set of preference weights that have been empirically derived. The most commonly applied set of preferences was developed in the UK using the time trade-off (TTO) method (Dolan 1997). General population 'value sets' have been derived for other countries (Kind 2003) and a set of TTO-based preference weights for the US adult population is in development.

The second part of the EQ-5D is a 20 cm VAS that has end points labelled 'best imaginable health state' and 'worst imaginable health state' anchored at 100 and 0, respectively. Respondents are asked to indicate how they rate their own health by drawing a line from an anchor box to that point on the VAS which best represents their own health on that day. Hence, the EQ-5D produces three types of data for each respondent: (1) a profile indicating the extent of problems on each of the five dimensions, (2) a population preference-weighted health index score based on the descriptive system, and (3) a self-rated assessment of health status based on the VAS. The two main pages of the EQ-5D take about a minute to complete.

Measurement properties

A study by Dorman et al. (1998) assessed the three-week test-retest reliability of the EQ-5D in a group of stroke patients. For the five dimensions, kappa coefficients ranged from 0.63 to 0.80. Intraclass correlation coefficients for the VAS and index scores were both 0.86, suggesting excellent reproducibility.

Brazier et al. (1993) tested the EQ-5D's construct validity by examining hypothesized relationships between the EQ-5D and other variables. They found expected distributions of EQ-5D scores for sociodemographic variables, health services use, and the diagnosis of a chronic physical problem. However, the associations were weaker and less often significant than those found with the SF-36. In addition, the EQ-5D had substantially greater ceiling effects. Johnson and Coons (1998) also provided evidence for the construct validity of the EQ-5D index and VAS scores, but the EQ-5D scores were less sensitive than SF-12 component summary measures to differences associated with slight morbidity.

Evidence for the responsiveness of the EQ-5D VAS was provided by König et al. (2002) in patients being treated for inflammatory bowel disease; however, the EQ-5D index score was not found to be responsive to clinically important change. Tidermark et al. (2003) found the EQ-5D index score to be highly responsive (slightly more so than the SF-36) in patients undergoing surgical procedures for displaced femoral neck fractures.

Alternate forms and translations

The EQ-5D is available as a self-administered form that asks about health 'today'. No information on supported alternative administration approaches has been reported in the literature. There are over 50 official language versions of EQ-5D; more are completed and awaiting official ratification by the EuroQol Group's Translation Committee. For further information visit http://www.euroqol.org.

SF-6D – background and description

With the dominance of the SF-36 among the profile measures, there has been significant interest in deriving a health index score from it to enable its incorporation into economic evaluation involving QALYs. As mentioned earlier, Ware et al. (1994) and Hays et al. (1993) developed physical and mental summary scores for the SF-36; however, they did not develop an overall summary or index score. In order to address this limitation, Brazier and colleagues (1998) undertook the development of a preference-based index that utilized health state classifications derived from the SF-36 items.

As Brazier et al. (1998) noted, the number of possible combinations of items and levels in the SF-36 would result in millions of health states. Hence, there was a need to create a simplified health state classification system based on selected SF-36 items. The resulting classification system has six dimensions (Table 5.2.2). The initial version of the SF-6D was based on 20 of the SF-36 items and defined 9,000 possible health states with two to six levels for each of the six dimensions.

However, Brazier et al. (2002) felt that the initial SF-6D, as well as the associated statistical models for predicting values for the health states it defined, had significant limitations. As a result, they undertook a much more extensive development process to create the current SF-6D. It is based on 11 SF-36 items and, with four to six levels for each of the six dimensions, it defines 18,000 possible health states. A UK general population study was conducted to elicit preferences for a sample of the SF-6D health states using a standard gamble technique. Based on extensive econometric modelling of the observed/elicited preferences, a model was constructed that is recommended for estimating mean preferences for all possible SF-6D health states.

Measurement properties

The SF-6D is the newest of the measures discussed in this chapter. There are vast amounts of evidence supporting the measurement properties of the underlying SF-36; however, evidence is just beginning to emerge for the SF-6D. Bosch *et al.* (2002) compared the responsiveness of the SF-6D with the HUI2 and HUI3 in patients treated for intermittent claudication. They concluded that the SF-6D was responsive to observed patient improvement, but less so than the HUI2 or HUI3. In a study of rheumatoid arthritis patients, Russell *et al.* (2003) reported that the SF-6D was responsive to treatment effect, though to a lesser extent than the EQ-5D.

Unlike the other preference-based measures, which have defined health states ranging in value from 1 (full health) to 0 (death) or lower (e.g., –0.59 when using the UK preference weights for the EQ-5D or –0.36 for the HUI3), the SF-6D has a more restricted range (i.e., 1 to 0.30 when using the valuation model recommended by the developers). This may impact its ability to detect change in persons with very poor health (Kopec and Willison 2003).

Alternate forms and translations

Because the SF-6D is based on 11 items from the SF-36, all the administration approaches and translations available for the SF-36 can be used. The advantages this brings are considerable, due to the substantial amount of SF-36 data that has been collected around the world. For further information contact John Brazier, Ph.D. (j.e.brazier@sheffield.ac.uk).

Conclusions

The purpose of this chapter was to introduce the reader to six generic health status measures. Of the instruments reviewed, the SF-36 is the most commonly used health status measure in the world today; however, this does not indicate that it is the best general instrument to use in every situation. The decision to use one instrument over another, to use a combination of two or more, to use a profile and/or a preference-based measure, or to use a generic measure along with a targeted measure should be driven by the purpose of the measurement. In addition, the choice should depend on a variety of other factors, including the characteristics of the population (e.g., age, health status, language/culture) and the setting in which the measurement is undertaken (e.g., clinical trial).

References

Barr, R. D., Petrie, C., and Furlong, W., *et al.* (1997). Health-related quality of life during post-induction chemotherapy in children with acute lymphoblastic leukemia in remission: An influence of corticosteroid therapy. *International Journal of Oncology*, **11**, 333–339.

Beaton, D. E., Hogg-Johnson, S., and Bombardier, C. (1997). Evaluating changes in health status: reliability and responsiveness of five generic health status measures in workers with musculoskeletal disorders. *Journal of Clinical Epidemiology*, **50**, 79–93.

Blanchard, C., Feeny, D., and Mahon, J. L., *et al.* (2003). Is the Health Utilities Index responsive in total hip arthroplasty patients? *Journal of Clinical Epidemiology*, **56**, 1046–1054.

Bombardier, C., Ware, J. E., and Russell, I. J., *et al.* (1986). Auranofin therapy and quality of life in patients with rheumatoid arthritis: results of a multicenter trial. *American Journal of Medicine*, **81**, 565–578.

Bonomi, A. E., Patrick, D. L., Bushnell, D. M., and Martin, M. (2000). Validation of the United States' version of the World Health Organization Quality of Life (WHOQOL) instrument. *Journal of Clinical Epidemiology*, **53**, 1–12.

Bosch, J. L., Halpern, E. K., and Gazzelle, G. S. (2002). Comparison of preference-based utilities of the Short-Form 36 Health Survey and Health Utilities Index before and after treatment of patients with intermittent claudication. *Medical Decision Making*, **22**, 403–409.

Bowling, A. (1997). *Measuring health: a review of quality of life measurement scales*, 2nd edn. Buckingham: Open University Press.

Boyle, M. H., Furlong, W., and Torrance, G. W., *et al.* (1995). Reliability of the Health Utilities Index-Mark III used in the 1991 cycle 6 General Social Survey Health Questionnaire. *Quality of Life Research*, **4**, 249–256.

Brazier, J., Jones, N., and Kind, P. (1993). Testing the validity of the Euroqol and comparing it with the SF-36 health survey questionnaire. *Quality of Life Research*, **2**, 169–180.

Brazier, J., Usherwood, T., Harper, R., and Thomas, K. (1998). Deriving a preference-based single index from the UK SF-36 Health Survey. *Journal of Clinical Epidemiology*, **51**, 1115–1128.

Brazier, J., Roberts, J., and Deverill, M. (2002). The estimation of a preference-based measure of health from SF-36. *Journal of Health Economics*, **21**, 271–292.

Brooks, R. and the EuroQol Group (1996). EuroQol: the current state of play. *Health Policy*, **37**, 53–72.

Conner-Spady, B. and Suarez-Almozar, M. E. (2003). Variation in the estimation of quality-adjusted life years by different preference-based instruments. *Medical Care*, **41**, 791–801.

Coons, S. J., Rao, S., Keininger, D. L., and Hays, R. D. (2000). A comparative review of generic quality of life instruments. *Pharmacoeconomics*, **1**, 13–35.

Dolan, P. (1997). Modeling valuations for EuroQol health states. *Medical Care*, **35**, 1095–1108.

Dorman, P., Slattery, J., and Farrell, B., *et al.* (1998). Qualitative comparison of the reliability of health status assessments with the EuroQol and SF-36 questionnaires after stroke. *Stroke*, **19**, 63–8.

Essink-Bot, M. L., Krabbe, P. F. M., and Bonsel, G. J., *et al.* (1997). An empirical comparison of four generic health status measures. *Medical Care*, **35**, 522–537.

EuroQol Group (1990). EuroQol – a new facility for the measurement of health-related quality of life. *Health Policy*, **16**, 199–208.

Fanshel, S. and Bush, J. W. (1970). A health status index and its application to health services outcomes. *Operations Research*, **18**, 1021–1066.

Feeny, D., Furlong, W., and Torrance, G. W., *et al.* (2002). Multiattribute and single-attribute utility functions for the Health Utilities Index Mark 3 system. *Medical Care*, **40**, 113–128.

Guyatt, G. H., Feeny, D. H., and Patrick, D. L. (1993). Measuring health-related quality of life. *Annals of Internal Medicine*, **118**, 622–629.

Hays, R. D. and Morales, L. S. (2001). The RAND-36 measure of health-related quality of life. *Annals of Medicine*, **33**, 350–357.

Hays, R. D., Sherbourne, C. D., and Mazel, R. M. (1993). The RAND 36-Item Health Survey 1.0. *Health Economics*, **2**, 217–227.

Horsman, J., Furlong, W., Feeny, D., and Torrance, G. (2003). The Health Utilities Index (HUI): concepts, measurement properties and applications. *Health and Quality of Life Outcomes*, **1**, 54.

Johnson, J. A. and Coons, S. J. (1998). Comparison of the EQ-5D and the SF-12 in an adult US sample. *Quality of Life Research*, **7**, 155–166.

Kaplan, R. M. and Anderson, J. P. (1996). The General Health Policy Model: an integrated approach. In B. Spilker (ed.) *Quality of life and pharmacoeconomics in clinical trials*, 2nd edn, pp. 309–22. Philadelphia: Lippincott-Raven.

Kaplan, R. M., Sieber, W. J., and Ganiats, T. G. (1997). The Quality of Well-being Scale: comparison of the interview-administered with a self-administered questionnaire. *Psychology and Health*, **12**, 783–791.

Kind, P. (2003). Guidelines for value sets in economic and non-economic studies using EQ-5D. In R. Brooks, R. Rabin and F. de Charro (eds) *The measurement and valuation of health status using the EQ-5D: a European perspective*, pp. 29–41. Dordrecht: Kluwer Academic Publishers.

König, H.-H., Ulshöfer, A., and Gregor, M., *et al.* (2002). Validation of the EuroQol questionnaire in patients with inflammatory bowel disease. *European Journal of Gastroenterology & Hepatology*, **14**, 1205–1215.

Kopec, J. A. and Willison, K. D. (2003). A comparative review of four preference-weighted measures of health-related quality of life. *Journal of Clinical Epidemiology*, **56**, 317–325.

McDowell, I. and Newell, C. (1996). *Measuring health: a guide to rating scales and questionnaires*, 2nd edn. New York: Oxford University Press.

Mullen, P. A., Lohr, K. N., Bresnahan, B. W., and McNulty, P. (2000). Applying cognitive design principles to formatting HRQOL instruments. *Quality of Life Research*, **9**, 13–27.

O'Brien, B. J., Spath, M., Blackhouse, G., Severens, J. L., Dorian, P., and Brazier, J. (2003). A view from the bridge: agreement between the SF-6D utility algorithm and the Health Utilities Index. *Health Economics*, **12**, 975–981.

O'Carroll, R. E., Smith, K., and Couston, M., *et al.* (2000). A comparison of the WHOQOL-100 and the WHOQOL-BREF in detecting change in the quality of life following liver transplantation. *Quality of Life Research*, **9**, 121–124.

Orenstein, D. M., Nixon, P. A., and Ross, E. A., *et al.* (1989). The Quality of Well-Being Scale in cystic fibrosis. *Chest*, **95**, 344–347.

Patrick, D. L., Bush, J. W., and Chen, M. M. (1973). Methods for measuring levels of well-being for a health status index. *Health Services Research*, **8**, 228–245.

Patrick, D. L. and Deyo, R. A. (1989). Generic and disease-specific measures in assessing health status and quality of life. *Medical Care*, **27**, S217–232.

Pyne, J. M., Sieber, W. J., David, K., Kaplan, R. M., Rapaport, M. H., and Williams, D. K. (2003). Use of the quality of well-being self-administered version (QWB-SA) in assessing health-related quality of life in depressed patients. *Journal of Affective Disorders*, **76**, 237–247.

Russell, A. S., Conner-Spady, B., Mintz, A. J., Mallon, C., and Maksymowych, W. P. (2003). The responsiveness of generic health status measures as assessed in patients with rheumatoid arthritis receiving infliximab. *Journal of Rheumatology*, **30**, 941–947.

Sieber, W. J., David, K. M., Adams, J. E., Kaplan, R. M., and Ganiats, T. G. (2000). Assessing the impact of Migraine on health-related quality of life: an additional use of the Quality of Well-being Scale—Self Administered. *Headache*, **40**, 662–671.

Stewart, A. L., Sherbourne, C. D., and Hays, R. D., *et al.* (1992). Summary and discussion of MOS measures. In A. L. Stewart and J. E. Ware (eds) *Measuring functioning and well-being: the Medical Outcomes Study approach*, pp. 345–71. Duke University Press, Durham, NC.

Taft, C., Karlsson, J., and Sullivan, M. (2001). Do SF-36 summary component scores accurately summarize subscale scores? *Quality of Life Research*, **10**, 395–404.

The WHOQOL Group (1995). The World Health Organization Quality of Life Assessment (WHOQOL): position paper from the World Health Organization. *Social Science and Medicine*, **41**, 1403–1409.

The WHOQOL Group (1998). Development of the World Health Organization WHOQOL-BREF quality of life assessment. *Psychological Medicine*, **28**, 551–558.

Tidermark, J., Bergström, G., Svensson, O., Törnkvist, H., and Ponzer, S. (2003). Responsiveness of the EuroQol (EQ-5D) and the SF-36 in elderly patients with displaced femoral neck fractures. *Quality of Life Research*, **12**, 1069–1079.

Torrance, G. W., Boyle, M. H., and Horwood, S. P. (1982). Application of multiattribute utility theory to measure social preferences for health states. *Operations Research*, **30**, 1043–1069.

Ware, J. E., Kosinski, M., and Keller, S. D. (1994). *SF-36 Physical and mental health summary scales: a user's manual.* Boston, MA: The Health Institute.

Ware, J. E., Kosinski, M., and Keller, S. D. (1996). A 12-item short-form health survey: construction of scales and preliminary test of reliability and validity. *Medical Care*, **34**, 220–233.

Ware, J. E. and Gandek, B. (1998). Overview of the SF-36 health survey and the international quality of life assessment (IQOLA) project. *Journal of Clinical Epidemiology*, **51**, 903–912.

Ware, J. E., Kosinski, M. A., and Dewey, J. E. (2000). *How to score version 2 of SF-36® Health Survey.* Lincoln, RI: QualityMetric Incorporated.

Ware, J. E., Kosinski, M. A., Dewey, J. E., and Gandek, B. (2001). *How to score and interpret single-item health status measures: a manual for users of the SF-8 Health Survey.* Lincoln, RI: QualityMetric Incorporated.

5.3

Practical considerations in the measurement of HRQoL in child/adolescent clinical trials

Jeanne M. Landgraf

All of man's strength and all his weakness go to make up the authority of any particular opinion which he may utter. Man is strong or weak with all his strength and weakness combined.

Thoreau, Journal February 16, 1854

Introduction

Compared to adults, children and youth have historically been considered 'healthy and resilient'. The tacit implication of this perception and the inherent complexities of engaging minor aged subjects in medical research often led to their exclusion from many health-related quality of life studies and randomized clinical trials. Increasingly, however, studies are specifically targeting children and youth.

This increased activity may be due in part to the convergence of a number of independent factors, including an intellectual shift in how health is defined. It is now largely accepted that 'health' is not simply the absence of physical disease, but also includes positive social and emotional functioning and well-being. In the early 1990s the American Medical Association (Gans *et al.* 1990) and the Office of Technology Assessment (1991) published seminal reports underscoring a growing concern that the occurrence of mental health, and social and behavioral problems among children and youth was understudied, and that little information was available with regard to the impact of these issues on the everyday health-related quality of life (HRQoL) for this special population.

Coincident to these seminal publications, development of both generic and condition/disease-specific quality of life measures for children and youth began in earnest. By the mid to late 1990s, a number of measures became available, but were utilized primarily in academic-based clinical research studies. The scientific work was quite substantive and resulted in several publications summarizing the content, development process, psychometric properties and other empirical findings for both generic and condition/disease-specific measures developed exclusively for children and youth (Drotar 1998; Eiser and Morse 2001a; Koot and Wallander 2001,

Rodrigue *et al.* 2000). The advent of these resource publications represented an important milestone for the field, and underscored the depth and breadth of the measures available. More importantly, by synthesizing the information they made it much easier for the researcher to understand the strengths and limitation of the measures, thereby facilitating more informed decision-making with regard to appropriate selection and use.

Two recent federal mandates have contributed significantly to the use of pediatric instruments within randomized clinical trials – The Pediatric Exclusivity Provision that was part of the 1997 Food and Drug Administration Modernization Act and The Best Pharmaceuticals for Children Act (Matza *et al.* 2004; Roberts *et al.* 2003). These regulations provided significant financial incentives to the pharmaceutical industry to study the effects of drugs on children approved for adults, but commonly given to children. These studies have centered on key issues such as safety, efficacy, pharmacokinetics, and/or pharmacodynamics. According to a recent publication (Roberts *et al.* 2003) between summer 1998 and spring 2002, the Food and Drug Administration requested studies on 242 adult drugs commonly used in children, and 53 of these drugs were granted exclusivity in exchange for conducting the studies.

In the past, trials have been of great value in highlighting directions for new treatments. The current emphasis – even for life-threatening conditions such as cancer or cystic fibrosis – is now on improvements in quality of life (Eiser 2003). The focus has also extended to child-centered investigations. A PubMed literature search conducted in April 2003 using the key words 'clinical trials' and 'child's quality of life' produced 163 published articles in the past five years – 61 of which have been published in the past two years. The trials were conducted across a broad spectrum of diagnoses/conditions and utilized both generic and condition-specific measures to assess the child's health-related quality of life.

As the name suggests, generic instruments are designed to assess the broad impact of a condition, whereas condition or disease-specific instruments are designed to capture particular aspects of life that are affected by an explicit physical, emotional or behavioral issue. Historically, conditions/diseases in children and adolescents have been defined using a categorical or diagnostic approach. Thus, for example, instruments have been developed across a broad array of chronic conditions such as asthma (French *et al.* 1994; Juniper *et al.* 1996a 1996b), attention-deficit/hyperactivity disorder (Landgraf *et al.* 2002), cancer (Armstrong *et al.* 1999; Bhatia *et al.* 2002; Goodwin *et al* 1994), Crohn's disease (Rabbett *et al.* 1996), diabetes (Ingersoll and Marrero 1991), migraine/severe headaches (Langeveld *et al.* 1997, 1999), spina bifida (Parkin *et al.* 1997), and pediatric enuresis (Landgraf *et al.* 2003).

It is important to note that a complementary non-categorical approach has also been proposed and used in epidemiological studies to define the conceptual boundaries for the term 'chronic health condition' (Stein *et al.* 1993, 1997) and to assess their prevalence, service use and cost within the public health arena. An excellent overview of the non-categorical approach is available elsewhere (Ireys 2001). Wider adoption of this perspective may result in the future development and application of new, more broadly defined measures that assess core aspects of HRQoL common across an array of chronic issues in children and adolescents as opposed to separate and unique condition/diagnosis-specific measures.

The superiority and merits of generic and specific measures – however the latter are defined and operationalized – have long been debated (Patrick and Deyo 1989; also see Chapter 5.4 of this book). To date, however, few if any studies have specifically addressed the trade-offs in precision with regard to generic child HRQoL measures versus condition/disease specific complements and the relationship of self-reported HRQoL to more traditional clinical markers such as severity or Forced Expiratory volume in 1 second (FEV_1) in asthmatics (McGrath *et al.* 1999). No doubt the debate will linger until further empirical evidence is known about the relative tradeoffs in precision and the degree of correlation (if any) between clinical parameters and self-reports in children/adolescents.

It has been recommended that generic measures be supplemented with specific disease-targeted instruments (Bungay and Ware, 1993; Eiser and Morse 2001a; Landgraf *et al.* 1996, 1999; Seid *et al.* 1999; Spieth 2001). In their 2001 review, Eiser and Morse noted that approximately 15 studies used a 'battery approach' to assessing quality of life. As the name infers, this method uses a compilation of independently developed batteries within the same study to create a questionnaire. Each of the modules is scored and reported independently. For example, a single study might utilize a behavior scale such as the Child Behavior Checklist (Achenbach 1979), a family scale such as the Family Adaptability, Cohesion, Evaluation Scales (Olson *et al.* 1985), a self-esteem scale such as the Piers–Harris (Piers 1969) and cognitive/intellectual functioning index like the Wechsler Intelligence Scale for Children (Kaufman 1979).

It is not always feasible to use the battery approach, or to include both generic and condition/disease-specific forms in a single study, as this adds to respondent burden and cost. Irrespective of respondent burden and cost, the overall selection of an appropriate instrument requires careful consideration and will depend on the target condition, information about the psychometric properties of the measure, including sensitivity to change, and other specific aspects of the trial itself.

A core set of standards should be used to evaluate the scientific merits of a measure – whether generic or condition/disease specific – and guide in its selection and use. These fundamental psychometric characteristics include reliability, validity and responsiveness – an aspect of validity that is of particular importance to clinical trials. The reader is guided to section one of this book (Hays and Revicki Chapter 1.3) and other resources for a comprehensive review of these principles as they pertain to the development and evaluation of HRQoL measures (Fayers and Machin 2000) and to measures in general (Nunnally and Bernstein 1994; Pedhazur and Pedhazur Schmelkin 1991; Thorndike *et al* 1991).

As noted in an earlier publication (Landgraf and Abetz 1996) and reiterated more recently by others (Eiser and Morse 2001a; Matza *et al.* 2004; Spieth 2001) there are several issues beyond reliability and validity that must also be considered when selecting an instrument for use with children or adolescents. These additional practical issues are also relevant to the selection of adult measures and include appropriateness of items and concepts, applicability of measures among different ethnic/race/cultural groups, instrument length and completion time, age and readability, use of pictures and mode of administration, response options, respondent selection, and interpreting scores and identifying meaningful differences.

The purpose of this chapter is to briefly identify characteristics of common generic HRQoL instruments within the context of these particular considerations. A summary of information across the general measures is presented in Table 5.3.1.

Due to space constraints, only generic instruments for which there is published information about reliability and validity are incorporated into the chapter. For example, the Nordic Quality of Life Questionnaire (Lindstrom and Eriksson 1993) is mentioned in the review by Eiser and Morse (2001a); however, information about reliability/validity were 'under evaluation' and the instrument is not currently listed in an online quality of life measures database link for several professional organizations, including the International Society for Quality of Life Research. Also excluded from the chapter is Eiser and Morse's reference to a generic instrument by Collier (1997) for which there currently does not appear to be a peer reviewed publication. The reader is encouraged to consult Koot and Wallander (2001), Rodrigue *et al.* (2000) and the Eiser and Morse technical report (2001a) for comprehensive reviews of both generic and condition/disease-specific measures.

Measures and their key citations

The following measures are cited throughout the text. They were selected because they were developed specifically for children and youth. Key citations for each measure – as they relate only to the principles specifically discussed in the chapter – are also noted:

- ◆ Child Health and Illness Profile Adolescent Edition (AE) and Child Edition (CE): CHIP-AE and CHIP CE (Rebok *et al.* 2001; Starfield *et al.* 1993, 1995; Riley *et al.* 2004a)

- ◆ Child Health Questionnaire Parent Form (PF) and Child Form (CF) – CHQ PF50, PF28 and CHQ CF87 – (Aitken *et al.* 2002; Asmussen *et al.* 2000; DeVeaugh-Geiss *et al.* 2002; Hepner and Sechrest 2002; Landgraf and Abetz 1997; Landgraf *et al.* 1996, 1998, 1999; McGrath *et al.* 1999; Michelson *et al.* 2001; Nixon-Speechly *et al.* 1999; Raat *et al.* 2002; Waters *et al.* 1999).

- ◆ Child Quality of Life Questionnaire – CQOL – (Graham *et al.*1997)

- ◆ Dartmouth COOP Picture Charts – COOP – (Wasson *et al.* 1994, 1995).

- ◆ Exeter Health-Related Quality of Life Measure – EHRQL – (Eiser *et al.* 1999, 2000)

Table 5.3.1

Characteristic	CHIP	CHQ	COOP	CQOL	EHRQL	FS11R	HAY	MEASURE HUI2/3	KINDL	PEDSQL	QOLP-AV	TACQOL	WCHMP	16/17D
Age	6-11(CE) 11-17 (AE)	5-18 (PF) 10-18 (CF)	12-21	9-15	6-11	0-16	7-13	2-18 0-old age	10-16	2-18	14-20	6-15	0-5	12-15 8-11
Concepts														
Behavior	X	X											X	
Bodily pain		X		X				X				X		
Cognitive							X	X				X		
Communication			X	X		X								
Disorders/physical complaints	X						X							
Emotional well-being	X	X	X	X		X			X	X	X			X
Family	X	X	X	X										
General Health	X	X	X										X	
Health habits	X		X											
Parental impact		X	X											
Physical/self care	X	X	X	X		X	X	X	X	X	X			X
Satisfaction/self worth	X	X					X				X			X
School	X	X	X							X				X
Social	X	X	X	X			X		X	X	X			X
Spiritual well-being											X			

Continued

Table 5.3.1 (Continued)

Characteristic	CHIP	CHQ	COOP	CQOL	EHRQL	FS11R	HAY	HUI2/3	KINDL	PEDSQL	QOLP-AV	TACQOL	WCHMP	16/17D
								MEASURE						
Ethnicity/gender findings	X	X			X	X		X	X	X				
Format														
Likert	X	X	X	X		X	X		X	X	X	X	X	
Categories of response								X			X		X	X
Visual analog scale				X										
Graphics (YES)	X		X					X	X					X
Mode of administration														
Computer and paper-pencil	X	X	X		X				X					
Norms/benchmarks	X	X						X		X				
Readability statistics	X	X								X				
Recall period	4 wks	4 wks	month	month	NS	2 wks	7 days	AP·	week	month	NS	weeks	NS	AP
Reliability														
Internal consistency	X	X	X		X	X	X		X	X	X	X	X	
Test-retest	X	X	X				X	X	X			X		X

Respondent

Child only		X		X				X	X
Child and Proxy	X	X	X		X		X	X*	X
Proxy only			X					X	X

Validity

Concurrent		X	X				X		X
Construct	X	X	X		X		X	X	X
Convergent	X	X	X			X	X		
Clinical	X	X		X	X		X	X	X
Criterion	X	X					X		X
Predicitve						X			
Responsivenss		X				X			

CE and AE = child edition and adolescent edition; PF and CF = parent form; NS = none specified; AP = at present state; * HUI2 (clinician/parent and child self-report begins age 8 and older; HUI3 is parent report only for children).

- Functional Status II(R) – FSII(R) – (Lewis *et al.* 1989; Stein and Jessop 1990)
- Health Utilities Index – HUI2 and HUI3 – (Barr *et al.* 1997; Feeny *et al.* 1992; 1995; 1996; 1998; Furlong 1996; Juniper *et al.* 1997; Le Galps *et al.* 2002; Lutetkin and Gold 2002; Nixon-Speechly *et al.* 1999; Raat *et al.* 2002; Saigal *et al.* 1994; Verrips *et al.* 2001)
- How are You? – HAY – (Bruil 1999)
- KINDL (Ravens-Sieberer *et al.* 1998)
- Pediatric Quality of Life Questionnaire – PedsQL – (Varni *et al.* 1999, 2001, 2003)
- Quality of Life Profile Adolescent Version – QOLP-AV – (Raphael *et al.* 1996)
- TACQOL (Theunissen *et al.* 1998; Vogels *et al.* 1998)
- Warwick Child Health and Morbidity Profile – WCHMP – (Spencer and Coe, 1996)
- 16 Dimensions, 17 Dimensions – 16D, 17D – (Apajasalo *et al.* 1996a, b).

General HRQoL measures and guidelines for selection and use

Defining HRQoL

Several formal approaches have been used to define quality of life – philosophical, economic, sociological, psychological, and medical (Lindstrom and Koehler 1991). Given these diverse perspectives, it is not surprising that a formal, standardized definition of the term 'quality of life' remains relatively elusive. The issue is further complicated because the terms 'health status' and 'functional status' are often used interchangeably with quality of life, but as yet no one has been successful in drawing a clear conceptual distinction between them (Eiser and Morse 2001a). Despite these differences, it is commonly accepted that the concept 'health-related quality of life' refers to the subjective evaluation of one's ability to perform usual tasks and their impact on one's everyday physical, emotional and social well-being.

Items and Concepts

The most critical design characteristic for instrument selection with child/adolescent samples is whether the instrument was developed using a developmentally grounded conceptual framework. Adapting items from an adult instrument by rewording them to be more child-relevant is not sufficient. The instrument must be relevant at both the concept level and the item level.

Self-esteem and the ability to get along with others are important aspect of one's adolescent development and can be found in many pediatric HRQoL instruments. Although it has been suggested that self-esteem should be included in adult measures (Stewart and Hays 1997), the concepts are not generally captured in adult HRQoL instruments. Despite this and other conceptual limitations, measures specifically developed for the adult population such as the SF-36 (Ware *et al.* 1993) and the

Quality of Well-Being Scale (Bradlyn *et al.* 1993) have sometimes been used in studies with children and/or adolescents.

It is essential to note that pediatric measures have benefited from the careful scientific work conducted in adults, and the majority of published instruments mirror the *measurement* approach used in adult work by adopting their architectural framework, including categorical response scales and corresponding methods of scoring and interpretation. However, their *conceptual* framework is unique to children/adolescents.

Several pediatric instruments have a direct lineage to adult measures. For example, the Dartmouth COOP Charts complements the picture charts initially developed for adults (Nelson *et al.* 1987, 1990a, b). The FSIIR was modeled on the SIP (Bergner *et al.* 1981). The HUI is applicable across children and adult populations (Feeny *et al.* 1996). The 16D, 17D were based on the 15D (Sintonen and Pekurinen 1993). The CHQ adopted an architectural approach similar to the SF-36 (Ware *et al.* 1993) by utilizing both global items and multi-item scales. It is interesting to note that the CHQ used a graduated response continuum for all items whereas a dichotomous approach (i.e., yes, no response) was used in the original SF-36 (Ware *et al.,* 1993) but later revised in subsequent iterations (i.e., SF-26v2) to include only graduated response options.

The conceptual framework for each of the pediatric HRQoL measures with lineage to adult instruments has undergone rigorous independent testing and evaluation. The COOP charts were developed by reviewing content from 15 different instruments (Wasson *et al.* 1994). The behavior scale in the FSII(R) was constructed using 18 resource documents such as the National Health Examination Survey and the Denver Prescreening Developmental Questionnaire (Stein and Jessop 1990). The 16 and 17 D utilized a multidisciplinary panel of experts to review items and parents and a sample of boys were asked to respond to the content of the measure as well (Apajasalo *et al.* 1996a, b). Content for the CHQ was also derived from existing pediatric measures and additional concepts were added based on observation and input from families and grounded theories of child development and language acquisition (Landgraf *et al.* 1996, 1999). The conceptual structure of the CHQ has been tested and replicated across different pediatric subgroups and cultures within the US and elsewhere (Hepner and Sechrest 2002; Raat *et al.* 2002; Waters *et al.* 1999). Preference scores have been examined for the HUI in France and the Netherlands (Le Galps *et al.* 2002; Raat *et al.* 2002).

It is also noteworthy to mention the conceptual distinction of two measures. In contrast to the other instruments, the PedsQL was derived from several pediatric oncology studies that included the use of a cancer-specific instrument (Varni *et al.* 1999). The HAY (Bruil 1999) is a general instrument but the measure also includes items specific to asthma, diabetes, epilepsy and juvenile rheumatoid arthritis.

Additionally, some instruments may contain items that are not applicable to a particular child age group or culture. For example, the HAY (Bruil 1999) includes an item about riding bicycles, an activity that is very common in the Netherlands (country of origin) but may be less so in other countries. Issues such as this could be reconciled during the translation and cross-cultural validation process by selecting comparable but more neutral examples. An instrument may also refer to 'playing at recess', which would not be appropriate for older adolescents attending high school. Thus, it is important to review any instrument for face validity and acceptability to the age group being targeted.

Domains identified in general measures ranged from three (QOLP-AV) to 17 (17D) and have yet to be proposed for the EHRQL (Eiser and Morse 2001a). In addition to the number of concepts, there is also great inconsistency in the labels that are used to identify them. Thus, it is challenging to understand the conceptual advantages of one measure versus another. It would appear based on the commonality – as evidenced below – that at a minimum the measure should capture the child/adolescents' emotional, physical and social well-being. Selection of the appropriate instrument will depend in part of the nature of the trial. For example, pain may be important for clinical studies testing a new therapy for AIDS or cancer. Behavior (e.g., the ability to get along with peers), school and social functioning and family impact are essential for studies that focus on issues such as attention-deficit/hyperactivity disorder. It may also be that a concept is not captured and in this case it may be appropriate to include an independent battery or module.

As mentioned previously, there is no standard for defining the unique conceptual areas captured across each measure. For example, the CHIP identifies concepts such as discomfort and achievement – labels that are not used in other measures. As such, in the absence of systematic review of the actual content of each measure, it is challenging for novice users and others to easily identify commonalities and differences with regard to the breadth of concepts measured and their definition.

With regard to items and concepts, questionnaires are often transferred onto a case report form for the purpose of conducting a clinical trial. It is important that the measure be reproduced with great precision. Items should not be reordered and scales should not be rearranged. For continuity, scales should remain intact and all items associated with a given scale should be presented on the same page if at all possible.

The following conceptual labels and the measures wherein they can be found are not meant to be definitive. They are meant as a point of reference to illustrate the degree of variation across the pediatric HRQoL instruments measures with regard to the concepts they are designed to measure.

- behavior: CHIP; CHQ; WCHMP
- bodily pain: CHQ; CQOL; HUI2 & 3; TACQOL
- cognitive: HAY; HUI2 & 3; TACQOL
- communication: COOP; CQOL; FSII(R);
- disorders/physical complaints: CHIP; HAY
- emotional well-being: CHIP; CHQ, COOP; CQOL: FSII(R); PedsQL; QOLP-AV; 16 &17D

+ family: CHIP; CHQ; CQOL; COOP

+ general health: CHIP; CHQ; WCHMP

+ health habits: CHIP; COOP

+ parental impact: CHQ

+ physical/mobility/self-care/vision/hearing: CHIP; CHQ; COOP; CQOL; FSII(R); HAY; HUI2 & 3; KINDL; PedsQL; QOLP-AV; TACQOL; 16&17D

+ satisfaction/self worth: CHIP; CHQ; HAY; 16&17D

+ school: CHIP; CHQ; COOP; PedsQL, 16&17D

+ social: CHQ; COOP; CQOL; HAY; KINDL; PedsQL; QOLP-AV; 16&17D

+ spiritual well-being: QOLP-AV

Psychometric findings

A measure needs to be 'acceptable' for the targeted mode of completion and display face validity. Most HRQoL measures are comprised of multi-item scales or sets of items that reflect a particular construct. It is critical, therefore, to independently demonstrate the internal consistency of items for each multi-item scale used in a given measure. Internal consistency reliability is most often assessed using Cronbach's Alpha. It has been proposed that test–retest should be provided only as a complement to internal consistency (Perrin 1995) and is appropriate and necessary as method for the evaluation of single items (Nunnally and Bernstein 1994).

Validity is an iterative process and there are a variety of approaches that have been adopted from disciplines such as education and psychology and applied to the health assessment field. Basically, a measure must provide empirical evidence that a score yields information about an intended construct and these findings must be replicated across multiple settings and samples. Further, in general, endorsement across the full range of possible responses for each scale within the questionnaire should be observed and missing data should be minimal (Stewart *et al*, 1992; Ware *et al.* 1997).

Findings concerning reliability and validity of the generic pediatric HRQoL measures continue to emerge. To date, the majority of the measures have been evaluated based on score differences between healthy and chronic condition groups. Further work is needed by independent investigators to explore the application of the measures and their ability to detect clinically meaningful differences across different settings and study designs. For many of the pediatric instruments, published findings concerning reliability and validity suggest that that they are scientifically robust, but further substantive validity work is needed for the QOLP-AV, the 16 & 17D and the WCHMP (Spieth 2001). Based on data from their initial study, developers of the COOP charts recommend it be used only as a screening tool because it lacks the precision of longer measures (Wasson *et al.* 1994).

Noticeably absent from the validity work published thus far for commonly used measures is empirical evidence of responsiveness – an important feature for measures to be used in the clinical trial context. The absence of findings is due in part to the limited application of the instruments, focused on cross-sectional studies, but it is also a reflection of the current state of the art. As the field continues to evolve and instruments are used more routinely within clinical trials and other intervention-based studies, it is expected that publications about responsiveness (i.e., change over time) – such as the ones by Barr *et al.* (1997), Juniper *et al.* (1997), DeVeaugh-Geiss *et al.* (2002), and Michelson *et al.* (2001) – will begin to emerge. Each application increases our understanding with regard to a measure's strength and limitations and provides useful information for interpreting the meaning of scores. Following is a brief listing of the HRQoL measures by psychometric category:

Reliability

- Internal consistency: CHIP; CHQ; COOP; EHRQL; FHSII(R); HAY; KINDL; PedsQL; QLP-AV; TACQOL; WCHMP
- Test–retest: CHIP; COOP; CQOL; HUI2 & 3; KINDL; WCHMP; 16 & 17D

Validity

- Concurrent: CHQ; COOP; FHSII(R); KINDL
- Construct: CHIP; CHQ; FHSII(R); HAY; HUI2 & 3; PedsQL; QLP-AV; WCHMP; 16 & 17D
- Convergent: CHIP; CHQ; COOP; CQOL; KINDL; TACQOL
- Clinical: CHIP; CHQ; COOP; EHRQL; HUI2 & 3; KINDL; PedsQL; TACQL; 16 & 17D
- Criterion: CHIP; CHQ; WCHMP
- Predictive: HUI2 & 3
- Responsiveness: CHQ; HUI2 & 3

Ethnicity and applicability

The applicability of items and constructs in children and their respective proxies when English is not the language spoken at home is also very important to understand. As early as 1994, Lewit and Baker noted that the cultural ethnicity of children was undergoing a dramatic shift. In a recent report by the U.S. Census Bureau using data from 2000, roughly 18 per cent or 47 million resident over five years of age reported speaking a language other than English at home (U.S. Census Bureau 2003) and the U.S. federal government has made a commitment to reduce racial and ethnic disparities in health (AHRQ 2000).

Separate item scaling analyses and internal consistency reliabilities have been reported by ethnic, age and gender subgroups for the CHQ (Landgraf *et al.* 1996, 1999; Landgraf and Abetz 1997) and published information about differences in scale scores by ethnicity are available for this measure as well as the CHIP, FSIIR, HUI2 & 3 and PedsQL. Publications regarding ethnicity are available for the following instruments:

◆ CHIP (Starfield *et al.* 1993, 1995; Riley *et al.* 2004a)

◆ CHQ (Asmussen *et al.* 2000; Hepner & Sechrest 2002; Landgraf *et al.* 1996, 1999; Landgraf and Abetz 1997; Landgraf and Abetz 1998),

◆ FSII(R) (Lewis *et al.* 1989; Stein and Jessop 1989)

◆ HUI2&3 (Furlong, 1996; Lutetkin and Gold 2002).

◆ PedsQL (Varni *et al.* 2001, Varni *et al.* 2003).

These publications suggest that developers are cognizant of the need to better understand the impact of important background information of self- and proxy-reported quality of life among children and adolescents. A recent unpublished 2003 report by Olson and colleagues from the American Academy of Pediatrics, suggests that the work conducted thus far is encouraging but inconclusive and will undoubtedly increase as the field continues to mature.

Questionnaire length and response time

There are inherent constraints within the clinical trial context that may impact the selection of an appropriate quality of life instrument. The most notable restriction is the busy pace of the clinical setting wherein most patients are recruited for participation and asked to complete questionnaires. Because of this, the overall length of the questionnaire and the ease of completion are important considerations in the selection process. Questionnaires that require the use of a trained interviewer may add to the expense of a study, and therefore may not be the most suitable method of administration for the busy clinic setting.

While a coarse measure may be sufficient for large samples (Nunnally and Bernstein 1994), the trade-offs between brevity and comprehensiveness are especially problematic in pediatric trials due to the low prevalence of many chronic conditions (Landgraf and Abetz 1996). The COOP, CQCL and the 16 & 17D capture each concept using single items. The use of global items has been criticized as being less precise than more extensive multi-item instruments (McHorney *et al.* 1992). Thus, while their length is attractive, the lack of precision and sensitivity could be a potential disadvantage in clinical trials involving small samples of patients. It has also been noted that some measures, while being more extensive, (i.e. they use multiple items – such as the PedsQL, HUI2, HIU3) may not address the full range of functioning needed for a particular condition and may also be less suitable for use (Eiser and Morse 2001a). The ideal measures then will be will be brief, use multiple items to assess a specific concept, and capture the full range of functioning across a broad conceptual platform.

The issue of instrument length and response time has not been formally addressed within the field of quality of life assessment (Eiser and Morse 2001a). In the adult arena, it is generally accepted that most respondents can complete 3–5 items per. It has been estimated in the educational field that it takes the average person about 30–45 seconds to respond to a multiple-choice type question (Thorndike *et al.* 1991). Taking into account the general stamina, and attentive ability of the respondent, and the amount of time usually spent waiting in the office it may be reasonable to assume that a questionnaire that requires only about 10–15 minutes or less would be the most suitable for use within the clinic setting. The respondent should be reasonably free from distractions, as this will facilitate the ease of completion and may help to reduce the number of missing responses that might occur due to disruptions.

Most of the identified measures fall within the suggested 10–15 timeframe. The exceptions are the published full-length versions of the CHIP-AE (Starfield *et al.* 1993; Starfield *et al.* 1995), the parent version of the child CHIP (Riley *et al.* 2004b), the child self-report CHQ-CF87 (Landgraf *et al.* 1996, 1999; Landgraf and Abetz, 1997), the HAY (Bruil 1999) and the 17D (Apajasalo *et al.* 1996). On average, these full-length forms take approximately 20–30 minutes to complete. It should be noted that the full-length versions of the CHIP and the CHQ were purposefully created as a questionnaire from which shorter more practical forms are extrapolated.

Age and readability

There is considerable variability with regard to the targeted age for which the most common pediatric HRQoL instruments can be used. Some child measures have been developed for use across a broad age spectrum from infants/toddlers to older adolescents (FSII (R) 0–16; HUI2 & 3 2–18; PedsQL 2–18). However, the majority of instruments are targeted for young children to middle/late adolescents 5/6–17/18 years (CHIP; CHQ; COOP; CQOL; EHRQoL; HAY; KINDL; TACQOL; 16D; 17D) while several also include individuals at the cusp of adulthood 19–21 years (COOP; QOLP-AV). It is important to note that there is a separate measure for children and adolescents for the CHIP (CE and AE, respectively) and that the PedsQL has multiple versions based on developmental age groupings. Thus, the use of multiple measures within the same study may add complexity to the study design and some burden to the office staff administering the forms in a busy clinical setting. Following are the measures and their targeted age range:

- CHIP CE: 6–11 AE: 11–17
- CHQ: 5–18; self rpt age 10
- COOP: 12–21
- CQOL: 9–15
- EHRQL: 6–11
- FSII(R): 0–16
- HAY: 7–13

- HUI2: 2–18 ; self rpt age 8 & HUI3: birth–old age
- KINDL: 10–16
- PedsQL 2–18; self rpt age 8
- QOLP-AV: 14–20
- TACQOL: 6–15
- WCHMP: 0–5
- 16D: 12–15 & 17D: 8–11

Although the appropriate age range for an instrument is specified at the outset of development, detailed information about the required reading comprehension level is less available. The information is essential to inform others about the cognitive ability needed to comprehend and respond to questions and is necessary irrespective of whether the child is self-reporting or a proxy respondent is used to answer on behalf of the child. It is becoming more and more critical as developed countries are becoming increasingly populated with non-native speakers – all of whom should be eligible to participate in surveys and studies but are often indirectly excluded because of language barriers.

Readability can be assessed using any number of methods, but is generally based on the complexity of the syntax including use of active/passive tense, the average number of words per sentence, and the number of sentences per paragraph (Flesch 1948; Fry 1977; Lapp and Flood 1978; Privette and David 1986). A readability statistic is provided with commonly used word processing programs, for example Microsoft word yields Flesch reading ease score and Flesch–Kincaid grade level scores. Readability statistics have only been formally reported for the CHIP (Riley *et al.* 2004b), the CHQ (Landgraf *et al.* 1999) and the PedsQL (Varni *et al.* 1999). Readability computations are also available for the CAHPS® 2.0 – a satisfaction instrument that contains both child and adult core surveys (Morales *et al.* 2001).

Other factors such as questionnaire layout, print size, use of white space versus text, and clarity of instructions can also impact the ease with which someone can read and understand a question and provide a response. These factors should be considered and weighed against the benefits and strengths of a particular measure, the target condition, trial design and the intended respondent.

Use of pictures

The use of faces to represent points along a continuum have been the focus of early investigations outside the field (Chernoff 1973; Hadorn *et al.* 1992) and preliminary findings are available appropriately in the adult arena for the COOP picture charts (Nelson *et al.*1987, 1990a, b). In a sample of 177 patients, Larson and colleagues (1992), observed that the figures, which are a unique hallmark of the COOP measure, did not influence responses. They cautioned, however, that further work was needed to reach definitive conclusions. Additional work examining differences in scores for global items with and without pictures relative to conceptually equivalent multi-item scales has also been reported in the adult field by McHorney and colleagues (1992).

The use of figures is more common in pediatric measures because visual representation (i.e., graphics or illustrations) enhances reading comprehension and makes it easier for very young children to complete questionnaires. A child is often asked to select a picture that best describes how he/she feels about an unrelated concept as a quick way to internally illustrate that the child understands the picture responses. Item scaling analysis and internal logic checks for consistency (Landgraf and Abetz 1997) can confirm that the measure has been understood. Riley and colleagues (2004a) build extensively on this approach by including cognitive interviewing in their studies and the use of 'gold standard' tests to assess cognitive ability concurrently.

Instruments that utilize graphics or illustrations include the CHIP; COOP; KINDL; and the 17D. Some pediatric instruments utilize figurative illustrations to define all points along the response continuum (Christie *et al.* 1993), while others use illustrations at only the anchor points and include a scaled response – circles that increase or decrease in size (Riley *et al.* 2003; Rebok *et al.* 2001). Use of pictures may help to make the task of completion more enjoyable (Eiser *et al.* 1999; Valla *et al.* 2000; Wasson *et al.* 1994). Limited work by Rebok and colleagues (2001) suggests that there are no effects on age, gender or race using cartoon character used in the CHIP – AE. Verrips and colleagues (2001) examined the impact of administration modality on scores using the HUI. While these studies represent significant steps with regard to measurement in the child arena, findings may not be generalizable because the studies were limited in scope and specific to their respective instruments only.

Instruments are generally developed using traditional paper-pencil format. However, Internet-based or computerized versions are becoming more and more common and are currently available for the CHIP, CHQ, EHRQL, and the KINDL as part of the original development plan or as an added administrative feature.

The introduction of personal computers, the Internet, web-based designs and other technologies such as cellular phones, wireless and personal digital assistant (PDAs) are also beginning to influence how data is collected and reported, especially within clinical trials. As the field of pediatric health assessments continues to advance and different technologies are refined, further scientific work to assess potential differences based on mode of administration and use of graphics seems warranted. Similar work has been performed with regard to personality assessment in the field of industrial and organizational psychology (Chee *et al.* 2002).

Recall period

There is tremendous variability in the recall time period used across the common generic pediatric instruments. Time intervals range from the past four weeks to the omission of any specific time period. An interval of the past four weeks has been recommended in the adult work to provide a reasonably stable sample of events yet allow for accuracy (Stewart *et al.* 1992). Unfortunately, the design protocol for some clinical studies may not complement the standard four-week format used in many of the standardized child HRQoL instruments. Additionally, some conditions may be more acute in nature (e.g., otitis media) thereby requiring the use of a brief time referent such as 'the past week' or 'past few days'. It may be possible to modify the time referent of a standardized measure to create an 'acute' version, as has been done in the adult field for the SF-36 (Ware *et al.* 1993), but any modifications would need to be approved by the developer and the psychometric properties would need to be carefully examined independently and then compared against findings achieved for the original instrument (Keller *et al.* 1997). It is also worth noting that for some adult instruments like the SF-36, about half of the items do not have a specified time frame.

As noted by Eiser and Morse (2001a), the pediatric field could benefit from further study with regard to the optimum recall time period. Most likely, findings will depend on the age of the child, his or her comprehension abilities, and whether the measure is designed to assess quality of life in general terms or is focused on a particular condition/disease.

It should also be noted that even within a standard time frame such as four weeks there was variation in how the time referent is worded. For example, one measure uses the 'past four weeks' whereas another uses 'past month'. Some measures use numerals (4) versus actual words (four), which could impact readability/comprehension. Following is a brief summary of the measures available by time referent:

- Several weeks or longer: 'Past 4 weeks' (CHIP; CHQ); 'Past month' (COOP; CQOL; PedsQL); 'In recent weeks' (TACQOL)
- 1 week or less: 'Past seven days' (HAY); ' The last week' (KINDL)
- 2 weeks: FSII(R)
- Present state: HUI2 & 3; 16 & 17D
- None reported: EHRQL; QOLP-AV; WCHMP

Response options

There are no published standard or definitive guidelines for selecting the appropriate number of response options. A multiple category response continuum provides for greater variability than the use of a dichotomous option (yes, no). However, the selection of an appropriately corresponding response gradation will depend on the nature and construction of the question itself. Questions can ask about frequency (how often); intensity (how much) or endorsement (how satisfied). It has been suggested in the adult literature that five to seven categories provide for optimal assessments, and that inconsistencies in reporting may arise with use of a response option beyond seven categories (Stewart *et al.* 1992).

As noted by Eiser and Morse (2001a) with few exceptions (Apajasalo *et al.* 1996a, b) few authors have specifically noted the degree of difficulty encountered by children in understanding categorical response options common to many scales. Low alpha coefficients or response inconsistencies may be sufficient proxy indicators in this regard. Some work has been performed with regard to the type and number of circles, hatch marks etc used for visual analog scales (Rebok *et al.* 2001) and for different types of measures (Juniper *et al.* 1997). Unfortunately, there is little empirical work in the pediatric field with regard to the use of response options and children's ability to understand and use them across different ages. Following is a brief summary of the measures in terms of response options:

- 3 points only: FSII(R)
- 4 points only: HAY; WCHMP
- 5 points only: COOP; KINDL, PedsQL (varies with age) QOLP-AV
- Mixed points: CHIP (3–5); CHQ (4–6); TACQOL (3–4)
- 7 points: CQOL
- Other: EHRQL uses a 2 part visual analogue scale; HUI2 & 3 uses 3–5 statements and the 16 & 17D use 5 'choices' – words and statements to reflect different levels of functioning.

Respondent

One of the more compelling issues with regard to self-assessment in pediatric trials is the selection of the appropriate respondent. The decision is guided by many factors including feasibility, cost, the particular disease/condition being investigated, the specific focus of the trial, and whether or not a given measure is available as an age appropriate child-completed and/or proxy-completed instrument.

Not surprisingly, debate still lingers about young children's abilities to self-rate how they are doing and feeling (Eiser and Morse 2001b). Increasingly though, evidence continues to emerge (Rebok *et al.* 2001; Riley *et al.* 2004a; Shahinfar and Levitt 2000; Valla *et al.* 2000) confirming earlier findings that children can provide reliable and valid self-assessments about physical symptoms, emotional well-being and self-esteem (Landgraf and Abetz 1996, 1997; Levi and Drotar 1999; Saigal *et al.* 1995; Theunissen *et al.* 1998).

Obtaining reports from children directly and their identified proxy is the ideal strategy, but it is not always possible to do so outside the research setting. Both perspectives are important, but can raise challenging issues with regard to analyses and interpretation of findings. For example, should data from multiple reporters be analyzed separately or combined? What if there is a lack of concordance or a significant difference in scores between the proxy and the child? Who should be considered the 'gold standard' when reporting findings? In the absence of clear guidelines, the answer to these questions must be carefully evaluated in the context and parameters of each unique study and the measure being used. The important point is to consider the breadth and depth of information that may be lost or gained by asking either the child or his/her proxy to report on HRQoL.

It is also important to understand that the use of a proxy carries with it some inherent challenges. It is often tacitly assumed that if a proxy is needed he/she will most likely be the child's parent. However, this may not always be the case. Increasingly, extended family members such as grandparents, aunts and uncles are raising children themselves or playing a substantive role in providing their care. Thus, it is important to understand the structure or make-up of each child's home and care environment to determine the most appropriate respondent. A key question to understand is who will be the most likely candidate to consistently bring the child to the clinic during the trial. In some instances it may be that there is no consistency and thus the child may be the more appropriate respondent.

Gender differences among parents and/or caregivers can also confound findings. For example, it has long been reported that fathers, relative to mothers, will rate children as having fewer behavioral or psychiatric problems (Jensen et al. 1988; Reynolds et al. 1985; Rothbart et al. 1966). Few studies, though, have systematically studied gender differences with regard to HRQoL. Some differences in parent and child gender effects were observed for the CHIP–CE (Riley et al. 2004a); the CHQ (Landgraf et al. 1996, 1999; Landgraf and Abetz 1998) and the PedsQL (Varni et al. 2003). Findings in this regard were not observed for the HUI (Furlong 1996).

The design of some trials and the stamina and health condition of the child may necessitate the use of a proxy respondent. Careful consideration should be made with regard to the appropriate selection of the proxy. The same proxy should be used throughout the trial once he or she has been identified at the child's enrollment into the study and a baseline HRQoL assessment has been obtained. This will assure that any differences over time are not inadvertently affected by a change among proxy reporters for a given child.

Following is a brief summary of the measures available by category of respondent:

+ Self-administered – Child/adolescent only: COOP; EHRQL; KINDL; QOLPV-AV; 16D
+ Both child/parent versions: CHIP; CHQ; CQOL; HAY; PedsQL: TACQOL
+ Interview: FSII(R) (parent); WCHMP (parent); 17D (child)
+ Other: HUI2 (clinician/parent and child self-report begins age 8 and older; HUI3 is parent report only for children).

Interpretation of scores and identifying meaningful differences

A critical but often overlooked aspect of a measurement concerns the interpretation of scores. Norms and confidence intervals for each measure would be advantageous in guiding others about the interpretation of quality of life scores and their clinical significance (Spieth 2001). It has particularly noted that the interpretation of QOL results is predominantly subjective (Fayers and Machin 2000). Given this and the increased use of instruments among individuals without specific measurement training, published guidelines about the meaning of scores seems essential. For example, patient-specific reports are available for the CHQ that include useful interpretive information for the novice user, such as norm-based scores and scores observed at the different percentiles for the U.S. sample of children.

Many of the commonly used general measures listed at the outset of this chapter use the Likert summative scoring approach (Likert 1932). The exceptions are the HUI (Feeny *et al.* 1992, 1995, 1996, 1998), the 16D (Apajasalo *et al.* 1996a), the 17D (Apajasalo *et al.* 1996b) and the EHRQL (Eiser *et al.* 1999, 2000). As defined by their authors, these preference-based measures ask the respondent to rate an attribute by selecting a single response from a list of five or six statements representing different levels of functioning. The EHRQL uses a visual analogue scale.

The summative multi-item approach to scale development is most commonly used because it allows for a conventional scoring method wherein individual responses to a set of items (known as a scale) are tallied and a mean is calculated to represent a given construct or concept (e.g. self-esteem). Quality of life instruments are multidimensional and generally utilize different response categories across the concepts that are measured. Thus, to put all scale scores on the same possible range, the raw mean score is transformed linearly to a 0–100 percent of total possible range. This is a relatively common convention and in most instances a higher score is usually interpreted as 'better' or 'higher' health-related quality of life.

Notable advances have been made with regard to scoring and interpretation for the CHIP, CHQ, HUI2 & 3 and the PedsQL. A taxonomy for adolescent health profile types is available for the CHIP-AE (Riley et al 1998a, 1998b) and is useful for interpreting the meaning of scores.

The CHIP-CE (Riley *et al.* 2004a), CHQ-PF (Landgraf *et al.* 1996, 1998, 1999), and the PedsQL (Varni *et al.* 1999, 2001, 2003) allow for individual concept-specific scale scores (i.e., physical functioning) and summary scores. The CHQ and the PedsQL refer to the latter as the 'physical' and 'psychosocial' summary scores. The CHIP refers to the summaries as 'domain scores.' The summary for the PedsQL physical score is equivalent to the eight-item physical functioning scale and is presented on a 0–100 continuum with a higher score indicated better health. The PedsQL psychosocial summary – also presented on a 0–100 continuum – is derived by obtaining an overall mean value for items answered in the three corresponding psychosocial subscales (emotional, social and school functioning).

The CHQ summaries are derived using factor weights (principal components orthogonal rotation) from a U.S. representative sample. The sample was selected using a two-staged area probability approach. The primary sampling units used were Standard Metropolitan Areas stratified by region, age, and race before selection.

The units of selection at the second stage were block groups stratified according to race and income. Both the CHIP-CE (Riley *et al.* 2004a) domains and subdomains (scales) and the summaries for the CHQ-PF are transformed as a linear T-score (mean score is 50 and the standard deviation is set to 10). In this way it is possible to better understanding the meaning of scores and potential differences.

The HUI provides an overall 'utility score'. The health states and utility scoring have undergone rigorous study and evaluation across multiple samples of patients (Feeny *et al.* 1996).

Condition/disease specific modules have been developed for the core PedsQL instrument (Varni 1999, 2001) and there is new information about scores and psychometric performance from a large population based study in California (Varni *et al.*, 2003). Age and gender-specific norms and benchmarks for some clinical conditions such as asthma, ADHD, juvenile rheumatoid arthritis, epilepsy, psychiatric disorders are available for the CHQ (Landgraf *et al.*, 1996, 1999).

Collectively, the body of work about the general instruments identified in this chapter – their psychometric properties, practical assets, scoring and interpretation of scores – illustrates the tremendous advances that have been realized in the child health assessment field in a relatively short period of time. Lessons learned during innovative field tests and empirical data highlight the many exciting challenges that await further study. But as others have noted (Eiser and Morse 2001a; Koot and Wallander 2001), the collective work also underscores several shortcomings and limitations to the measurement work conducted thus far.

Future direction

Self-reflection is an important precursor to personal growth. Introspection is no less valid in academic-based research. To move forward it is important to understand what has been gained, what needs further work, and what is practical and worthy of achievement. Therein, a specific direction will begin to emerge. Perhaps the most compelling question that lies before us is also the simplest – what do we know about the health-related quality of children and adolescents? Despite substantive work to date it is not possible to actually answer the question, because of the variation both in the content of the measures currently being used and the nature/focus of the investigations. Perhaps this is simply because the vast majority of work has focused exclusively on the evaluation of measures as opposed to assessing the outcome of care and treatment across and within groups of children/adolescents. At a minimum, to move forward will require consensus about the most appropriate and universal conceptual framework against which health-related quality of life can be defined. For example, most of the measures appear 'functionally' focused – is the child limited in physical or social attributes? Can the child accomplish activities at home or at school? Does the child display 'appropriate' behavior? Does the child take unnecessary risks? Does the child get along with others, at work and at home? But is there a perspective aside from physical emotional or social functionality that should also be considered? Do concepts such as hope, spirituality, creativity, self-expression or self-expectation have any relevance in a health-related quality of life instruments?

Aside from theoretical discussions, the field could benefit from practical application of existing measures. First, it is no longer a question of 'Can children answer for themselves and at what age'? Both the child's perspective and the caregiver's view are important. Thus, the more compelling question is 'What is the best way to reconcile discrepancies across reporters?' In this regard, it may be helpful to understand from behavioral psychologists how divergent information is used during the diagnostic screening process for emotional and behavioral problems. Much will depend on the purpose of the investigation. For example, when developing a treatment plan it might be advantageous to know the degree of discrepancy between the child/adolescent and his or her proxy. The information could be used as part of an overall education plan and assist the practitioner in understanding whether additional supportive or ancillary services might be needed for the family.

Alternatively, depending on the agent being used in a clinical trial, it might be advantageous to get direct reports from both older children/adolescents and their parent/proxy on separate issues. For example, the child/adolescent may be the optimal reporter with regard to internal changes, such as the impact of the new treatment on self-esteem or emotional well-being. However, treatment may also indirectly benefit the family/parent/proxy (less stress at home, less worry about the child) and it would be important to capture this from someone directly affected such as the parent/caregiver.

Second, to better understand the health of young people there needs to be greater consensus with regard to the terminology and age classifications used across the measures, so that it might be possible to conduct a meta analysis of findings and draw more definitive conclusions. A tremendous amount of work has been conducted but it is challenging to 'wrap one's arms around it'. Related to this, new measures need to focus on the older youth – those who are in the critical transition between high school/college and the 'working world' generally 18 to 22 years of age.

Third, to assist in a broader understanding of health, it may make sense to shift from the development of condition/disease-specific measures to those that are non-categorical. As an important first step, it might be worth exploring conceptual similarities across common chronic conditions by convening the different developers as opposed to trying to derive the similarities through content or construct analysis. Would non-categorical measures be dissimilar from generic instruments?

Fourth, our understanding of health among children and adolescents could be enriched if there was a concerted effort across all measures to derive clinically meaningful differences in addition to statistical significance. Considerable advances have been made with regard to scoring and precision, but further work is needed to convey the complexity of these advances and what they mean in everyday terms to the lay users who are not part of the academic scientific community.

Fifth, we need to understand the relationship between traditional clinical markers and health-reported quality of life from both the perspective of the child/adolescent and his or her caregiver and the use of general as well as specific measures. Sixth, it is important to further integrate new technology (the Internet, etc.) into instrument development. To date most work has been limited to data collection in the school settings or clinics. The intention should not be focused exclusively on how technology may impact scores, but to use emergent technologies as a viable method for obtaining reports from youth across a broader array of settings, in an effort to try and reach those that do not typically get recruited for trials or studies. Finally, it would be useful to know the trade-offs in precision between generic and specific measures. In addition, it would useful to know about trade-offs across general measures – especially those that utilize a different approach to measurement. There have been some studies looking at mutual concurrent validity in this regard (Raat *et al.* 2002), but further work is needed.

Clearly, these ideas are ambitious and will require the concerted effort of both developers and users within the traditional randomized clinical trial setting and elsewhere. The outcome, though, may yield that which currently eludes us all – a more useful and informed understanding of the health of children/adolescents and the quality of their everyday life.

References

Achenbach, T. M. and Edelbrrok, C. S. (1979). The Child Behavior Profile II: boys aged 12–16 and girls aged 6–11 and 12–16. *J Consult Clinic Psychol*, **47**, 223–33.

AHRQ (Agency for Healthcare Research and Quality) (February 2000). Addressing racial and ethnic disparity in health care. Fact Sheet. Maryland: AHRQ Publication No. 00-P041. *http://www.ahrq.gov/research/disparit.htm* (last accessed 15 September 2003).

Aitken, M. E., Tilford, J. M., and Barrett, K. W., *et al.* (2002). Health status of children after admission for injury. *Peds*, **2**, 110(2), 337–342.

Apajasalo, M., Sintonen, C., and Holmberg, C., *et al.* (1996a). Quality of life in early adolescence: a sixteen-dimensional health related measure (16D). *Qual Life Res*, **5**(2), 205–211.

Apajasalo, M., Rautonen, J., and Holmberg, C., *et al.* (1996b). Quality of life in pre- adolescence: a seventeen-dimensional health related measure (17D). *Qual Life Res*, **5**(6),532–538.

Armstrong, F. D., Toledano, S. R., and Miloslavich, K., *et al.* (1999). The Miami Pediatric Quality of Life Questionnaire: parent scale. *J Cancer*, **S12**, 11–17.

Asmussen, L., Olson, L. M., Grant, E. N., Landgraf, J. M., Fagan, J., and Weiss, K. B. (2000). Use of the Child Health Questionnaire in a sample of moderate and low-income inner-city children with asthma. *Am J Respir Crit Care Med*, **162**(4), 1215–1221.

Barr, R. D., Petrie, C., Furlong, W., Rothney, M., and Feeny, D. (1997). Health-related quality of life during post-induction chemotherapy in children with acute lymphoblastic leukemia in remission: an influence of corticosteroid therapy.' *Int J Onc*, **11**, 333–339.

Bergner, M., Bobbitt, R. A., and Carter, W. B., *et al.* (1981). The Sickness Impact Profile: Development and final revision of a health status measure. *Med Care*, **19**, 787–805.

Bhatia, S., Jenney, M. E., and Bogue, M., *et al.* (2002). The Minneapolis-Manchester Quality of Life Instrument, reliability and validity of the adolescent form. *J Clin Onc*, **29**(24), 4692–4698.

Bradlyn, A. S., Harris, C. V., Warner, J. E., Ritchery, A. K., and Zaboy, K. (1993). An investigation of the validity of the Quality of Well-being Scale with pediatric oncology patients. *Health Psych*, **12**, (3), 246–250.

Bruil, J. (1999). *Development of a Quality of Life Instrument for Children with Chronic Illness.* Leiden: Leiden University.

Bungay, K. and Ware, J. E. (1993). *Measuring and Monitoring Health-related Quality of Life. Current concepts.* Kalamazoo: The Upjohn Company.

Chee, C. S., Drasgow, F., and Roberts, B. (2002). The equivalence of Internet and paper-and-pencil personality assessments. Paper presented at the annual meeting of the Society for Industrial and Organizational Psychology. 12–14 April 2002. Toronto Canada.

Chernoff, H. (1973). The use of faces to represent points in k-dimensional space graphically. *J Am Stat Assoc*, **68**, 361–368.

Christie, M. J., French, D., Sowden, A., and West, A. (1993). Development of child-centered disease-specific questionnaires for living with asthma. *Psychosom Med*, **55**(6), 541–548.

Collier, J. (1997). Developing a generic child quality of life questionnaire. *British Psychological Society, Health Psychology Update*, **28**, 12–16.

DeVeaugh-Geiss, J., Conners, C. K., and Sarkis, E. H., *et al.* (2002). GW320659 for the treatment of Attention-Deficit/Hyperactivity Disorder in Children. *J Am Acad. Child Adolesc. Psychiatry*, **41**(8), 914–920.

Drotar, D. (ed.) (1998). *Measuring Health-related Quality of Life in Children and Adolescents: implications of research and practice.* Mahwah, NJ: Lawrence Erlbaum Associates.

Eiser, C. (March 2003). Use of measures in evaluation and clinical trials. Paper presented at the American Academy of Pediatrics Invited Conference entitled, 'Critical Challenges in Developing and Applying Health Status and Outcomes Measures'. Schamburg, Illinois 24015 March 2003.

Eiser, C. and Morse, R. (2001a) Quality-of-life measures in chronic diseases of childhood. *Health Technol Assess*, **5**(4).

Eiser, C. and Morse, R. (2001b). Can parents rate their child's health-related quality of life? Results from a systematic review. *Quality of Life Res*, **10**(4), 347–357.

Eiser, C., Vance, Y. H., and Seamark, D. (2000). The development of a theoretically driven measure of quality of life for children aged 6–11 years. *Child Care Health Dev*, **26**, 445–456.

Eiser, C., Cotter, I., Oades, P., Seamark, D., and Smith, R. (1999). Health-related quality-of-life measures for children. *In J. Cancer*, S12, 87–90.

Fayers, P. M. and Machin, D. (2000). *Quality of Life Assessment Analysis and Interpretation.* Chichester: John Wiley & Sons, Ltd.

Feeny, D., Furlong, W., Barr., Torrance, G. W., Rosenbaum, P., and Weitzman, S. (1992). A comprehensive multiattribute system for classifying the health status of survivors of childhood cancer. *J Clin Oncol*, **10, 6**, 923–928.

Feeny, D. F., Furlong, W., Boyle, M., and Torrance, G. W. (1995). Multi-attribute health status classification systems, Health Utilities Index. *PharmacoEcon*, **7**, 490–502.

Feeny, D. F., Furlong, W., Boyle, M., and Torrance, G. W. (1996). Health utilities index. In B. Spilker (ed.) *Quality of Life and Pharmacoeconomics in Clinical Trials*, pp. 239–252. Philadelphia: Lipincott-Raven Publishers.

Feeny, D., Furlong, W., and Barr, R. D. (1998). Multiattribute approach to the assessment of health-related quality of life, Health Utilities Index. *Med Pedia Onc*, **31**(S), 54–59.

Flesch, R. F. (1948). A new readability yardstick. *J Applied Psych*, **32**, 221–233.

French, D. J., Christie, M. J., and Snowden, A. J. (1994). The reproducibility of the Childhood Asthma Questionnaires, measures of quality of life for children with asthma aged 4–16 years. *Q Life Res*, **3**, 215–224.

Fry, E. (1977). Fry's readability graph, clarifications, validation and extension to level 17. *J Reading*, Dec, 242–252.

Furlong, W. J. (1996). Variability of utility scores for health states among general population groups. MSc thesis, McMaster University.

Gans, J. E., Blyth, D. A., Elster, A. B., and Gaveras, L. L. (1990). *America's Adolescents, how healthy are they?* Chicago, IL: American Medical Association, Department of Adolescent Health.

Goodwin, D. A. J., Boggs, S. R., and Graham-Pole, J. (1994). Development and validation of the Pediatric Oncology Quality of Life Scale. *Psychol Assess*, **6**, 321–328.

Graham, P., Stevenson, J., and Flynn, D. (1997). A new measure of health-related quality of life for children, preliminary findings. *Psychol Health*, **12**(5), 655–665.

Hadorn, D. C., Hays, R. D., Uebersax, J., and Haber, T. (1992). Improving task comprehension in the measurement of health status preferences, a trial of informational cartoon figures and paired-comparison tasks. *J Clin Epidemiol*, **45**, 233–243.

Hays, R. and Revicki, D. (2004). Reliability (test-retest), sensitivity and responsiveness, validity. In P. Fayers and R. Hays (eds) *Quality Life Assessment in Clinical Trials*, pp. 25–39. Oxford: Oxford University Press.

Hepner, K. A. and Sechrest, L. (2002). Confirmatory factor analysis of the Child Health Questionanire Parent Form 50 in a predominantly minority sample. *Qual Life Res*, **11**, 763–773.

Ingersoll, G. M. and Marrero, D. G. (1991). A modified quality-of-life measure for youths, psychometric properties. *Diabet Educ*, **17**(2), 114–118.

Ireys, H. (2001). Epidemiology of childhood chronic illness, issues in definitions, service use, and costs. In H. M. Koot and J. L. Wallander (eds) *Quality of Life in Child and Adolescent Illness*, pp.123–150. Brunner-Routledge, East Sussex and Taylor and Francis Inc., New York.

Jensen, P. S., Traylor, J., and Xenakis, S. N., *et al.* (1988). Child psychopathology rating scales and interrater agreement. 1. parents' gender and psychiatric symptoms. *Journal of the American Academy of Child and Adolescent Psychiatry*, **27**, 442–450.

Juniper, E. F., Guyatt, G. H., Feeny, D. H., Ferrie, P. J., Griffith, L. E., and Townsend, M. (1996a). Measuring quality of life in the parents of children with asthma. *Q Life Res*, **5**, 27–34.

Juniper, E. F., Guyatt, G. H., Feeny, D. H., Ferrie, P. J., Griffith, L. E., and Townsend, M. (1996b). Measuring quality of life in children with asthma. *Q Life Res*, **5**, 35–46.

Juniper, E. F., Guyatt, G. H., Feeny, D. H., Griffith, L. E., and Ferrie, P. J. (1997). Minimum skills required by children to complete health-related quality of life instruments for asthma, comparison of measurement properties. *Euro Resp J*, **10**, 2285–2294.

Kaufman, A. S. (1979). *Intelligence testing with the WISC-R.* New York: Wiley and Sons.

Keller, S. D., Bayliss, M. B., Damiano, A., Goss, T., Hsu, M. A., and Ware, J. E. (1997). Comparison of responses to SF-36 health survey questions with one-week and four-week recall periods. *J Health Serv Res*, **32**(3), 67–384.

Koot, H. M. and Wallander, J. L. (2001). *Quality of Life in Child and Adolescent Illness.* Brunner-Routledge, East Sussex and Taylor and Francis, Inc., New York.

Landgraf, J. M. and Abetz, L. (1996). Measuring health outcomes in pediatric populations, issues in psychometrics and application. In B. Spilker (ed.) *Quality of Life and Pharmacoeconomics in Clinical Trials*, pp. 793–802. Philadelphia: Lipincott-Raven Publishers.

Landgraf, J. M. and Abetz, L. A. (1997). Functional status and well-being of children representing three cultural groups, initial self reports using the CHQ-CF87. *J Psych & Health*, **12**, 839–854.

Landgraf, J. M. and Abetz, L. (1998). Influences of sociodemographic characteristics on parental reports of children's physical and psychosocial well-being, early experiences with the Child Health Questionnaire. In D. Drotar (ed.) *Measuring Health-related Quality of Life in Children and Adolescent: Implications for research and practice*, pp. 105–26. Mahwah, NJ: Lawrence Erlbaum.

Landgraf, J. M., Abetz, L., and Ware, J. E. (1996, 1999). The Child Health Questionnaire User Manual. First printing Boston, MA: New England Medical Center; second printing Boston, MA: Health Act.

Landgraf, J. M., Maunsell, E., and Nixon-Speechley, K. N., *et al.* (1998). Canadian-French, German and United Kingdom Versions of the Child Health Questionnaire (CHQ-PF50), Methodology and Preliminary Item Scaling Results. *Qual of Life Res*, **7**(5), 433–445.

Landgraf, J. M., Rich, M., and Rappaport, L. (2002). Measuring quality of life in children with Attention-deficit/Hyperactivity disorder and their families. *Arch Pediatr Adolesc Med*, **56**, 384–391.

Landgraf, J. M., Abidari, J., Cilento, B. G., Cooper, C. S., Schulman, S. L., and Ortenberg, J. (2003). Coping, commitment, and attitude, quantifying the everyday burden of enuresis on children and their families. *Pediatrics*, in Press.

Langeveld, J. H., Koot, H. M., and Passchier, J. (1997). Headache intensity and quality of life in adolescents, how are changes in headache intensity in adolescents related to changes in experienced quality of life? *Headache*, **37**(1), 37–42.

Langeveld, J. H., Koot, H. M., and Passchier, J. (1999). Do experienced stress and trait negative affectivity moderate the relationship between headache and quality of life in adolescents? *J Pediatr Psychol*, **24**(1), 1–11.

Lapp, D. and Flood, J. (1978). *Teaching Reading to Every Child*. New York: McMillan.

Larson, C. O., Hays, R. D., and Nelson, E. C. (1992). Do the pictures influence scores on the Dartmouth COOP Charts? *Q Life Res*, **V1**, 247–49.

Le Galps, C., Buron, C., Costet, N., Rosman, S., and Slama, G. (2002). Development of a Preference-Weighted Health Status Classification System in France, the Health Utilities Index. *Health Care Management Science*, **V5**(1), 41–51.

Levi, R. B. and Drotar, D. (1999). Health-related quality of life in childhood cancer, discrepancy in parent-child reports. *In J. Cancer*, **S12**, 5–64.

Lewis, C. C., Pantell, R. H., and Kieckhefer, G. M. (1989). Assessment of chidlren's health status, field test of new approaches. *Med Care*, **27**(3), S54–65.

Lewit, E. G. and Baker, L. G. (1994). Race and ethnicity changes in children. In R. Behrman (ed.) *The Future of Children: Critical health issues for children and youth. Volume* **3**, pp. 13–44. Los Angeles, CA: David and Lucille Packard Foundation.

Likert, R. (1932). A technique for the measurement of attitudes. *Arch Psychol*, **140**, 5–55.

Lindstrom, B. and Eriksson, B. (1993). Quality of life among children in Nordic countries. *Q Life Res*, **2**(1), 23–32.

Lindstrom, B. and Koehler, L. (1991). Youth, disability and quality of life. *Pediatrician*, **18**(2), 121–128.

Lutetkin, E. I. and Gold, M. R. (2002). Comprehensibility of measures of health-related quality of life in minority and low-income patients. *J National Med Assoc*, **94**(5), 327–335.

Matza, L. S., Swenson, A. R., Flood, E. M., Secnik, K., and Leidy, N. K. (2004). Assessment of health-related quality of life in children, recommendations and review of conceptual and methodological issues. *Value In Health* **7**, 79–92.

McGrath, M. M., Bukstein, D. A., Buchner, D. A., Guzman, G. I., Landgraf, J. M., and Goss, T. F. (1999). Assessment of the relationship between disease severity and general and disease-specific health-related quality of life in pediatric asthma patients. *Amb Child Health*, **5**, 249–261.

McHorney, C. A., Ware, J. E., and Rogers, W., *et al.* (1992). The validity and relative precision of MOS short-and-long form health status scales and Dartmouth COOP charts. *Med Care*, **30**(Suppl.), 253–265.

Michelson, D., Faries, D., Wernicke, J., *et al.*, and the Atomoxetine ADHD Study Group (2001). Atomoxetine in the treatment of children and adolescents with Attention-Deficit/Hyperactivity Disorder, A randomized, placebo-controlled, dose-response study. *Pediatrics*, **108**(5), 1–9.

Morales, L. S., Weidmer, B., and Hays, R. D. (2001). Readability of CAHPSÒ 2.0 child and adult core surveys. In M. L. Cynamon and R. A. Kulka (eds), *Seventh Conference on Health Survey Research Methods*, pp. 83–90. Hyattsville, Maryland: DHSS Publication No. (PHS) 01–1013.

Nelson, E. C., Wasson, J., and Kirk, A., *et al.* (1987). Assessment of function in routine clinical practice, description of the COOP Chart Method and preliminary findings. *J Chron. Dis*, **40**, 55S–63SS.

Nelson, E. C., Landgraf, J. M., and Hays, R. D., *et al.* (1990a). The functional status of patients, How can it be measured in physicians' offices? *Med Care*, **28**, 1111–1126.

Nelson, E. C., Landgraf, J. M., and Hays, R. D., *et al.* (1990b). The COOP function charts, a system to measure patient function in physicians' offices. In M. Lipkin (ed.) *Functional Status Measurement in Primary Care*, pp. 97–131. New York: Springer-Verlag.

Nixon Speechly, K., Maunsell, E., and Desmeules, M., *et al.* (1999). Mutual concurrent validity of the Child Health Questionnaire and the Health Utilities index, an exploratory analysis using survivors of childhood cancer. *Int J Cancer*, S12, 95–105.

Nunnally, J. C. and Bernstein, I. H. (1994). *Pyschometric Theory*, 3rd edn. New York: McGraw-Hill, Inc.

Office of Technology Assessment (1991). *Adolescent Health. Vol 1, Summary and policy options*. Washington, DC: U. S. Government Printing Office.

Olson, D. H., Porter, J., and Lavee, Y. (1985). *FACES III, Family Adaptability, Cohesion, Evaluation Scales*. St. Paul, MN: University of Minnesota Press.

Parkin, P. C., Kirpalani, H. M., and Rosenbaum, P. L., *et al.* (1997). Development of a health-related quality of life instrument for use in children with spina bifida. *Qual Life Res*, **6**(2), 123–132.

Patrick, D. L. and Deyo, R. A. (1989). Generic and disease-specific measures in assessing health status and quality of life. *Med Care*, **27**, S217–232.

Pedhazur, E. and Pedhazur Schmelkin, L. (1991). *Measurement, Design, and Analysis*. Hillsdale, NJ: Lawrence Erlbaum.

Perrin, E. B. (1995). SAC Instrument Review Process. *Medical Outcomes Trust Bulletin*, **3**(4), 1–8.

Piers, E. V. (1969). *Manual for the Piers-Harris children's self concept scale*. Nashville, TN: Counsellor Recording and Tests.

Privette, G. and David, S. (1986). Reliability and readability of a questionnaire peak performance and peak experience. *Pysch Rep*, **58**, 491–494.

Rabbett, H., Elbadri, A., and Thwaites, R., *et al.* (1996). Quality of life in children with Crohn's disease. *J Pediatr Gastroenterol Nutr*, **23**(5), 528–533.

Raat, H., Bonsel, G. J., Essink-Bot, M. L., Landgraf, J. M., and Gemke, R. J. B. J. (2002). Reliability and validity of comprehensive health status measures in children; The Child Health Questionnaire in relation to the Health utilities Index . *J Clin Epi*, **55**(1), 67–76.

Raphael, D., Rukholm, E., Brown, I., and Hill-Bailey, (1996). The quality of life profile – adolescent version, background, description and initial validation. *J Adolesc Health*, **19**(5), 366–375.

Ravens-Sierber, U. and Bullinger, M. (1998). Assessing health-related quality of life in chronically ill children with the German KINDL, first psychometric and content analytical results. *Qual Life Res*, **7**(5), 399–407.

Rebok, G., Riley, A., and Forrest, C., *et al.* (2001). Elementary school-aged children's reports of their health, A cognitive interviewing study. *Q Life Res*, **10**(1), 59–70.

Reynolds, W. M., Anderson, G., and Bartell, N. (1985). Measuring depression in children, a multimethod assessment investigation, *J Abnorm Child Psychol*, **13**, 513–526.

Riley, A. W., Green, B. F., Forrest, C. B., Starfield, B., Kang, M., and Ensminger, M. (1998a). A taxonomy of adolescent health, development of the adolescent health profile-types. *Med Care*, **36**(8), 1228–1236.

Riley, A. W., Forrest, C. B., Starfield, B., Green, B., Kang, M., and Ensminger, M. (1998b). Reliability and validity of the adolescent health profile-types. *Med Care*, **36**(8), 1237–1248.

Riley, A. W., Forrest, C. B., Starfield, B., Rebok, G., Green, B. F., and Robertson, J. (2004). The Parent Report Form of the CHIP-Child edition, Reliability and Validity. *Medical Care*, **42**(3), 210–220.

Roberts, R., Rodriquez, W., Murphy, D., and Crescenzi, T. (2003). Pediatric Lebeling; Improving the safety and efficacy of pediatric therapies. *JAMA*, **290**(7), 905–911.

Rodrigue, J. R., Geffken, G. R., and Streisand, R. M. (2000). *Child Health Assessment, A handbook of measurement techniques*. Boston, MA: Allyn and Bacon.

Rothbart, M. K. and Maccoby, E. E. (1966). Parent's differential reactions to sons and daughters. *J Pres Soc Psychol*, **4**, 237–243.

Saigal, S., Feeny, D., Furlong, W., Rosenbaum, P., Burrows, E., and Torrance, G. (1994). Comparison of the health-related quality of life of extremely low birthweight children and a reference group of children at age eight years. *J Pediatrics*, **125**(3), 418–425.

Saigal, S., Furlong, W. J., Rosenbaum, P. L., and Feeny, D. H. (1995). Do teens differ from parents in rating health-related quality of life? A study of premature and control teen/parent dyads. *Pediatr. Res*, **37**, 271A.

Seid, M., Varni, J. W., Rode, C. A., and Katz, E. R. (1999). The Pediatric Cancer Quality of Life Inventory, a modular approach to measuring health-related quality of life in children with cancer. *Int J Cancer*, **S12**, 71–76.

Shahinfar, N. A. and Levitt, (2000). Preschool children's exposure to violence, relation of behavioral problems to parent and child reports. *Am J Orthopsych*, **70**, 115–125.

Sintonen, H. and Pekurinen, M. (1993). A fifteen-dimensional measure of health-related quality of life (15D) and its applications. In S. R. Walker and R. M. Rosser (eds) *Quality of Life Assessment, Key issues in the 1990s*, pp. 185–95. Dordrecht: Kluwer Academic Publishers.

Spencer, N. J. and Coe, C. (1996). The development and validation of a measure of parent-reported child health and morbidity, the Warwick Child Health and Morbidity Profile. *Child Care Health Dev*, **22**(6), 367–379.

Spieth, L. E. (2001). Generic health-related quality of life measures for children and adolescents. In H. M. Koot and J. L. Wallander (eds) *Quality of Life in Child and Adolescent Illness*, pp.49–88. Brunner-Routledge, East Sussex and Taylor and Francis Inc., New York.

Starfield, B., Bergner, M., and Ensminger, M., *et al.* (1993). Adolescent health status measurement, development of the Child Health and Illness Profile. *Pediatrics*, **91**(2), 430–435.

Starfield, B., Riley, A., and Green, B., *et al.* (1995). The adolescent child health and illness profile, a population-based measure of health. *Med Care*, **33**(5), 553–566.

Stein, R. K. and Jessop, D. J. (1989). Measuring health variables among Hispanic and non-Hispanic children with chronic conditions. *Med Care*, **104**(4), 377–384.

Stein, R. E. K. and Jessop, D. J. (1990). Functional status II(R), a measure of child health status. *Med Care*, **28**(11), 1041–1055.

Stein, R., Coupey, S., Bauman, L., Westbrook, L., and Ireys, H. (1993). Framework for identifying children who have chronic conditions, the case for a new definition. *J of Pediatrics*, **122**, 342–347.

Stein, R., Westbrook, L., and Bauman, L. (1997). The questionnaire for identifying children with chronic conditions, a measure based on a noncategorical approach. *Pediatrics*, **99**, 513–521.

Stewart, A. L. and Hays, R. D. (1997). Conceptual, measurement, and analytic issues in assessing health status in older populations. In T. Hickey & M. Speers (eds) *Public Health and Aging*, (pp. 163–189. Baltimore, MD: The Johns Hopkins University Press.

Stewart, A. L., Hays, R. D., and Ware, J. E. (1992). Methods of constructing health measures. In A. L. Stewart and J. E. Ware (eds), *Measuring Functioning and Well-being, The medical outcomes study approach*, pp. 67–85. Durham, NC: Duke University Press.

Theunissen, N. C., Vogels, T., and Koopman, H. M., *et al.* (1998). The proxy problem, child report versus parent proxy report in health-related quality of life research. *Q Life Res*, **7**(5), 387–397.

Thorndike, R. M., Cunningham, G. K., Thorndike, R. L., and Hagen, E. P. (1991). *Measurement and Evaluation in Psychology and Education*. New York: Macmillan Publishing Company.

U. S. Census Bureau (released February **25**, 2003). Summary Tables on Language Use and English Ability, 2000 (PHC-T-20). Last accessed September 2003. *http, //www/census/gov/population/www/cen2000/phc-t20.html*

Valla, J.W., Bergeron, L., and Smolla, N. (2000). The Dominic-R, a pictorial interview for 6-to-11 year old children. *J Am Acad Child Adoles Psychiatry*, **39**(1), 85–93.

Varni, J. W., Seid, M., and Rode, C. A. (1999). PedsQL, measurement model for the Pediatric Quality of Life Inventory. *Med Care*, **37**, 126–139.

Varni, J. W., Seid, M., and Kurtin, P. (2001). PedsQL, reliability and validity of the Pediatric Quality of Life Inventory Version 4.0 generic core scales in healthy and patient populations. *Med Care*, **39**(8), 800–12.

Varni, J. W., Burnwinkle, T. M., Seid, M., and Skarr, D. (2003). The PedsQL 4.0 as a pediatric population health measure, feasibility, reliability and validity. *Amb Peds*, **3**, 329–341.

Verrips, G. H. W., Stuifbergen, M. C., and den Ouden, D. L., *et al.* (2001). Measuring health status using the Health Utilities Index, agreement between raters and between modalities of administration.' *J Clin Epi*, **54**(5), 475–481.

Vogels, T., Verrips, GH., and Verloove-Vanhorick, S. P., *et al.* (1998). Measuring health-related quality of life in children, development of the TACQOL parent form. *Q Life Res*, **7**(5), 457–465.

Ware, J. E., Snow, K., Kosinski, M., and Gandek, B. (1993). *SF-36 Health Survey Manual and Interpretation Guide*. Boston, MA: The Health Institute, New England Medical Center.

Ware, J. E., Harris, W. J., Gandek, B., Rogers, B., and Ray Rease, P. (1997). *MAP-R for Windows, Multitrait/multi-item analysis program-revised user's guide*. Boston, MA: Health Assessment Lab.

Wasson, J. H., Kairys, S. W., Nelson, E. C., Kalishman, N., and Baribeau, P. (1994). A short survey for assessing health and social problems of adolescents. *J Fam Pract*, **38**(5), 489–494.

Wasson, J. H., Kairys, S. W., and Nelson, E. C. (1995). Adolescent health and social problems, a method for detection and early management. *Arch Fam Med*, **4**, 51–56.

Waters, E., Wright, M., Wake, M., Landgraf, J. M., and Salmon, L. (1999). Measuring the health and well being of children and adolescents, A preliminary comparative evaluation of the Child Health Questionnaire (CHQ-PF50). *Amb Child Health*, **5**, 131–141.

Developing disease-targeted HRQoL measures for neurologic conditions

Barbara G. Vickrey

Introduction

The 'Decade of the Brain' in the 1990s ushered in the development of an unprecedented number and variety of new neurotherapeutics. Research efforts focused on basic neuroscience and translation of those findings into novel drugs, devices, and procedures. For the first time, therapies directly targeting the primary disease process were developed for conditions like multiple sclerosis, Alzheimer's disease, amyotrophic lateral sclerosis, and migraines; a new wave of medical and surgical therapies became available for epilepsy, stroke, and Parkinson's disease. Future advances in our understanding of the mechanisms underlying neural growth and regeneration should lead to breakthroughs in treatment of spinal cord injury and many neurodegenerative conditions. Societal investment in clinical trials for neurological conditions – for example, from the National Institutes of Health and other federal agencies, the pharmaceutical industry, private foundations, and other sources – has been substantial. The need for clinical trials is expected to continue to grow as the large body of basic neuroscience research continues to expand our knowledge of the pathophysiology and genetics of neurologic disease (Sung *et al.* 2003).

The benefit of a new therapy is best judged using data from carefully conducted studies – typically randomized controlled trials (RCTs)– measuring the most relevant outcomes. Until recently, mortality, disease symptoms or manifestations and laboratory and radiologic findings comprised the entire reported outcomes (Holloway and Dick 2002). Reports on the impact of treatments on patients' perceptions of their physical, mental, and social health – their health-related quality of life (HRQoL) – were relatively rare (Vickrey 1999). For example, clinical trials in epilepsy typically used a 50 per cent reduction in seizure frequency as the sole or primary outcome, yet recent studies incorporating patient-oriented outcomes like HRQoL have demonstrated little impact of seizure reduction on HRQoL unless complete freedom from seizures is achieved (Birbeck *et al.* 2002).

The 'burden' of neurologic disease and special issues in measuring HRQoL for neurologic conditions

Neurologic disorders encompass conditions affecting the brain, spinal cord, and peripheral nerves. Among the more common neurological disorders are stroke, seizure disorders, peripheral neuropathy, dementia, and Parkinson's disease, with prevalence estimates ranging from 200 to 650 cases per 100,000. Dementia and head injury are among the most costly neurologic diseases from a societal perspective (Lewin-ICF 1992).

Manifestations of neurologic disease are protean. Because the very essence of the individual can be affected – particularly among those disorders affecting the brain – measurement of HRQoL introduces some particular challenges. For example, stroke can affect the ability to comprehend language, and dementia invariably affects cognition. These impairments may limit or preclude the ability of persons with those conditions to reliably provide self-report information, the preferred source of HRQoL data (McDowell and Newell 1996). In addition, persons with disorders affecting the central or peripheral nervous system have a diverse range of symptoms and disease manifestations, courses (episodic, static, slowly progressive, rapidly progressive/terminal), and age groups affected (children, adults, elderly).

Generic vs. disease-targeted measures

Over the last decade, HRQoL measures have been developed that are targeted at neurologic conditions: epilepsy, multiple sclerosis, peripheral neuropathy, Parkinson's disease, stroke, and others (Fischer *et al.* 1999; Jenkinson *et al.* 1995; Vickrey *et al.* 2000, 1992; Williams *et al.* 1999). In addition, a number of neurology clinical trials have included HRQoL measures. These studies have used either generic HRQoL measures – measures applicable to populations without a specified disease – or a combination of generic and disease-targeted measures.

In a previous chapter (Chapter 1.1), the definitions and perceived advantages and disadvantages of generic versus disease-targeted HRQoL instruments were described. A generic measure is relevant to individuals generally rather than specific to one condition. Many generic HRQoL measures have been used in HRQoL studies of persons with neurologic diseases, including the SF-36, the Nottingham Health Profile, the Sickness Impact Profile, and others (Longstreth *et al.* 1992; Riazi *et al.* 2003; Karlsen *et al.* 2000). For some studies and neurologic diseases, these measures were used because no disease-targeted measures were available; the primary advantage of use of generic measures has been the ability to make comparisons of HRQoL to that of people with other conditions (Figure 5.4.1; Vickrey *et al.* 1994) or to the general US population (Wagner *et al.* 1996).

Disease-targeted HRQoL measures are tailored to a particular disease and may include 'generic' HRQoL domains that are particularly relevant to that disease as well as disease-*specific* items or scales. An example of a disease-specific item in an

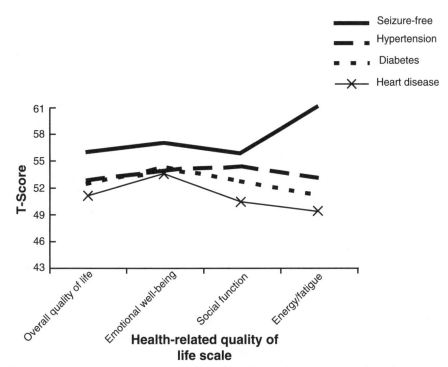

Fig. 5.4.1 HRQoL scores of adults now seizure-free after undergoing surgery for refractory epilepsy compare to adults with hypertension, diabetes, and heart disease (adjusted for age and gender).

epilepsy-targeted HRQoL measure is 'How much of the time during the past four weeks have you worried about having another seizure?' The potential advantage of disease-targeted measures is that the ability to measure change in the targeted subgroup may be enhanced (Birbeck *et al.* 2000). As recommended by Hays in Chapter 1.1, one approach to development of an HRQoL measure that leverages the advantages of both types of instruments is to select a generic core measure, and develop a disease-targeted 'supplement' or additional component. Examples of approaches for doing this for epilepsy and for peripheral neuropathy follow.

Example: development of an HRQoL measure for epilepsy

Epilepsy is a chronic neurologic condition affecting all ages (children, adults, elderly). The lifetime prevalence is about 0.5 per cent. Epilepsy is characterized by a propensity to have recurrent seizures. The most common kinds of seizures are episodes – usually brief, lasting seconds to minutes – of altered awareness or complete loss of consciousness. Some seizures are characterized by auras, a sensory sensation or experience (like a smell or an abdominal sensation, or déjà vu) that may occur alone or may be followed by altered awareness and/or loss of consciousness. (The cause of most seizures is unknown, but seizures themselves reflect abnormal, rhythmic discharges of neurons in the brain).

The most common treatment for epilepsy is medication, but for about one-quarter of persons with epilepsy, medication is ineffective and seizures are considered medically refractory. In those situations, some individuals may undergo brain surgery, most commonly, removal of the temporal lobe region of the brain, because a common form of epilepsy is manifest as seizures that originate from this region. Despite the fact that temporal lobectomy had been conducted for nearly 50 years, as of the early 1990s, many questions about the impact of this treatment on patients' HRQoL remained unanswered. There were anecdotal reports that the surgery might have effects (e.g., on memory or language) that adversely impacted HRQoL. In addition, it was observed that some persons with resolution of their seizures were unable to achieve better HRQoL because of the prolonged duration of epilepsy prior to surgery, which adversely affected employment and educational attainment in a way that seizure control in adulthood did not readily ameliorate. Finally, it was evident that investigators from different epilepsy surgery centers used different classification systems for reporting seizure outcomes after surgery, and it was not clear which of those systems were the most 'valid' reflections of epilepsy surgery outcome.

To address these questions, a measure of HRQoL applicable to adults with medically refractory epilepsy eligible for consideration for surgical treatment was needed (Vickrey et al. 1992). Investigators in the early 1990s interested in studying this question developed a list of desired characteristics for such an outcome tool: reliable, valid, comprehensive yet feasible to administer and obtainable by self-report. Investigators wanted to be able to compare the HRQoL of epilepsy surgery patients to that of other chronic conditions and to the general population, to evaluate whether patients 'cured' of their epilepsy had better HRQoL than that of persons with other chronic medical conditions and had HRQoL comparable to an age- and gender-adjusted sample representative of the general population. On review of existing generic HRQoL measures and literature regarding HRQoL impacts of epilepsy, it was clear that a generic HRQoL measure would not capture all the dimensions of HRQoL relevant to persons who undergo surgery for epilepsy. Thus, a decision was made to develop an additional, epilepsy-targeted component.

The generic core measure selected was the SF-36, tapping HRQoL dimensions of general health perceptions, energy/fatigue, social function, emotional well-being, role limitations due to emotional health problems, role limitations due to physical health problems, physical function and pain. A review of the literature on HRQoL issues additionally relevant to persons undergoing epilepsy surgery and discussions with clinicians caring for persons undergoing epilepsy surgery identified these additional HRQoL dimensions: cognitive function, role limitations due to memory, speech, or language problems, epilepsy-targeted health perceptions, and overall quality of life. Some of these dimensions were generic but not covered by the SF-36, for example, overall quality of life. Other dimensions were epilepsy-targeted, like role limitations due to memory, speech, or language problems. Finally, the epilepsy-targeted health perceptions items were specific to epilepsy, for example, 'I seem to get seizures a little easier than other people with epilepsy' (response choices range from 'definitely true' to 'definitely false').

Item analyses

The field test instrument included 57 items (the SF-36 items and 21 supplemental items) and was administered by mail survey to 224 persons who had previously undergone an epilepsy surgery evaluation, with responses from 200 (response rate = 89 per cent). In addition to these HRQoL items, the survey included questions about seizure occurrence in the prior 12 months and the Profile of Mood States (POMS), to assist in evaluating construct validity. Multi-trait scaling analyses of the 57 items were conducted to examine item discrimination across scales (Hays and Hayashi 1990). Eighty-six per cent of correlations of field test items with their hypothesized scales were more than two standard errors greater than correlations of the items with other scales in the measure. However, two items were dropped due to low correlations with their originally hypothesized scale. The final HRQoL instrument included 55 items and thus was named the Epilepsy Surgery Inventory (ESI)-55. Table 5.4.1 lists the 11 scales in the measure, the number of items in each scale derived from SF-36 items, and the number of items specifically developed for the epilepsy surgery HRQoL measure.

Scale score variability and reliability

Means, standard deviations, and percentage of patients scoring at the possible minimum and maximum scores were determined to examine variability and whether there were 'floor' or 'ceiling' effects on any scale. Internal consistency reliability of the 11 multi-item scales was assessed, and Cronbach's alpha ranged from 0.68 to 0.88 and was considered adequate for group comparisons (Nunnally 1978).

Factor analysis of scales and development of summary scores

Factor analysis of the eleven ESI-55 scales was conducted to evaluate higher order dimensions of HRQoL and which scales contributed to each. Several number of factor criteria were examined (e.g., scree test, parallel analysis) and it was decided that a three-factor solution was appropriate. These factors appeared to represent mental health, physical health, and cognitive/role limitations. Interfactor correlations ranged from 0.56 to 0.64, indicating moderate relationships yet sufficiently distinctive factors. Table 5.4.1 indicates on which factors each scale predominantly loaded. Formulas for summary HRQoL scores for each of these three factors were derived from factor analysis weights.

Table 5.4.1 Epilepsy Surgery Inventory (ESI)-55 Scales, number of items derived from the generic core measure and from the epilepsy-targeted supplement, and higher-order HRQoL Dimension (from factor analyses of scales)

Scale	No. of SF-36 Items	No. of Supplement Items	Total no. of Items	Higher order HRQoL Domain
Health perceptions	5	4	9	Mental = physical
Physical function	10	0	10	Physical
Pain	2	0	2	Physical
Energy/fatigue	4	0	4	Mental>physical
Overall quality of life	0	2	2	Mental
Emotional well-being	5	0	5	Mental
Cognitive function	0	5	5	Cognitive/role
Role limitations due to emotional problems	3	2	5	Cognitive/role
Role limitations due to physical problems	4	1	5	Cognitive/role = physical
Role limitations due to memory, speech, language problems	0	5	5	Cognitive/role
Social function	2	0	2	Mental = cognitive/role
Change in health	1	0	1	n/a

Construct validity

One assessment of construct validity was examination of Pearson product-moment correlations between selected ESI-55 scales and POMS scales. A priori hypotheses were that correlations would be significantly higher between the emotional well-being and other mental health dimension scales of the ESI-55 and the POMS scales than correlations of the physical health scale (and other physical health dimension scales) of the ESI-55 and POMS scales. This hypothesis was confirmed. For example, the Pearson product-moment correlation between the POMS Depressed scale and the ESI-55 Emotional Well-being scale was –0.68, whereas the correlation between the POMS Depressed scale and the ESI-55 Physical Function scale was –0.25. The former correlation was significantly larger than the latter (Steiger 1980).

Another evaluation of construct validity was analysis of associations between post-operative seizure control and HRQoL. It was hypothesized that better seizure control would be associated with higher (better) ESI-55 scores. Post-surgical patients were categorized into three groups: completely seizure-free, having only auras without seizures, and having one or more seizures in the prior year. One-way ANOVA linear trend F-ratios were determined for associations between these three categories of seizure control and mean scores for each of the eleven ESI-55 scales. As hypothesized, seizure-free patients had significantly higher scores on all scales than patients who continued to have seizures. Patients having only auras scored in-between on all scales. The ESI-55 scale that most highly discriminated across all three categories of seizure control – with the highest linear trend F-ratio (=45) out of the eleven analyses – was the nine-item health perceptions scale. This scale included both the generic SF-36 health perceptions scale items and four epilepsy-targeted or specific items. The investigators also calculated the linear trend F-ratio for the five item SF-36 health perceptions scale. These items are a subset of the nine items in the ESI-55 health perceptions scale. The linear trend F-ratio was still high (F-ratio = 30), but two-thirds the magnitude of the linear trend F-ratio for the scale with the additional four epilepsy-targeted items, indicating that these items add important content and discriminatory power to the health perceptions scale of the disease-targeted HRQoL measure.

Example: development of an HRQoL measure for peripheral neuropathy

In 2002 the Scientific Advisory Committee of the Medical Outcomes Trust published recommendations including that focus groups and interviews with patients be conducted before developing an HRQoL tool, so that its content is grounded in the conceptualization of HRQoL impacts from the patient's perspective (Aaronson *et al.* 2002). Such focus groups should purposely include a broad range of impairments, cultural groups, age groups and both genders. As an example of the value of this recommendation, persons with mobility impairments may conceptualize and value their health state differently from those without them; without such data prior to development, a measure may not be relevant in a target population (Hays *et al.* 2002).

Peripheral neuropathies can have a wide range of metabolic, toxic, degenerative, infectious, and genetic causes. The common pathophysiology is damage of peripheral nerves, with clinical manifestations ranging from pain and sensory loss in limbs to weakness and impaired autonomic nervous system functioning. Some neuropathies are acute while others are chronic and progressive. Development of an HRQoL measure for persons with peripheral neuropathy was informed by existing literature, but also required collection of primary data via focus groups and interviews of persons with peripheral neuropathy, to identify the range of relevant HRQoL domains (Vickrey *et al.* 2000). This was because the existing literature on HRQoL impacts of neuropathy was relatively sparse, and because the evolving standards for development of HRQoL measures included collection of data directly from persons affected with the condition in the instrument development stage.

Investigators purposely recruited for focus groups men and women with peripheral neuropathy having a range of severity and from diverse cultural and age groups.

Table 5.4.2 Descriptive statistics and reliability of peripheral neuropathy HRQoL measure (from Table 1 of Vickrey et al, 2000)

Scale or Item	Number of items	Mean[a]	Standard Deviation	Minimum score	Maximum score	% of patients scoring at floor	% of patients scoring at ceiling	Cronbach's Alpha	Test–retest Reliability[b] (n = 42)
Physical functioning	11	73.0	25.7	7	100	0.0	18.8	0.93	0.83
Role limitations – physical health	6	65.8	33.3	3	100	0.0	31.3	0.87	0.72
Pain	7	65.5	21.9	15	100	0.0	6.3	0.91	0.84
Energy/fatigue	5	56.8	23.4	4	100	0.0	1.3	0.93	0.80
Upper extremities	6	91.9	11.2	42	100	0.0	37.5	0.80	0.84
Balance	8	79.2	19.1	18	100	0.0	18.8	0.89	0.77
Self-esteem	6	79.9	16.9	42	100	0.0	15.0	0.81	0.82
Emotional well-being	7	71.4	17.2	20	94	0.0	0.0	0.91	0.83
Stigma	3	93.5	14.8	50	100	0.0	78.8	0.88	0.42
Cognitive functioning	3	76.8	20.1	20	100	0.0	20.0	0.88	0.68
Role limitation – emotional	3	66.7	38.6	0	100	15.0	51.3	0.76	0.61
General health perceptions	7	58.6	20.3	18	100	0.0	1.3	0.81	0.77
Sleep	5	71.1	18.4	19	100	0.0	3.8	0.67	0.63
Social functioning	9	80.5	19.6	19	100	0.0	17.5	0.89	0.69

Health distress	3	68.3	25.5	7	100	0.0	11.3	0.93	0.79
Sexual function	2	68.7	34.2	0	100	10.1	40.5	0.76	0.72
Physical health summary score [c]	—	50.0	10.0	26.3	64.6	0.0	0.0	0.97	0.83
Mental health summary scores [c]	—	50.0	10.0	28.2	64.3	0.0	0.0	0.95	0.82
Satisfaction with sexual function	1	55.1	38.0	0	100	20.5	25.0	n/a	0.79
Overall health	1	70.5	17.7	20	99	0.0	0.0	n/a	0.56

Vickrey et al. (2000) p. 101., copyright Sage Publications Inc. Reprinted by permission of Sage Publications, Inc.

[a] Means and standard deviations at baseline QOL.

[b] The test-retest reliability estimate is the intraclass correlation from a two-way random effects model. When n = 42, only patients who completed both the baseline and first follow-up and answered that their health has been 'about the same' at the first follow-up compared to three months previously are included in the analysis. Mean test-retest interval = 91 days. While this criterion for stability is not optimal, it yields test-retest reliability estimates that are likely to be conservative.

[c] The overall, physical, and mental health summary scores were converted to T-scores; these summary scores included contributions across all scales and were based on factor analyses and regression analyses.

[d] Internal consistency reliability of the physical and mental health summary scores was estimated with Mosier's formula (Mosier 1943).

Three focus groups that included a total of 22 adults recruited from the practices of three different specialists and from academic and community practices in southern California were held. Protocols were developed that included open-ended questions about the perceived HRQoL impacts of peripheral neuropathy. Summaries of the focus groups were generated by an experienced moderator, with the aid of audiotapes of each group.

Analyses of these focus group summaries revealed that in addition to domains addressed by most generic measures, peripheral neuropathy appeared to have significant impacts on HRQoL areas including self-consciousness, self-esteem, stigma, sleep, social isolation and health distress, among others. Field test items were developed by supplementing a generic core measure, the SF-36, with items drawn from several different existing measures tapping these domains, for example the Rosenberg Self-Esteem Scale (Rosenberg 1965) and additional items developed *de novo*. Items that were created included those addressing the impact of neuropathy on daily activities, work, sleep, social activities, and other dimensions (balance, fear of falling, ability to handle objects with hands) that these focus group data suggested were affected by having a peripheral neuropathy. Examples of items from the neuropathy-targeted component are 'Because of your peripheral neuropathy, how much pain in your hands have you had during the past four weeks?' and 'How true or false is the following statement for you: I worry about falling in front of other people.'

The final field test measure had 162 items in total and was administered at baseline and at three and six months to 80 adults participating in a multi-center, randomized trial of a neuropathy treatment. To evaluate construct validity, data on ratings of neuropathy symptoms, neurological examination findings, and electrophysiologic studies of velocity of transmission along peripheral nerves were analyzed in relation to the HRQoL data.

The initial step in development of the measure was to evaluate placement of items into scales and to reduce the number of items to a target length of approximately 100, which was felt to be a maximum feasible length for use in subsequent clinical research studies. Items were placed into hypothesized scales based on their content. In addition to using iterative multi-trait scaling analysis as described for development of the epilepsy-targeted HRQoL measure above, because of the large number of items, factor analyses of subgroups of selected items were performed to assess the underlying dimensionality of these subsets. The final measure included 97 items: the 36 items of the SF-36 and 61 neuropathy-targeted items. Ninety-one items were distributed across a total of 16 multi-item scales, and there were six single items.

Analogous to the ESI-55, some SF-36 scales were expanded to incorporate neuropathy-targeted/specific items; some neuropathy-targeted scales were entirely comprised of new items or items adapted from other measures (Table 5.4.3). This peripheral neuropathy-targeted HRQoL measure was longer than the ESI-55 because of the desire to be comprehensive in coverage of domains uncovered during the focus groups.

Table 5.4.3 Multiple sclerosis-targeted HRQoL scale scores and number of days in the past month unable to work or attend school because of health

Scale	Disability days due to health		F^c	Relative Validity[d]
	None N = 60–61	At least One day N = 17		
Physical functioning	78.0[a]	55.7[b]	11.4	9.6
Role limitations – physical health	74.8[a]	38.6[b]	20.1	16.9
Pain	70.0[a]	52.0[b]	10.4	8.7
Energy/fatigue	61.3[a]	43.8[b]	8.4	7.1
Upper extremities	94.0[a]	85.8[b]	6.4	5.4
Balance	83.2[a]	65.4[b]	13.3	11.2
Self-esteem	83.1[a]	66.9[b]	14.1	11.8
Emotional well-being	75.7[a]	55.5[b]	23.8	20.0
Stigma	96.9[a]	80.9[b]	8.1	6.8
Cognitive functioning	80.8[a]	62.0[b]	13.6	11.4
Role limitations – emotional	76.0[a]	37.3[b]	15.8	13.3
General health perceptions	63.2[a]	44.7[b]	12.7	10.6
Sleep	74.9[a]	60.5[b]	9.3	7.8
Social functioning	86.5[a]	58.8[b]	25.2	21.2
Health distress	71.6[a]	57.6[b]	4.1	3.5
Sexual function	71.0	58.3	1.2	1.0
Physical health summary score	52.6[a]	42.0[b]	18.8	15.8
Mental health summary score	52.8[a]	40.2[b]	27.6	23.2

[a,b] Means within a row with different superscripts differ significantly ($p < 0.05$; t-test).

[c] F-ratio = T-squared, from t-test of difference in means

[d] Relative validities were calculated as the ratios of the F-ratios of each scale to the F-ratio of the scale with the smallest F-ratio (the sexual function scale), set to 1.

Modified from table 4 of Vickrey *et al.* 2000. Copyright Sage Publications Inc., reprinted by Permission of Sage Publications, Inc.

Future research plans include exploration of a subset of items from the longer neuropathy-targeted measure that capture much of the information as the longer instrument, but is briefer and might thus be more feasible to use in certain applications.

Exploratory factor analyses provided support for two underlying dimensions for the scales, yielding physical and mental health dimensions. Correlation between these dimensions was 0.57. Factor scores from this factor analysis solution were used to derive physical and mental health summary scores for the peripheral neuropathy measure.

Descriptive statistics to evaluate scale score variability, internal consistency reliability, and test–retest reliability among subjects meeting criteria as stable over two points in time were calculated for individual scales and for the summary scores (Table 5.4.3). Reliability estimates for the two summary scores were generated using Mosier's formula (Mosier 1943).

To evaluate construct validity, a number of hypothesized associations between HRQoL and clinical and sociodemographic variables were analyzed. An example of one of these analyses in shown in Table 5.4.4, where patients were categorized into two groups according to whether or not they had any disability days due to health problems in the prior 30 days. F-ratios for each scale and for the two summary scores were generated from T-squared of the t-test of the difference in mean HRQoL scores across the two groups. Relative validity was calculated as the ratio of the F-ratio for each scale relative to the F-ratio of the scale having the smallest F-ratio, which was set to 1 (Liang *et al.* 1985). For this particular analysis of construct validity, relative validity was highest for the Mental Health Summary Score.

In another analysis of construct validity, Spearman correlations were determined between the Mental and Physical Health Summary Scores, and peripheral neuropathy symptom measures, neurologic examination measures, and electrophysiologic measures of peripheral nerve function (Table 5.4.4). Strongest correlations were observed with symptom measures, with lesser or no correlations with the neurologic examination or electrophysiologic tests. This indicates that the HRQoL measure is providing additional information beyond that of examination of electrophysiologic findings. Physical Health Summary scores were more highly associated with these clinical measures than were Mental Health Summary scores.

Value of information obtained using disease-targeted HRQoL measures for neurologic conditions

One of the putative advantages of disease-targeted measures is that they may be more responsive to change over time for a particular condition, because they encompass particularly relevant constructs to persons with a particular disease. Examples of how disease-targeted HRQoL measures for four different neurologic conditions provided additional information beyond that of a generic measure follow.

Parkinson's disease

The Parkinson's Disease Questionnaire (PDQ)-39, originally developed in the UK, is a 39-item, self-administered measure that includes items tapping eight HRQoL areas: mobility, activities of daily living, emotional well-being, stigma, social support, cognitions, communication and bodily discomfort (Damiano *et al.* 1999). Generation of items was drawn from semi-structured interviews with 20 outpatients with PD (Peto *et al.* 1995). In an analysis of the two measures, the SF-36 did not cover all areas of

Table 5.4.4 Relationships between peripheral neuropathy-targeted HRQoL summary scores and neurologic symptoms, neurologic examination findings, and electrophysiologic tests (N range from 75 to 79); Table 5 of Vickrey et al. 2000, copyright Sage Publications, Inc. Reprinted by Permission of Sage Publications Inc.

HRQoL scale	Symptoms			Neurologic Examination			Electrophysiologic tests	
	Sensory symptoms	Motor symptoms	Autonomic symptoms	Sensory exam	Strength exam	Reflexes	Sural nerve conduction amplitude	Peroneal nerve conduction amplitude
Mental health summary								
Spearman correlation	−0.11	−0.15	−0.25	0.09	−0.11	0.08	0.04	−0.06
p-value	0.35	0.19	0.02	0.45	0.32	0.49	0.71	0.59
Physical health summary								
Spearman correlation	−0.46	−0.47	−0.24	−0.23	−0.18	−0.06	0.04	−0.004
p-value	0.0001	0.0001	0.03	0.04	0.11	0.58	0.74	0.97

HRQoL relevant to PD. The PDQ-39 was designed to fill the identified gap (Jenkinson *et al.* 1995).

Peripheral neuropathy

Analysis of the 'added value' of the neuropathy-targeted component of the previously described HRQoL measure for peripheral neuropathy has also been evaluated. Associations between disability days due to health and the SF-36 Physical Health Summary Score revealed an F-ratio of 9.7, nearly half the magnitude of the F-ratio for the Physical Health Summary Score of the peripheral neuropathy targeted measure (= 18.8). In another example, statistically significant associations were found between the peripheral neuropathy-targeted mental health summary scores and autonomic symptoms ($P = 0.02$; Table 5.4.4); however, associations of the SF-36 mental health summary score and autonomic symptoms were non-significant (Vickrey *et al.* 2000).

Epilepsy

To assess whether an epilepsy-targeted HRQoL measure is more responsive (able to detect HRQoL change over time) than a generic measure, two epilepsy-targeted measures and a generic measure were administered to patients participating in an antiepileptic drug trial (Birbeck *et al.* 2000). Data were collected at baseline and at a 28-week follow-up. Subjects had a mean age of 38 years, were 48 per cent male, and had a baseline seizure frequency of 3.6 per month. One external criterion for change, defined at study onset, was a two-category or greater improvement in patients' self-ratings of their overall condition. These ratings were obtained at baseline and at the 28-week follow-up. Forty-eight patients whose ratings were unchanged at baseline and follow-up were classified as unchanged. There were 27 patients who met the criterion to be classified as 'changed'.

The HRQoL measures that were administered included the Quality of Life in Epilepsy (QOLIE)-89, the QOLIE-31, the SF-36, and the SF-12. The QOLIE-89 is an 89-item measure of HRQoL for persons with epilepsy that includes the SF-36 as a generic core. Four summary scores, including an epilepsy-targeted summary score, can be derived from the QOLIE-89. The QOLIE-31 has no complete generic core measure and includes a subset of 31 of the 89 items in the QOLIE-89. Findings were that the epilepsy-targeted HRQoL measures yielded large or medium-to-large effect sizes, whereas effect sizes for the generic measures were small or medium (Table 5.4.5). Similar findings were observed using a different external criterion for change based on change in seizure occurrence from baseline to follow-up.

Multiple sclerosis

The added value of multiple-sclerosis targeted components to a generic measure was demonstrated in a study of 170 adults with multiple sclerosis who responded to a mailed survey, out of 227 consecutive referrals to a multiple sclerosis clinic (Vickrey *et al.* 1997). Reflecting the epidemiology of multiple sclerosis, 72 per cent of subjects

Table 5.4.5 Effect sizes of epilepsy-targeted and generic HRQoL measures based on longitudinal data from 27 persons with epilepsy meeting criterion for 'changed'

Measure	Effect size	Interpretation
Epilepsy-targeted:		
QOLIE-89 epilepsy-targeted	0.80	large
QOLIE-31 Overall score	0.74	large/medium
Generic:		
SF-36 Mental composite	0.41	medium
SF-12 Physical composite	0.17	small

were female, average age was 45 years, and average duration of multiple sclerosis was 9.4 years. Subjects completed paper-pencil versions of the SF-36, the MS Activities of Daily Living measure (Gulick 1988), a multiple sclerosis-targeted measure that has four scales (motor, communication, social activity, intimacy), and the health distress scale from the Medical Outcomes Study (Stewart *et al.* 1992). The health distress scale is a generic scale but was identified as being particularly relevant to people with multiple sclerosis and thus included in the study as a disease-targeted scale.

To analyze whether multiple sclerosis-targeted measures provided additional information beyond that of the generic measure, associations between the generic measure and two criterion variables (level of mobility; overall multiple sclerosis symptom severity in the prior year) were assessed. These associations were determined by regressing each criterion variable onto the eight SF-36 scales using forward stepwise regression until all variables entering at $P < 0.15$ were included. In the second stage of this analysis, forward stepwise linear regression was carried out, with 'forced' inclusion of the eight SF-36 scales, then forward stepwise regression of a set of additional, multiple sclerosis-targeted scales (including the MS ADL Scales and the health distress scale), until all variables entering at $P < 0.15$ were included in the model. Results were that R-square for each of the models that allowed inclusion of multiple sclerosis-targeted scales were higher than for the corresponding model in which no disease-targeted scales were included. In each of the second stage models, two multiple sclerosis-targeted scales were significantly associated with each criterion variable in final models (Table 5.4.6).

Gaps in HRQoL measurement for neurologic conditions and future directions

Proxy assessment of HRQoL

For neurologic disorders like Parkinson's disease (PD) or Alzheimer's disease (AD) and other dementias, cognitive impairment may develop or progress over time, within the

Table 5.4.6a Associations between generic and multiple sclerosis-targeted HRQoL scales and level of mobility in multiple sclerosis

Criterion variable	Level of mobility	
	Generic scales only in model	Generic and MS-targeted scales allowed in model
Adjusted R-square	0.51	0.70
Generic scale, p-values:		
Physical Function	<0.0001	<0.0001
MS-targeted scales:		
Motor	N/A	<0.0001
Social	N/A	0.04

Table 5.4.6b Associations between generic and multiple sclerosis-targeted HRQoL scales and symptom severity in prior year

Criterion variable	MS symptom severity in prior year	
	Generic scales only in model	Generic and MS-targeted scales allowed in model
Adjusted R-square	0.34	0.44
Generic scale, p-values:		
Physical function	<0.0001	0.01
Social function	0.02	not significant
MS-targeted scales:		
Motor	N/A	<0.0001
Health distress	N/A	0.0004

time frame of many clinical trials. While a sizeable minority of patients with PD has dementia, most do not; however, cognitive impairment may develop over time within the time frame of longitudinal research studies. Information on equivalence of HRQoL information provided by patients and by proxy informants (Andresen *et al.* 2001; Sneeuw *et al.* 2002) is necessary so that generic and disease-targeted HRQoL outcome measures can be used in PD and dementia clinical research studies. It is desirable to understand the agreement between patients and proxies to allow investigators to plan future studies that might incorporate HRQoL reports from both sources, minimizing loss of information due to missing data, when a respondent's ability for self-report declines over time. Information on factors (for example severity, cognitive level, age, education, frequency of contact) affecting agreement between patients and proxies is also needed.

Incorporation of patients' perspectives of HRQoL impacts of neurologic disease

For several less common neurologic conditions, disease-targeted HRQoL measures have not been developed, or have minimal or no grounding in patient's conceptualization of their HRQoL. Research support is needed to elicit such data and to compare the performance of disease-targeted measures relative to generic measures in persons with these conditions.

Item banks

A comprehensive item bank provides the flexibility of administering the fewest number of items to each study participant that will yield the maximum information about their HRQoL. In contrast to a 'one size fits all' fixed-length survey, an item bank makes it possible to tailor the administration of items so that they match each individual's location on the underlying attribute. For example, asking someone whether he or she has felt happy most of the time in the last 4 weeks is likely to be uninformative if they have already reported thoughts of committing suicide during this time interval. Similarly, asking individuals if they can dress themselves would probably be a waste of time, once you know they have no limitations in performing vigorous activities. By combining information about the difficulty of each item in the bank with progressively better (more precise) estimates of a person's location on the underlying continuum, it is possible to administer the best tailored survey for each individual (see Chapter 1.5).

Modes of administration

In addition to more traditional paper-pencil and interviewer modes of administration, newer technologies like web-based surveys, use of pen-tablet personal computers, interactive voice recognition telephone interviews, and others are increasingly being incorporated into clinical research studies. During 2002, 22 per cent of all clinical trials used some form of electronic data capture, and the projection for 2003 is 30 per cent (Clinical Data Interchange Standards Consortium and CenterWatch.Survey, 2/03). As the clinical research field moves toward increasing use of multimodal electronic data capture, evaluation of data quality by different modes will be essential to prevent exclusion of otherwise eligible patients from clinical trials. Thus, evaluation of properties and burden of disease-targeted tools to measure HRQoL for neurologic conditions via multiple modes is needed.

References

Aaronson, N. K., Alonso, J., Burnam, A., Lohr, K. N., Patrick, D. L., Perrin, E., and Stein, R. E.K. (2002). Assessing health status and quality of life instruments: attributes and review criteria. Scientific Advisory Committee of the Medical Outcomes Trust. *Quality of Life Research,* **11,** 193–205.

Andresen, E. M., Vahle, J. V., and Lollar, D. (2001). Proxy reliability: Health-related quality of life (HRQoL) measures for people with disability. *Quality of Life Research*, **10**, 609–619.

Birbeck, G. L., Hays, R. D., Cui, X., and Vickrey, B. G. (2002). Seizure reduction and quality of life improvements in people with epilepsy. *Epilepsia*, **43**, 535–538.

Birbeck, G. L., Kim, S., Hays, R. D., and Vickrey, B. G. (2000). Quality of life measures in epilepsy: how well can they detect change over time? *Neurology*, **54**, 1822–1827.

Damiano, A. M., McGrath, M. M., Willian, M. K., Snyder, C. F., LeWitt, P. A., Reyes, P. F., Richter, R. R., and Means, E. D. (2000). Evaluation of a measurement strategy for Parkinson's disease: Assessing patient health-related quality of life. *Quality of Life Research*, **9**, 87–100.

Fischer, J. S., LaRocca, N. G., Miller, D. M., Ritvo, P. G., Andrews, H., and Paty, D. (1999). Recent developments in the assessment of quality of life in multiple sclerosis (MS). *Multiple Sclerosis*, **5**, 251–259.

Gulick, E. E. (1988). The self-administered ADL scale for persons with multiple sclerosis. In D. F. Waltz and O. L. Strickland (eds) *Measurement of Nursing Outcomes, Volume I: Measuring Client Outcomes*, pp. 128–159. New York: Springer Publishing Co.

Hays, R. D. and Hayashi, T. (1990). Beyond internal consistency reliability: Rationale and user's guide for the Multitrait Analysis program on the microcomputer. *Behavior Research Methods, Instruments, and Computers*, **22**, 167.

Hays, R. D., Hahn, H., and Marshall, G. (2002). Use of the SF-36 and other health-related quality of life measures to assess persons with disabilities. *Arch Phys Med Rehabil*, **83**, S4–S9.

Holloway, R. G. and Dick, A. W. (2002). Clinical trial end points: on the road to nowhere? *Neurology*, **58**, 679–86.

Jenkinson, C., Peto, V., Fitzpatrick, R., Greenhall, R., and Hyman, N. (1995). Self-reported functioning and well-being in patients with Parkinson's Disease: Comparison of the Short-form Health Survey (SF-36) and the Parkinson's Disease Questionnaire (PDQ-39). *Age and Ageing*, **24**, 505–509.

Karlsen, K. H., Tandberg, E., Arsland, D., and Larsen, J. P. (2000). Health related quality of life in Parkinson's disease: a prospective longitudinal study. *J Neurol Neurosurg Psychiatry*, **69**, 584–589.

Lewin, I. C. F. (1992). *The Cost of Disorders of the Brain*. Washington, DC: The National Foundation for Brain Research.

Liang, M. H., Larson, M. G., Cullen, K. E., and Schwartz, J. A. (1985). Comparative measurement efficiency and sensitivity of five health status instruments for arthritis research. *Arthritis Rheum*, **28**, 542–547.

Longstreth, W. T. Jr, Nelson, L., Linde, M., and Munoz, D. (1992). Utility of the Sickness Impact Profile in Parkinson's disease. *J Geriatr Psychiatry Neurol*, **5**, 142–148.

McDowell, I. and Newell, C. (1996). *Measuring Health: A Guide to Rating Scales and Questionnaires*, 2nd edn. New York: Oxford University Press.

Mosier, C. I. (1943). On the reliability of a weighted composite. *Psychometrika*, **8**, 341–348.

Nunnally, J. (1978). *Psychometric Theory*, 2nd edn. New York: McGraw-Hill.

Peto, V., Jenkinson, C., Fitzpatrick, R., and Greenhall, R. (1995). The development and validation of a short measure of functioning and well-being for individuals with Parkinson's disease. *Quality of Life Research*, **4**, 241–248.

Riazi, A., Hobart, J. C., Lamping, D. L., Fitzpatrick, R., Freeman, J. A., Jenkinson, C., Peto, V., and Thompson, A. J. (2003). Using the SF-36 measure to compare the health impact of multiple sclerosis and Parkinson's disease with normal population health profiles. *J Neurol Neurosurg Psychiatry*, **74**, 710–714.

Rosenberg, M. (1965). *Society and the Adolescent Self-image.* Princeton: Princeton University Press.

Sneeuw, K. C., Sprangers, M. A., and Aaronson, N. K. (2002). The role of health care providers and significant others in evaluating the quality of life of patients with chronic disease. *J Clin Epidemiol,* **55,** 1130–1143.

Steiger, J. H. (1980). Tests for comparing elements of a correlation matrix. *Psychological Bulletin,* **87,** 245.

Sung, N. S., Crowley, W. F. Jr, Genel, M., Salber, P., Sandy, L., Sherwood, L. M., Johnson, S. B., Catanese, V., Tilson, H., Getz, K., Larson, E. L., Scheinberg, D., Reece, E. A., Slavkin, H., Dobs, A., Grebb, J., Martinez, R. A., Korn, A., and Rimoin, D. (2003). Central challenges facing the national clinical research enterprise. *JAMA,* **289,** 1278–1287.

Vickrey, B. G. (1999). Getting oriented to patient-oriented outcomes. *Neurology,* **53,** 662–663.

Vickrey, B. G., Hays, R. D., and Beckstrand, M. (2000). Development of a health-related quality of life measure for peripheral neuropathy. *Neurorehabilitation and Neural Repair,* **14,** 93–104.

Vickrey, B. G., Hays, R. D., Genovese, B. J., Myers, L. W., and Ellison, G. W. (1997). Comparison of a generic to disease-targeted measures of health-related quality of life in multiple sclerosis. *Journal of Clinical Epidemiology,* **50,** 557–569.

Vickrey, B. G., Hays, R. D., Graber, J., Rausch, R., Engel, J. Jr., and Brook, R. H. (1992). A health-related quality of life instrument for patients evaluated for epilepsy surgery. *Med Care,* **30,** 299–319.

Vickrey, B. G., Hays, R. D., Rausch, R., Engel, J., Jr., Sutherling, W., and Brook, R. H. (1994). Quality of life of epilepsy surgery patients compared to outpatients with hypertension, diabetes, heart disease, and/or depressive symptoms. *Epilepsia,* **35,** 597–607.

Stewart, A. L., Hays, R. D., and Ware, J. E. (1992). Health perceptions, energy/fatigue, and health distress measures. In Stewart A. L. and Ware J. E. (eds.) *Measuring Functioning and Well-Being: The Medical Outcomes Study Approach.* Durham, NC: Duke University Press.

Wagner, A. K., Bungay, K. M., Kosinski, M., Bromfield, E. B., and Ehrenberg, B,L. (1996). The health status of adults with epilepsy compared with that of people without chronic conditions. *Pharmacotherapy,* **16,** 1–9.

Williams, L. S., Weinberger, M., Harris, L. E., Clark, D. O., and Biller, J. (1999). Development of a stroke-specific quality of life scale. *Stroke,* **30,** 1362–1369.

Section 6

Beyond clinical trials

Values and valuation in the measurement of HRQoL

Paul Kind

Introduction

Value is intrinsic to all human activity in the sense that we strive to accumulate those things that give us satisfaction or pleasure and to avoid exposure to those that cause us distress or pain. The mechanisms that produce this state of affairs are complex, and shaped by diverse factors in our physical and social environment including our developmental experience. Whilst it is true that we lack an internal 'currency' with which to quantify the magnitude of any value, we nevertheless recognize that some things are of greater importance (have higher value) than others. In as much as our actions reflect our underlying preferences it could be said that they are ultimately expressions of our private values. Health is generally a highly valued attribute that has a significant impact on our capacity to engage in activities commensurate with a good quality of life. We encounter the influence of value in all aspects of our lives and inescapably so in the context of health and health care. The value that we attach to our own present and future health status helps to shape our health behaviours. The assessment made by others of our health status, including that made by health care professionals, may have far-reaching consequences in determining treatment. In some health care systems such assessments may even influence eligibility and entitlement. The degree to which our personal experience of ill-health and its impact on our functional capacity are perceived and understood by others is dependent on the way that they process such information, and this in turn incorporates aspects of their personal and professional value systems.

When we describe our own health we refer to those things which for us are the salient, most relevant and important aspects of our perception of our own condition. When we observe the health of others we may apply a wholly different framework. Health itself is a differentiated concept since we can and do distinguish between good and poor health. We may characterize the latter in terms of pain, fatigue, anxiety or physical incapacity. Good health goes beyond the mere absence of such problems. Measuring health status is to estimate the extent to which an individual possesses (good) health, and this requires an appropriate metric. Such a metric would allow us to resolve several important questions – is an individual in good or poor health, has their health (status) changed over time, what is the direction of any change, and ultimately, what is the magnitude of that change? Many metrics in the realm of science are calibrated in terms of standard units for which there are universally recognized definitions. Although systems may compete, conversion is often a simple and uncontentious matter; for example, in measuring temperature, conversion between °Celsius and °Fahrenheit is trivial. Standard definitions of health can be identified[1] but are often regarded as problematic. Intuition rather than definition guides our understanding and use of the concept we label 'health'. If definition is in doubt, then this uncertainty extends to health status as the descriptive or quantitative representation of the level of health possessed by an individual or group.

In its simplest form we might try to gauge health status in terms of a self-classification elicited in response to the question 'How are you?', for which three general categories of answer – positive, neutral, negative – are possible. Of course the question can be more broadly interpreted as relating to the respondent's (dis)satisfaction with their (ill)health status and it is this notion of bother, nuisance, or inconvenience that is the defining characteristic of what is termed health-related quality of life (HRQoL). The key differentiating property that distinguishes the measurement of HRQoL from the measurement of health status is that the former incorporates an element of value and it is the value attribute that permeates all aspects of the design and application of HRQoL measures. The act of defining HRQoL marks the start of a process that depends to a greater or lesser extent on the exercise of value.

Since it is the *value* attribute that underpins the HRQoL metric, it follows that it is *this* that should command attention when considering the design and application of measures that seek to represent HRQoL. What value is attached to the component dimensions of HRQoL? How are those values determined, and by whom? Ignoring such questions itself represents a statement of value – such questions count for naught. We effectively endorse the values embedded within any measure when we choose to ignore the question of value. Since value and valuation are critical to theory and practice of HRQoL measurement, it is surprising that they are so readily marginalized. This chapter seeks to redress that imbalance.

Measurement

Underpinning all forms of measurement is the capacity to describe. Tallying or counting, the simplest arithmetic operation, is made possible only when we are able to determine when items are the same or different. Items that match count – those that

---

[1] 'Health is a state of complete physical, mental and social well-being and not merely the absence of disease or infirmity.' World Health Organization (1948).

differ do not. A nominal classification of this type is qualitative in nature but provides a portal to all higher level measurement. Descriptive classification may appear a trivial form of measurement but such systems nevertheless have great usefulness. The International Classification of Diseases provides a useful mechanism for categorizing patients according to a standardized description of diagnosis. Information based on this classification allows us to characterize individual patients, to count the number of patients with the same classification, to compute the proportion of patients with any specific classification and to compare such data across health care systems, nationally and internationally. Although such nominal classifications lack a formal value component, they are an essential precursor of HRQoL instruments.

The simplest binary classification of health status (alive or dead) distinguishes two states, one of which is often (although not universally) regarded as preferable to the other. When such a descriptive classification allows us to not only distinguish between different categories, but further enables us to place categories in some sort of hierarchical order, then our measurement is of a more sophisticated form. In such an ordinal classification we are not only able to identify objects belonging to the same category, but we know something about the ordering of categories – whether one category dominates another. The ubiquitous 'none/mild/moderate/severe' classification used, for example, to categorize symptom severity contains just such information. Different patients categorized as 'moderate' are regarded as having a broadly similar level of symptom severity. Despite its qualitative status, such an ordinal system can find powerful application. For example, in the measurement of health outcomes such a classification can be used to indicate the direction of change. A patient with pre- and post-treatment assessments of respectively 'severe' and 'moderate' demonstrates, by inference, a positive change in symptoms. Quantitative measurement that generates data with true cardinal properties becomes possible once we are able to specify the units of measure. By assigning the numbers 1 to 4 to this symptom classification we confer a form of value or weighting to the basic descriptive system. This measurement process assigns 4 to the category 'severe' and 2 to the category 'mild'. Such interval scales can be used to quantifying the distance between points along the scale. Ratio scales, having both a defined unit of measure and a non-arbitrary zero, dominate this hierarchy of measurement types.

In the measurement of HRQoL we are concerned with the twin components of description and valuation that underpin all forms of measurement. We require a descriptive system that gives physical expression to the concept itself. A system of this sort would, as a minimum, list the dimensions that were identified as relevant in the measurement of quality of life. The real potential of HRQoL measurement can be realized once this descriptive system is linked to a valuation system that enables a numeric score to be assigned to those different HRQoL components. Stevens (1946) defines measurement as the assignment of numbers to objects according to some rule. Figure 6.1.1 provides a graphical representation of this process.

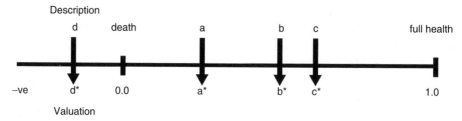

Fig. 6.1.1 Measurement – the correspondence between descriptive and valuation systems.

Using such a schematic, we might identify several health states – *a*, *b*, *c* and *d*. We know something about their relative 'severity' in that *c* is closer to full health than *a* or *b*. State *d* is worse than dead. Other things being equal, moving a patient from *b* to *c* would represent an improvement in their health status. Note that, at this juncture, the inferences we are able to draw from such a descriptive system are constrained because the system is ordinal in nature. We can identify the direction of change but not its magnitude. For us to quantify both the direction and the magnitude of change we need to have an indication of the value associated with health states *a* and *c*, in this case the distance between *b** and *c**. State *d*, being worse than dead, has a negative value since dead in this measurement system has a value of zero. Despite this negative value it is still possible to derive positive health gain from treatment if it results in moving a patient to any state to the right (i.e. moving towards full health).

In general terms, the measurement of health-related quality of life is concerned with the mapping of states of health described in some systematic fashion into a corresponding set of values. The rules whereby a given health state is assigned a particular value can and do vary, so that a single health state can attract more than value when observed under different circumstances. This situation arises in part as a consequence of the lack of agreed standards in defining and valuing HRQoL (and health status more generally).

Implicit values

The association between value and the measurement of HRQoL can be traced back to the earliest decisions taken by the instrument developers. Choices made by the developer influence the methods used to construct new measures. This is intrinsic to much of the science of HRQoL measurement – indeed to the practice of science in general. The conceptualization of HRQoL and its expression through a given descriptive system owes much to the private vision of the developer. Choices concerning those descriptive items to retain and those to reject may be partly driven by their psychometric properties, but the indicators of performance themselves require interpretation. The format of the instrument, including the way that items are presented, the type of responses elicited, their coding and processing are all matters determined by the developer. Any discussion of the justification for such matters is likely to be confined to the early

Description	Score
Normal	100
Normal activity; minor signs/symptoms	90
Subnormal activity; some signs/symptoms	80
Unable to work or to continue normal activities	70
Requires occasional assistance	60
Requires considerable assistance and frequent care	50
Disabled; requires special care	40
Severely disabled; hospitalised	30
Very sick; hospitalised with active support treatment	20
Moribund	10
Dead	0

Fig. 6.1.2 The Karnofsky Performance Scale.

stages of the development process, so that evidence bearing on these factors can be difficult to locate. However, the end-users have an obligation to familiarize themselves with such issues since in adopting any measurement system they are in effect endorsing any and all embedded values.

Even apparently simple measures used to represent HRQoL may depend on powerful assumptions regarding value. The Karnofsky Performance Scale (KPS) (Karnofsky *et al.* 1948), described in Figure 6.1.2, has been widely used in oncology studies.

The (KPS) is an instrument that categorizes patients' functional status on a scale characterized by end points with descriptive categories 'normal' and 'dead'. The lower limit imposes the constraint that no functional state can be worse than being dead – a position that probably reflected Karnofsky's personal viewpoint, but may or may not accord with the views of today's patients for whom KPS observations are recorded. More troubling in such a system is the conversion of textual descriptions into corresponding index 'scores'. In this case values of 100 and 0 are attached to the two anchor categories of the scale. Intermediate states incur equal decrements of 10 points. This assumed equality of decrement is nothing more than a reflection of Karnofsky's private value system. The implications of this value system are rarely explored by the end-user. The category *Requires occasional assistance* with an index score of 60 has a value that is twice that of the category *Severely disabled; hospitalized* with an index score of 30. This implied relationship is effectively reinforced every time KPS is used.

The subtle infiltration of value can be seen in more sophisticated instruments in which the audit trail is less obvious. The RAND-MOS SF-36 contains two items that capture information regarding pain, each with its own response categories as shown below (Ware and Sherbourne 1992).

Pain item I (question 21)		Pain item II (question 22)	
Response 'score'		**Response 'score'**	
none	6	not at all	5
very mild	5	a little bit	4
mild	4	moderately	3
moderate	3	quite a bit	2
severe	2	extremely	1
very severe	1		

Within item I the response *severe* is valued as half that of *mild*. The unit of value is defined by the movement from *none* to *very mild*. Within item II *quite a bit* is assigned a 'score' that is half the value of *a little bit*. The unit value is defined by the difference between *not at all* and *a little bit*. The internal value structure within each item is of course fundamentally different, but the arithmetic operation enacted to derive a pain dimension 'score' appears simply to ignore this. The two item scales are given a new origin by subtracting 1 from the item response scale so that they run from 0 to 5 and 0 to 4 respectively. The sum of the 'scores' produced by the responses to questions 7 and 8 are then divided by 9 (the new maximum 'score') and converted into a percentage by multiplying by 100. Elevation to a scale with cardinal properties is thus effortlessly achieved. The embedded values that underpin this manoeuvre are henceforth lost from view. The arithmetic manipulation of response categories shrouds access to the underlying value system. No matter what subsequent numerical or statistical operation follows, the fact remains that the original scoring convention encapsulates the private, untested values of the instrument developer. As such, it can be argued that although the uncoded responses to the two pain questions do indeed constitute patient self-report, the subsequent transformation into a pain dimension 'score' is achieved by overlaying a set of values that have no corresponding legitimacy. Similar examples that demonstrate the role of implicit values are not difficult to locate in the literature. It is not the *existence* of this phenomenon that is potentially dangerous for the scientist as user of the HRQoL technology, so much as the lack of attention given to its impact on the performance of the technology itself.

Profile measures are sometimes preferred as a means of displaying concurrent observations across the component dimensions of HRQoL. The Nottingham Health Profile (Hunt *et al.* 1985) is but one example and produces subscale scores for six dimensions on the basis of yes/no responses to the 36 items that comprise the questionnaire. A typical means of displaying these subscale scores is shown in Figure 6.1.3, which is based

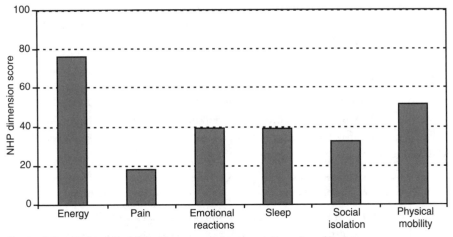

Fig. 6.1.3 Nottingham Health Profile – a sample presentation of profile data.

on data reported in an evaluation study of heart transplantation (O'Brien *et al.* 1987). The mean scores for emotional reaction and sleep in pre-transplant patients appear as virtually identical in the profile. Both are roughly half that of the energy dimension and twice that of pain. In reporting profile data of this type it is easy to unconsciously introduce the notion of that such mean scores are comparable across dimensions. The 40 per cent score for emotional reactions is simply the proportion of the maximum possible score for that dimension. In equating this percentage with that for sleep, we are in effect forcing on these dimensions an equal weighting that implies comparability where there is none. What this type of profile lacks is the explicit values associated with each dimension that would guide our interpretation of subscale scores. As they stand we are drawn to treat them as having equal value when they almost certainly do not. Of course if the relative weights of each dimension were known, then the profile could be readily converted into a single summary score.

There are other aspects of HRQoL measurement where valuation is implied through usage. In reporting the analysis of HRQoL data the performance of an instrument may be represented by its effect size – essentially the ratio between a mean change score and the variance in that score when initially measured. An effect size is considered 'good' if it exceeds a commonly recognized threshold value (Cohen 1988). Whilst this statistic conveys some useful information when applied to a given HRQoL measure used in different settings, the comparison of effect sizes across different HRQoL measures is legitimized only if the metric is considered to have universal value. An effect size statistic has relative, not absolute value. To suggest that one HRQoL instrument has a superior performance to another on the basis of a comparison of effect sizes is to entertain the notion that a unit change in the ratio has equal value across all measurement scales and in all therapeutic settings. As a statistical concept and when applied to value-free data this can work well enough, but when used to discriminate between value-based HRQoL data this is another matter altogether.

Explicit values

Probably the earliest evidence bearing on the explicit valuation of health outcomes comes from the Code of Hammurabi,[2] a detailed account of the payments due to medical practitioners (and the penalties imposed on them) as a consequence of their interventions. For example, number 216 states:

> If a physician make a large incision with an operating knife and cure it, or if he open a tumor (over the eye) with an operating knife, and saves the eye, he shall receive ten shekels in money.

It is worth noting that the 'value' of that outcome changes according to the position of the beneficiary within the socio-legal framework of society – a slave or ex-slave being worth less than a citizen. More recently, the monetary values associated with the consequences of treatment, accident or misfortune have been the subject of investigation. Rosser and Watts (1972) published an analysis of the financial settlements determined by English Courts of Law. Such settlements make explicit reference to loss of function, pain and suffering, and allocate specific sums of money under these two broad headings. That information was used to determine the relative value of each of 28 health states defined by a 7*4 matrix. Health status in this context was defined in terms of respectively disability and distress.

In general, the values of the components of any HRQoL descriptive system are not known unless and until they are formally investigated. A variety of methods for eliciting formal values for HRQoL instruments have been used including magnitude estimation (Kaplan *et al.* 1979; Rosser and Kind 1978), paired comparisons (McKenna *et al.* 1981; Kind and Rosser 1988) category rating (Blischke *et al.* 1975, Carter *et al.* 1976) and equivalence matching (Patrick *et al.* 1973; Rosser 1981). These methods have their origins in psychophysics and experimental psychology and draw on a significant body of knowledge obtained over more than half a century. A second group of valuation methods that originate in the economics discipline include Standard Gamble (SG) and Time Trade-Off (TTO), the one being developed as a proxy for the other. Both methods are formulated so as to derive estimates of utility – a form of preference measure that has particular relevance for economists since it embodies notions of sacrifice/exchange. The relationship between values derived by psychophysical methods and utilities remains the subject of dispute. It would be hugely advantageous were a simple mechanism to be found that enabled values obtained via one procedure to be transformed so as to match those resulting from a second procedure. However, no such remedy is yet to hand, although there some fairly consistent findings, for example, the relationship

[2] Multiple locations on the WWW, for example see http://www.wsu.edu/~dee/MESO/CODE.HTM

between values obtained from category rating and magnitude estimation methods has long been known to be curvilinear. Attempts to link category rating with SG or TTO utilities remain only partially successful. A single universal transformation of category rating data has yet to be identified so that the suggested use of category rating as a simpler proxy needs to be resisted. More troubling are the systematic differences that emerge when the values from competing procedures are compared. Utilities elicited using SG are typically higher than those obtained via TTO and both are higher than values derived using psychophysical methods. In such circumstances the choice of valuation methods (and hence the HRQoL value set) is as likely to be shaped by personal conviction as it is by any conventional theory. Some of these methods are further described in Chapter 6.2, while Chapter 6.3 explains the technique of discrete choice experiments.

Explicit values associated with the measurement of health-related quality of life are rarely found other than for generic instruments. A list of candidate instruments and measures is given in Table 6.1.1.

The Health Utilities Index (HUI), also described in Chapter 6.2, is typical of this group. A descriptive system based on eight dimensions each with five or six levels, it defines a universe of some 972,000 health states. The weight used to represent the (social) value of each of those health states is derived using a set procedure, the details of which have been widely published and cited. Although there can, and indeed is, debate about the specific valuation methods adopted or the analytic methods used to process the valuation data they generate, the procedures are fully documented and open to inspection and, potentially, replication. The social preference weights associated with the HUI are thus made *explicit* in a form that enables the end-user to be fully informed about their status. This highly desirable position is something of a rarity amongst HRQoL instruments, and is a design attribute that is shared by those instruments listed in Table 6.1.1. More commonly encountered is the instrument that is constructed in such a way that the rationale of its scoring system is obscured, so that the end-user must take on trust the procedures that led to its formulation. In its most extreme form, it must be accepted that some instruments used as quantitative measures of health-related quality of life lack the necessary measurement properties for legitimate use as cardinal measures.

For certain specific applications, most notably in respect of economic evaluation, the measurement of health-related quality of life is subject to additional requirements. Cost–utility analysis summarizes the consequences of health care in terms of quality-adjusted life years (QALYs). The QALY is a unit of measure that combines information on quantity and quality of life. The arithmetic product of these two elements effectively represents the area under the curve generated by plotting health-related quality of life against surviving life expectancy. The metric used to represent life expectancy is straightforward enough, but for the purposes of computing QALYs the measure of HRQoL should conform to the requirements identified by the Washington Panel on

Table 6.1.1 Generic HRQoL and associated valuation methods

	Reference	Category rating	Magnitude estimation	Equivalence matching	Paired comparisons	Visual analogue scale	Standard Gamble	Time Trade-Off
Quality of Well-being (QWB)	Patrick et al. 1973	✓	✓	✓				
Sickness Impact Profile (SIP)	Bergner et al. 1976	✓						
Rosser Index	Rosser and Watts 1972		✓	✓	✓		✓	
Nottingham Health Profile (NHP)	Hunt et al. 1985				✓			
15D	Sintonen 2001					✓		
Health Utilities Index (HUI)	Torrance et al. 1995					✓	✓	✓
EQ-5D	Brooks 1996				✓	✓		✓
Assesment of Quality of Life (AQoL)	Hawthorne et al. 1999							✓
SF-6D	Brazier et al. 1998					✓	✓	

Cost-Effectiveness in Health and Medicine (Gold *et al.* 1996). The HRQoL weights used to compute QALYs should of course be cardinal, and must have a single index format. Furthermore, the weights must lie on a scale that assigns values of 1 and 0 to full health and dead respectively. The consequences of these requirements taken together effectively rule out a whole class of HRQoL instrument. Any profile that lacks the capacity to be represented as a summary index necessarily fails to meet the requirements needed for cost–utility analysis. The Washington Panel proposed further restrictions as to the source of valuations for use in cost-effectiveness analysis. The valuations should represent the social preferences of the general population in the first instance, rather than being based on any particular patient subset. The list of potential instruments that might satisfy these requirements is probably confined to four of those given in Table 6.1.1. Hence for the specialist application of HRQoL measures in economic evaluation there are only a handful of instruments from which to choose. By contrast the range of condition-specific or targeted HRQoL measures is vastly wider. The widespread adoption of HRQoL measures in clinical studies has encouraged the use of generic measures as both clinical and economic outcome variables. However, the restricted qualifications imposed on data required for economic analysis should not be permitted to dictate the source or type of values deemed necessary for the evaluation of clinical outcomes. The route to weighted HRQoL data is mediated through the original response data that is based on the descriptive system that underpins any given instrument. It is entirely feasible to consider using different value sets for different purposes, rather than placing the requirements of health economists over those of researchers from other disciplines. Hence a generic HRQoL measure might be weighted using a 0–1 scale of social preferences for the purposes of cost–utility analysis, but those same data might be weighted using patient preferences to inform clinical decision-makers.

The choice of method used to determine explicit values in measuring health-related quality of life is a matter largely settled by consideration of the intended application to which those values are to be put. Resolving the question as to *whose* values should be used is another matter altogether. Amongst the different possible approaches to constructing quality of life measures the so-called individualistic approach is based on the concept that quality of life is 'what the individual says it is' (Joyce *et al.* 2003); see also Chapter 4.1. Proponents of this approach argue that the legitimate source of all information relating to quality of life is the individual person or patient him or herself. There is, of course, some limited force to this argument if the assessment of health outcomes is confined to the individual case, but in the opinion of this author it cannot be regarded as a practical approach in designing tools for use in clinical studies and in other circumstances where HRQoL data must be aggregated. It is sometimes suggested that since patients or those suffering from a particular condition have direct, first-hand experience they should form the definitive source of any HRQoL values. This is a somewhat dangerous counsel to follow, since the values elicited from an individual with substantial experience of a condition are likely to differ from those obtained from a newly diagnosed patient. Accommodation to a problem is likely to occur in many situations, so that what may be a highly valued component of HRQoL at the outset of illness may assume a more marginal consideration after some time. The presumed qualification of patients that rests upon their experience of ill-health is lost and becomes then a matter of degree of experience. In the context of particular disease settings it may be desirable to harvest values from a range of patients with difference levels of experience. The practical limitation of this approach becomes clearer if we seek to aggregate data across patients. Problem areas identified by one patient may not be mentioned by others. Furthermore, the value attached by different patients to the same problem obstructs the aggregation process. All this is not to say that the views of individual patients do not count – merely that their views represent one perspective among many possible. However, where generic HRQoL measures are concerned, another difficulty is encountered that further dilutes the argument in favour of patient values. Generic measures are by definition general purpose and designed to be used in a range of therapeutic and disease settings. It is inconceivable therefore that the views of any single patient group should be used to represent the perspective of those with experience of poor health. Indeed it can be safely argued that if we wish to tap the values of such individuals, we should survey the general population in whom such experience is naturally located.

Summary

The issue of value and valuation on the measurement of HRQoL may be easily avoided, but it should not be so lightly dismissed. We have no absolute metric with which to observe and report HRQoL, so that the practical use of instruments developed for use in this field is bedevilled by the volatility of the science itself. Values, whether implicit or explicit, are interwoven in the fabric of all HRQoL measures. The more telling challenge for us is not whether this matters in itself, but rather what are the likely consequences of adopting one instrument (and its set of related values) over another. It may yet turn out to be the case that the practical implications of using cardinal estimates of HRQoL are fairly resistant to the values used to obtain those quantitative data. If in fact it matters little whether we use the values from the old or the young, the sick or healthy, to estimate the worth of changes in HRQoL, then the choice as to which reference group to select becomes more obviously a matter for politicians than for research scientists. For us to reach some closure in this matter we must first be in a position to consider more systematically the effects of utilising different value sets, obtained from different reference groups, using different valuation methods – all applied to the same standard descriptive system. By way of preparation for that ultimate sensitivity analysis we also need to be more assertive in confronting the infiltration of concealed values in the construction and use of all measures of health-related quality of life.

References

Bergner, M., Bobbit, R. A., and Kressel, S., *et al.* (1976). The Sickness Impact Profile: conceptual formulation and methodology for the development of a health status measure. *International Journal of Health Services*, **6**, 393–415.

Blischke, W. R., Bush, J. W., and Kaplan, R. M. (1975). Approaches and techniques: successive interval analysis of preference measures in a health status index. *Health Services Research*, **10**, 181–198.

Brazier, J., Usherwood, T., Harper, R., and Thomas, K. (1998). Deriving a preference-based single index from the UK SF-36 health survey. *Journal of Clinical Epidemiology*, **51**, 115–128.

Brooks, R. G. (1996). EuroQol: the current state of play. *Health Policy*, **37**, 53–72.

Carter, W. B., Bobbitt, R. A., Bergner, M., and Gilson, B. S. (1976). Validation of an interval scaling: The Sickness Impact Profile. *Health Services Research*, **11**, 516–528.

Cohen, J. (1988). *Statistical Power Analysis for the Behavioral Sciences*, 2nd edn. Hillsdale, NJ: Lawrence Earlbaum Associates.

Gold, M. R., Siegel, J. E., Russell, L. B., and Weinstein, M. C. (1996). *Cost-effectiveness in Health and Medicine.* Oxford: Oxford University Press.

Hawthorne, G., Richardson, J., and Osborne, R. (1999). The Assessment of Quality of Life (AQoL) instrument: a psychometric measure of health related quality of life. *Quality of Life Research*, **8**, 209–224.

Hunt, S., McEwen, J., and McKenna, S. (1985). Measuring health status: a new tool for clinicians and epidemiologists. *Journal of the Royal College of General Practitioners*, **35**, 185–188.

Joyce, C. R., Hickey, A., McGee, H. M., and O'Boyle, C. A. (2003). A theory-based method for the evaluation of individual quality of life: the SEIQoL. *Quality of Life Research*, **12**, 275–280.

Kaplan, R. M., Bush, J. W., and Berry, C. C. (1979). Health status index: category rating versus magnitude estimation for measuring levels of well-being. *Medical Care*, **17**, 501–525.

Karnofsky, D. A., Abenmann, W. H., and Craver, L. F., *et al.* (1948). The use of nitrogen mustards in the palliative treatment of carcinoma. *Cancer*, **1**, 634–656.

Kind, P. and Rosser, R. M. (1988). The quantification of health. *European Journal of Social Psychology*, **18**, 63–77.

McKenna, S. P., Hunt, S. M., and McEwen, J. (1981). Weighting the seriousness of perceived problems using Thurstone's method of paired comparisons. *International Journal of Epidemiology*, **10**, 93–97.

O'Brien, B. J., Buxton, M. J., and Ferguson, B. A. (1987). Measuring the effectiveness of heart transplant programmes: quality of life data and their relationship to survival analysis. *Journal of Chronic Disease*, **40**, 137S–158S.

Patrick, D. L., Bush, J. W., and Chen, M. M. (1973). Methods for measuring levels of well-being for a health status index. *Health Services Research*, **8**, 228–245.

Rosser, R. M. (1981). A set of descriptions and a psychometric scale of severity of illness: an indicator for use in evaluating the outcome of hospital care. Doctoral thesis. London University.

Rosser, R. M. and Kind, P. (1978). A scale of valuations of states of illness: is there a social consensus? *International Journal of Epidemiology*, **7**, 347–358.

Rosser, R. M. and Watts, V. C. (1972). The measurement of hospital output. *International Journal of Epidemiology*, **1**, 361–368.

Sintonen, H. (2001). The 15D instrument of health-related quality of life: properties and applications. *Annals of Medicine*, **33**, 328–36.

Stevens, S. S. (1946). On the theory of scales of measurement. *Science* **103**, (2684), 677–680.

Torrance, G. W., Furlong, W., Feeny, D., and Boyle, M. (1995). Multi-attribute preference functions: Health Utilities Index. *Pharmacoeconomics*, **7**, 503–520.

Ware, J. E. and Sherbourne, C. D. (1992). The SF-36 Short Form health status survey: conceptual framework and item selection. *Medical Care*, **30**, 473–483.

World Health Organization. (1948). Constitution as adopted by the International Health Conference, New York, 19–22 June, 1946; signed on 22 July 1946 by the representatives of 61 States (Official Records of the World Health Organization, no. **2**, p. 100) and entered into force on 7 April 1948.

Preference-based measures: utility and quality-adjusted life years

David Feeny

Introduction

Preference-based measures are playing an increasingly important role in the assessment of health-related quality of life (HRQoL) as an outcome measure in clinical trials and other studies, in supporting decision analyses, and in supporting economic evaluations and health technology assessments of screening, prevention, and treatment interventions. The chapter will discuss the conceptual foundations of preference-based measures, describe the two basic approaches to preference-based measurement, summarize evidence on reliability, construct validity, responsiveness (longitudinal construct validity), and predictive validity, and briefly describe selected applications.

Conceptual Foundations

Health status and HRQoL are assessed for a variety of purposes including description, discrimination, evaluation, and prediction (Guyatt *et al.* 1993). Discrimination refers to the ability to distinguish among groups at a point in time (cross-sectional study). Evaluation refers to the ability to capture within-person change over time (prospective study). Prediction refers to the ability of one measure to predict another measure, for instance the ability of a "short form" of an instrument to predict the score on the corresponding "long form". Alternatively, prediction may refer to the ability of an assessment of HRQoL at one point in time to predict HRQoL in subsequent periods. Measures designed for one purpose may be less than ideal when used for other purposes.

Measures of health status provide descriptive information on the health of subjects at a particular point in time. Typically physical, mental, and social aspects of health are included. HRQoL goes beyond describing health status by including a valuation of the health state. Patrick and Erickson (1993, p 22) provide a prominent definition of HRQoL: "health-related quality of life is the value assigned to duration of life as modified by the impairments, functional states, perceptions, and social opportunities that are influenced by disease, injury, treatment, or policy." Preference-based measures provide one approach to the valuation of health states.

The measurement of HRQoL is based on a conceptual framework and a set of fundamental normative assumptions. It is important to be explicit about the underlying framework employed. One of the major conceptual foundations of preference-based measures is microeconomic theory and decision science (see for instance Becker 1965; Grossman 1972; Feeny 2000; basic references on utility theory in health applications include Torrance 1986; Torrance and Feeny 1989; and Feeny and Torrance 1989). (The psychometric foundations for preference-based measures are discussed in Chapter 6.1.)

To illustrate the framework, consider a very simple world in which there are two final consumption goods: health status and a composite "other" good (non-health goods, services, and leisure). Individuals have preferences over each of the two final goods. The utility function (Equation 1) summarizes preferences over combinations of health status and the composite good.

$$U = f(HS, C) \tag{1}$$

where U is utility;
HS = health status;
C = composite final consumption good.

Note that in this framework health status directly "enters" the utility function. This means that health status is a fundamental determinant of utility or the overall level of well being. Further, both final consumption goods (HS and C) are produced by the final consumer (within the household) using the time and goods purchased in the market. The health status production function is given in Equation (2).

$$HS = f(C, T_{hs}, MC, GE, PE, SE) \tag{2}$$

where C is defined above;
T_{hs} = time devoted to the production of health status;
MC = medical care;
GE = genetic endowment;
PE = physical environment;
SE = social environment.

Health status depends on the nature and amount of consumption of others goods (eating fresh fruits and vegetables versus using tobacco), time spent producing health status (regular exercise, sleep), medical care, one's genetic endowment, the nature of the physical environment (air and water quality, occupational exposures), and the social environment (degree of inequality, social support).

Two major approaches

There are two major families of preference-based measures: direct and multi-attribute (Guyatt *et al* 1993; Drummond *et al.* 1997). Direct measures involve asking patients to value health states. In contrast, in the multi-attribute, or indirect approach, patients complete health status questionnaires. A utility scoring function is then used to provide utility scores for the health states as assessed by the patients. The conventional scale for preference-based measures is anchored on 0.00 for dead and 1.00 for perfect health.

Direct Preference-Based Measures

In the direct approach the respondent is asked to place a value on a health state. Valuations are obtained using one or more of a variety of elicitation techniques. The three most common techniques are the visual analogue scale (VAS), standard gamble (SG), and time tradeoff (TTO).

In much of the decision science literature a distinction is made between value and utility scores. Both reflect preferences. Value scores are obtained under conditions of certainty. The VAS and TTO (discussed below) are therefore classified as value scores. Utility scores are obtained under conditions of uncertainty (risk). SG scores (discussed below) are therefore utility scores.

VAS. One of the most commonly used elicitation techniques is a VAS, often implemented with a prop known as the Feeling Thermometer (FT). (Descriptions of techniques for preference-elicitation surveys are found in Furlong *et al.* 1990.) The FT is a vertical line divided into 101 points, labeled from 0 to 100. Usually, the top anchor of the FT is labeled "Most Desirable" and the bottom anchor is labeled "Least Desirable". (See Figure 6.2.1.) The respondent is given a set of health states to value and asked to place the health states on the VAS both to reflect the rank order of the states and to ensure that the relative position of the states on the VAS reflects their strength of preference for the states.

The mix of health states being evaluated at the same time can affect scores for particular health states obtained using the VAS; the VAS is subject to context effects (Torrance *et al.* 2001; Streiner and Norman 1995). In response to this problem and to assist in the interpretation of scores, some investigators use the marker-state approach to provide a relevant context (Bennett and Torrance 1996). Health-state descriptions are developed for hypothetical health states that describe the range of experience of patients with a particular disease or problem. In general, the evidence is that scores for hypothetical marker states are stable over time (Llewellyn-Thomas *et al.* 1993; Feeny, Blanchard *et al.* 2003, in press; Jansen, Stiggelbout, Wakker *et al.* (2000); Laupacis *et al.* 1993; Saigal *et al.* 2003) and thus are useful in providing a relevant context.

The VAS is also subject to end-of scale aversion (Torrance *et al.* 2001; Streiner and Norman 1995). Respondents typically avoid putting states very close to the most desirable or least desirable ends of the scale. End-of-scale aversion can lead to lower scores for health states judged to be only marginally less desirable than the most desirable end of the scale. Similarly, higher scores are obtained for states ranked just above the least desirable end of the scale.

Measurement Properties, VAS, Construct Validity. In general, VAS scores perform as one might expect them to perform. Health states involving heavy burdens of morbidity are scored lower than those with more modest burdens. Typically the rank ordering of

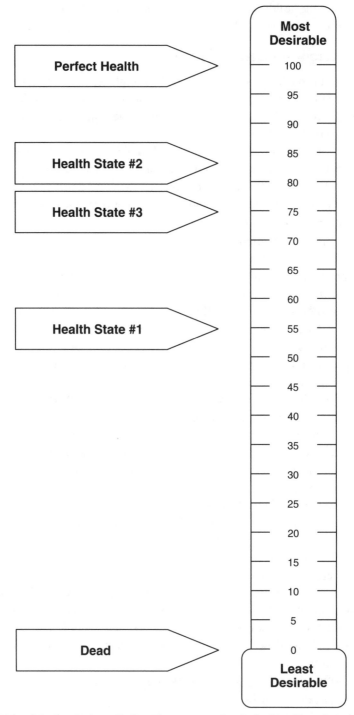

Fig. 6.2.1 Visual Analog Scale, or Feeling Thermometer, For Ordinal Ranking of Health States.

health states agrees across preference elicitation techniques. There are, however, studies in which rank orderings have been somewhat inconsistent across techniques. (Giesler *et al.* 1999).

Typically VAS scores correlate moderately (0.35 – 0.49) with TTO and SG scores (Torrance 1976; Green *et al.* 2000). TTO embody time preference; VAS scores do not. SG scores embody time and risk preferences; VAS scores do not. These underlying differences in the construct being measured account, in part, for the moderate level of association among scores. Similarly, SG scores for the same health state are typically greater than TTO which in turn are greater than VAS scores.

Reliability, VAS. The test-retest reliability of VAS scores over time intervals of one week to 3 months has been assessed in a variety of contexts (Torrance 1976; Green *et al.* 2000; Torrance 1986; O'Brien *et al.* 1994; Macran 2003). Correlations of 0.62 to 0.95 have been observed, with most ≥ 0.70, a level of test-retest reliability usually viewed as acceptable for group level comparisons (Hays *et al.* this volume, 1993; Revicki *et al.* 2000; McDowell and Newell 1996).

Responsiveness, VAS. In a number of contexts VAS scores appear to have been moderately to highly responsive using effect size or the responsiveness index as a measure of responsiveness. See for instance Bombardier *et al.* 1986; Feeny *et al.* 1998; Juniper *et al.* 1997; Macran 2003.

Practical Aspects, VAS. The VAS is seemingly easy to use. In practice, however, preference elicitation using the VAS, TTO, or SG often requires interviewer administration using well-trained and supervised professional interviewers (Furlong *et al.* 1990). Although many regard the VAS as more user-friendly than the TTO and SG, respondents in a number of studies have rated it as more difficult (Patrick *et al.* 1994). As the number of states on the VAS goes up, the number of pair-wise combinations increases rapidly, generating substantial cognitive demands. Ironically the choice-based techniques, the TTO and SG, may be less demanding. In interview settings, a rule of thumb for administration of the VAS is that each health state will take an average of five minutes (including the fixed time for instructions, introductions, etc.).

The SG. The SG is a choice-based technique for preference elicitation (Drummond *et al.* 1997; Torrance 1986). The respondent is given a choice between a specified period of time in an intermediately ranked-health state or a lottery. The lottery consists of the same period of time in perfect health (or some other state that is preferred to the intermediately ranked state) with probability p and dead (or some other state less preferred to the intermediately ranked state) with probability 1–p. (See Figure 6.2.2.) The probability p is varied until the respondent is indifferent between the lottery and the sure thing. The better the intermediately ranked state, the higher the probability that the respondent will require to be indifferent. The utility score for the intermediately ranked state is derived from the indifference probability.

The SG is directly tied to von Neumann-Morgenstern expected utility theory (von Neumann and Morgenstern 1944; Torrance 1986; Torrance and Feeny (1989); Feeny and

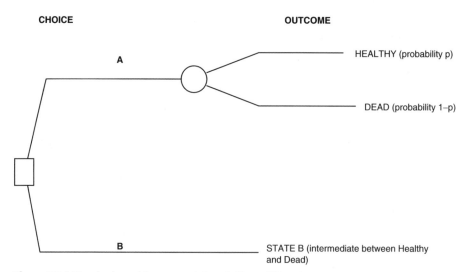

Figure 6.2.2 Standard gamble approach for eliciting utility values.

Torrance 1989; Feeny 2000). Expected utility theory assumes that people have stable well-formulated utility functions. Among the key axioms of expected utility theory are the requirements that utilities be transitive and that utilities are continuous. Continuity implies that if A is preferred to B and B is preferred to C (and thus, by transitivity, A is preferred to C), there exists a lottery with outcomes of A or C such that the subject is indifferent to the lottery versus B. The SG is based directly on the continuity axiom. Because of the explicit tie to theory, conceptually the SG is the gold standard for assessing preferences (and utilities) for health states.

The TTO. The TTO is another choice-based technique for preference elicitation (Drummond *et al.* 1997; Torrance 1976, 1986; Torrance *et al.* 1972). The respondent is given a choice between a specified period of time in perfect health or a specified period of time in a health state less than perfect health. (See Figure 6.2. 3.) The period of time in perfect health is then varied until a point of indifference is found between a longer period (t) in the health state being evaluated or a shorter period of time in perfect health (x). The value score for the health state is then x/t. Life in the state for t years is "equivalent" to x years in perfect health.

The SG is directly tied to expected utility theory. Conceptually the TTO can be linked to the same theory, by retaining all of the axioms of expected utility theory, and adding the additional requirement that utility in additional healthy time is linear with respect to time. In practice, the utility function appears to be concave with respect to healthy time, implying that TTO scores will typically be less than SG scores, an implication consistent with results from most empirical studies. Thus, from the conceptual point of view, the SG is less demanding in that it requires fewer assumptions.

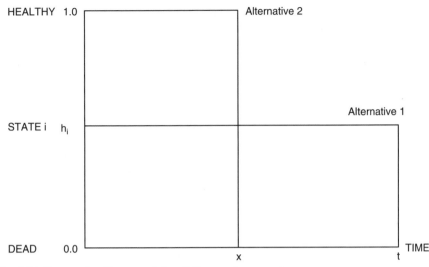

Fig. 6.2.3 Time trade-off approach for eliciting preference values.

Measurement Properties, SG and TTO. It is convenient to discuss evidence on the measurement properties for the SG and the TTO together.

Construct Validity, SG and TTO. In a wide variety of context the SG and TTO perform as one would expect them to perform. Ness *et al.*1999 constructed seven path states that described both treatment process and outcome associated with colorectal cancer. The ordering of mean SG scores agreed with *a priori* hypotheses. (See also Hayman *et al.* 1997.) Albertsen *et al.* (1998) report TTO estimates for health states associated with prostate cancer that conform to expectations about rank order. (See also Chapman *et al.* 1999; Ashby *et al.* 1994.)

However, it has sometimes been the case that patients undergoing therapy are unwilling to trade any time or risk of survival (O'Connor *et al.* 1987). If patients are unwilling to trade time or risk of survival, they assign a value of 1.00, the same as perfect health, to their current health state. Thus there will be no scope for improvement in score and this will attenuate the responsiveness of the TTO and SG (for an example using TTO in colorectal cancer see Stiggelbout *et al.* (1995); for evidence using TTO in the context of prostate cancer see Chapman *et al.* (1998); for evidence on TTO in the context of genetic testing for risk of breast cancer see Grann *et al.* (1998, 1999).

TTO has also been used to evaluate states associated with screening for breast cancer (Johnson *et al.* 1998; Hall *et al.* 1992). Because screening involves temporary (process) and outcome (chronic) states, more complicated preference-elicitation procedures have often been used. Subjects were asked to evaluate "path states" consisting of a sequence of events describing both the process and outcome of treatment (see also Kuppermann *et al.* 1997).

SG and TTO scores collected before decisions have been made have been shown to be consistent with subsequent choices. For instance Singer *et al.* 2003 found that patients who had low SG scores for their current health were much more likely to decide to be put on the waiting list for lung transplantation than patients with high SG scores (see also Carter *et al.* 1986; Heckerling *et al.* 1994).

Reliability, SG and TTO. In general, the test-retest reliability of the SG has been acceptable. O'Brien and Viramontes (1994) report an ICC of 0.82 for patients who assessed the same health states four weeks later. Green *et al.* (2000) in their review paper report a range of results from various studies with correlations of 0.53 to 0.82. Shiell *et al.* (2000) report ICCs between assessments of 0.78 (1 week after initial assessment), 0.72 (7 weeks later), and 0.70 (8 weeks later). ICCs for test-retest for SG scores for marker states (mean time between assessments of 5.2 months) of 0.65 to 0.83 are reported by Feeny *et al.* 2004a.

Similarly, in general, test-retest reliability for the TTO has been acceptable. Correlations of 0.63 to 0.81 have been observed for intervals of four to six weeks (Torrance 1986). Green *et al.* (2000) report correlations of 0.63 to 0.87 for intervals of 1 to 16 weeks. See also Ashby *et al.* 1994; Albertsen *et al.* 1998; Saigal *et al.* 2001; and Grann *et al.* 1999.

Responsiveness, SG and TTO. A number of analysts who have collected SG and TTO scores in longitudinal studies have found them to be moderately to highly responsive using a variety of measures of responsiveness such as effect size. In a study of total hip arthroplasty, Blanchard *et al.* 2003 provides evidence of moderate effect size (0.50 – 0.79; responsiveness) for the SG and a large effect size (≥0.80) for the Health Utilities Index Mark 3. In a double-blind placebo-controlled randomized clinical trial in arthritis of an oral gold compound, Bombardier *et al.* (1986) found that a direct preference measure (using SG, TTO, and VAS) was among the most responsive of the wide variety of measures employed in the study.

Practical Aspects, SG and TTO. The SG and TTO are choice-based techniques. Both involve complex cognitive processes and are more demanding than the completion of standardized health-status assessment questionnaires.

The traditional technology for obtaining SG and TTO scores is the in-person interview (Furlong *et al.* 1990). The quality of the data is enhanced by the use of scripts and props in interviews. Interviewers need to be well trained and carefully supervised and interviews should be audiotaped for quality assurance. A rule of thumb is that one should budget 5 minutes of interview time per health state to be evaluated using the SG or TTO.

More recently, computer-assisted interview techniques have been developed. Results to date are promising (Lenert and Kaplan 2000). However, there appears to be a lack of evidence on agreement between scores from computer-assisted and in-person interviews.

Clinically Important Differences/Change. SG and TTO scores are not assessed with great precision. For instance, respondents may find it difficult to distinguish differences in probabilities (for the SG) of less than 0.05. Differences in scores of 0.10 or larger are clearly important (Furlong *et al.* 1990). Many would regard differences in scores of 0.05 or larger as important.

Multi-Attribute Preference-Based Measures

In the direct approach to the assessment of HRQoL, patients are asked to assess and value their current health state. An alternative (and not mutually exclusive) approach is to use a multi-attribute system. The three most commonly used multi-attribute measures are the EuroQol EQ-5D (Essink-Bot *et al.* 1993; EuroQol 1990; Dolan 1997; Rabin and de Charro 2001), the Health Utilities Index (HUI) (Feeny *et al.* 1996; Feeny *et al.* 2002; Furlong *et al.* 2001), and the Quality of Well Being scale (QWB) (Patrick *et al.* 1973; Kaplan and Anderson 1996). Recently Brazier *et al.* 2002 have introduced the SF-6D, a multi-attribute system based on the Short Form 36 (Ware and Sherbourne 1992; Ware 1996). Table 6.2.1 summarizes the characteristics of each of the systems discussed.

In order to facilitate applications in assessing health status and to ensure the feasibility of estimating a multi-attribute utility function (scoring function), it is necessary to limit the number of attributes or dimensions of health status included in the system. In practice, the QWB has four dimensions; the EQ-5D includes five dimensions; HUI2 includes seven; HUI3 includes eight; and SF-6D includes six.

In the multi-attribute approach, respondents complete a health-status questionnaire that is similar to questionnaires for generic profile measures such as the RAND-36 (Hays and Morales 2001) and SF-36 (Ware and Sherbourne 1992; Ware 1996). The scoring systems for the multi-attribute measures are, however, based on a different paradigm. The scores for multi-attribute health states quantify the value attached to the health state based on preference-scores obtained from a random sample of the general population. In contrast, the psychometric-based scoring systems for the generic-profile measures describe the health status of the subject and provide information on the "location" of that health state in the distribution of health states experienced by patients with a particular disease and/or the distribution found in the general population.

The EQ-5D. The EQ-5D includes several components. First, there is a health-status classification system. Health status in the EQ-5D consists of five dimensions (or attributes): mobility, self-care, usual activity, pain/discomfort, and anxiety/depression. There are three levels defined for each dimension: no problem, some problem, or extreme problem. A standardized questionnaire based on the system is available. The health status of an individual at a point in time can be represented as a five-element vector, one level for each dimension (Kind 1996).

A score for that categorical information on health status can be obtained by using a scoring formula. The Dolan (1997) scoring system, the most commonly used one,

Table 6.2.1 Description of EuroQol EQ-5D, Health Utilities Index Mark 2 (HUI2) and Mark 3 (HUI3), Quality of Well-Being (QWB), and Short-Form 6D (SF-6D) Multi-Attribute Preference-Based Measures

Measure	Dimensions of Health Status and (Number of Levels)	Number of Unique Health States	Scoring	Function
EQ-5D	Mobility (3); Self-Care (3); Usual Activities (3); Pain/Discomfort (3); Anxiety/Depression (3)	243 plus unconscious, and dead	*Ad hoc* Modified	Linear Additive based on TTO scores from random sample of British population
HUI2	Sensation (4); Mobility (5); Emotion (5); Cognition (4); Self-Care (4); Pain and Discomfort (5); Fertility (3)	24,000 plus dead		Multiplicative Multi-Attribute based on SG Scores from random sample of parents in general population in Canada
HUI3	Vision (6); Hearing (6); Speech (5); Ambulation (6); Dexterity (6); Emotion (5); Cognition (5); Pain and Discomfort (5)	972,000 plus dead		Multiplicative Multi-Attribute based on SG Scores from random sample of general population in Canada
QWB	Mobility (3); Physical Activity (3); Social Activity (5); Symptom/ Problem Complex (27)	1,215 plus dead		Linear Additive based VAS scores from random sample of general population in the U.S.
SF-6D	Physical Functioning (6); Role Limitations (4); Social Functioning (5); Pain (6); Mental Health (5); Vitality (5)	18,000 plus dead	*Ad hoc* Modified	Linear Additive Based on SG scores from a random sample of the U.K. general population

is based on preference scores using the TTO obtained from a representative sample of adults in the United Kingdom. Because some states (for instance the state (3,3,3,3,3) with extreme problems in all five dimensions) were considered by respondents to be worse than dead, the scale runs from –0.59 to 1.00. Many refer to the scores derived from the scoring system as EQ-5D index scores. A modified linear additive functional form is used for the EQ-5D scoring function. This functional form implies that there are no important interactions in preferences among the dimensions of health status. Thus, the disutility of a moderate problem with mobility ("I have some problems in walking about") does not depend on the degree of problem (if any) with respect to anxiety/depression.

Another component of the EQ-5D system is a VAS on which respondents provide a rating of their own current health state. General measurement properties of the VAS have already been described so the use of the EQ-5D VAS will not be reviewed further here.

Measurement Properties, Content Validity, EQ-5D. The five dimensions of health status included in the EQ-5D are of general relevance and importance in virtually all health assessment contexts. The omission of cognition has been identified as a problem with the EQ-5D (Krabbe *et al.* 1999).

Construct Validity, EQ-5D. In general, there is evidence of the construct validity of the EQ-5D system in a variety of clinical applications (Brazier *et al.* 1996, 1999; Dorman *et al.* 1998; Essink-Bot *et al.* 1997; Trippoli *et al.* 2001). However, in the context of migraine patients, Essink-Bot *et al.* 1997 found that the SF-36 discriminated between groups better than a variety of other measures including the EQ-5D and Nottingham Health Profile. In several studies EQ-5D has substantially greater ceiling effects than the SF-36, HUI, or other generic measures (Coons *et al.* 2000; Macran *et al.* 2003; Essink-Bot *et al.* 1998). Suarez-Almazor and Conner-Spady 2001 provide evidence that mean direct TTO scores for two hypothetical health states associated with rheumatoid arthritis and mean TTO scores for the patient's current health did not agree with EQ-5D index scores for the same states.

Reliability, EQ-5D. Macran 2003 provides evidence from two studies indicating acceptable reliability. With respect to test-retest reliability, Dorman *et al.* (1998) report kappa coefficients of 0.63 to 0.80 for the five dimensions of EQ-5D in a group of stroke patients and an ICC of 0.86 for the index scores. In a review article Coons *et al.* (2000) cite a two-week test-retest ICC of 0.78 for index scores in patients with rheumatoid arthritis.

Responsiveness, EQ-5D. There is evidence that in a variety of types of applications EQ-5D is responsive to large changes in health status. A number of investigators have commented that the coarseness of the system with only three levels per dimension may limit responsiveness (Brazier *et al.* 1993, 1996, 1999; Lydick 2000). Brazier *et al.* (1999) found that EQ-5D was responsive to changes in health status associated with total knee replacement for osteoarthritis but was not responsive in detecting change in patients with osteoarthritis being treated in rheumatology clinics.

Clinically Important Differences/Change. The developers of the EQ-5D do not provide a statement concerning differences in EQ-5D index scores that are likely to be clinically important. Nonetheless, to assist in sample size calculations and related exercises, one can argue that any change in level within the EQ-5D system is clinically important. The smallest change in EQ-5D index score associated with a change in level is 0.036, implying that a difference of 0.036 or more in an index score is important.

Practical Aspects, EQ-5D. The EQ-5D is among the briefest of instruments. Missing values are more common with the EQ-5D VAS component of the system than with the health status classification system (Essink-Bot *et al.* 1997; Coons *et al.* 2000). In a pretest for the 1998 National Population Health Survey (NPHS) in Canada, Statistics Canada (Houle and Berthelot 2000) found that on average the EQ-5D took 1.5 minutes to complete (computer assisted telephone interviewer administration) with a 2.2% non-response rate (any item missing).

The HUI. There are three major versions of the HUI: HUI Mark 1 (Torrance *et al.* 1982), HUI Mark 2 (Feeny *et al.* 1992), and HUI Mark 3 (Feeny *et al.* 1995, 2002). In all three cases there is a health-status classification system, a questionnaire to obtain information within which to classify subjects according to that system, and a multi-attribute utility function to provide utility scores of health-related quality of life. Because HUI2 and HUI3 have superceded HUI1 in most applications, discussion will focus on HUI2 and HUI3.

HUI2 consists of seven attributes (dimensions or domains) of health status: sensation (vision, hearing, and speech), mobility, emotion, cognition, self-care, pain, and fertility. The original application of HUI2 was in the childhood cancer. Because some survivors experience sub- or infertility, fertility was included. However, in most applications fertility is omitted.

The scoring function for the HUI2 system is based on preference measurements using the VAS and SG obtained from a random sample of parents in the general population in Hamilton, Ontario, Canada (Torrance *et al.* 1995, 1996). (Because the original application of HUI2 was cancer in childhood, parents were selected as respondents.) The HUI2 scoring function employs a multiplicative functional form, a form that permits interactions in preferences among attributes. The parameter values imply that the attributes are preference complements. This means that the disutility associated with a loss of function in two attributes is less than the sum of the "individual" disutilities associated with the independent loss of the function for each attribute. Evidence on the ability of the HUI2 scoring function to "predict" direct SG scores obtained from patients, family members of patients, and members of control groups is found in Feeny *et al.* 2003; Feeny *et al.* 2004b; see also Gabriel *et al.* 1999 and Moore *et al.* 1999.

The HUI3 system was originally designed for the 1990 Ontario Health Survey. HUI3 includes eight attributes: vision, hearing, speech, ambulation, dexterity, emotion, cognition, and pain. There are five or six levels per attribute. HUI3 has been widely used in population health surveys in Canada including the 1994 and ongoing NPHS and the Canadian Community Health Survey.

The HUI3 scoring system is based on preferences scores obtained from a random sample of the general population in Hamilton, Ontario. As with the HUI2 function, the functional form is multiplicative (Feeny *et al.* 2002; Furlong *et al.* 1998). Evidence of the out-of-sample predictive validity of the HUI3 scoring function is found in Feeny *et al.* 2002. Respondents were randomized to the modeling survey or the direct survey. Preference scores provided by respondents to the modeling survey were used to estimate the multiplicative function. Respondents in the direct survey provided SG scores for 73 HUI3 health states. There was a high level of agreement, an intra-class correlation of 0.88, between directly measured scores and scores generated by the multiplicative function.

Measurement Properties, Content Validity, HUI. The attributes in HUI2 were chosen on the basis of their importance, as judged by members of the general population (Feeny *et al.* 1996; Furlong *et al.* 2001). HUI3 was in turn based on HUI2 but with modifications to enhance descriptive power and to obtain structural independence. Structural independence means that logically a person can be in any level for one attribute and any other level for another attribute. A consequence of the structural independence of the HUI3 system is that there is relatively little overlap (much less than in EQ-5D) among attributes (Houle and Berthelot 2000). Correlations among attribute levels in HUI3 ranged from 0.02 (vision and speech) to 0.35 emotion and cognition); in contrast results for EQ-5D ranged from 0.24 (self-care and anxiety/depression) to 0.64 (mobility and usual activities). Thus, in general each item on the HUI questionnaire provides new information.

Construct Validity, HUI. HUI2 and HUI3 have demonstrated construct validity in a wide variety of clinical and population health settings. HUI has distinguished the burden of morbidity in survivors of standard risk acute lymphoblastic leukemia (ALL) from that in survivors of high-risk ALL (Barr *et al.* 1993). HUI has also been able to distinguish the burden of morbidity as a function of the dose of radiation in survivors of brain tumors in both adult and pediatric patients (Barr *et al.* 1999; Whitton *et al.* 1997). There is a substantial body of evidence on the construct validity of HUI2 and HUI3 in childhood cancer (Pickard *et al.* 2003). Evidence for adult oncology includes Ramsey *et al.* (2000).

Grima *et al.* (2000) in a study of multiple sclerosis patients found that HUI2 was able to distinguish the stage of disease, as assessed by the expanded disability status scale. Similarly, Neumann *et al.* (1999, 2000) found that HUI2 and HUI3 were able to distinguish the stage of disease (as assessed by the clinical dementia rating, CDR) in Alzheimer patients. For instance, mean HUI3 scores for CDR 0.5 (questionable),

1 (mild), 2 (moderate), 3 (severe), 4 (profound), and 5 (terminal) were 0.47, 0.39, 0.19, 0.06, −0.08, and −0.23 (Neumann *et al.* 2000, p 418). Bayoumi and Redelmeier (1999) provide evidence of the construct validity of HUI2 in distinguishing among levels of severity in HIV infection and AIDS. Younossi *et al.* (2001) report evidence of the construct validity of HUI2 in distinguishing among patients with chronic liver disease by degree of severity. Grootendorst *et al.* (2000) provide evidence of construct validity for HUI3 in the context of a population health survey.

Reliability, HUI. Test-retest reliability for HUI3 has been examined in a population health survey (Boyle *et al.* 1995). Kappa values for attributes varied from 0.14 to 0.73 (median = 0.59), with most indicating substantial agreement. The ICC for overall scores (using the provisional scoring system) was 0.73. Evidence for reliability in clinical studies includes stable systemic lupus erythematosus (SLE) patients (Moore *et al.* 1999).

Responsiveness, HUI. HUI has been shown to be responsive in detecting changes in health status experienced by children on "maintenance" therapy for ALL (Furlong *et al.* 2001; Barr *et al.* 1997). Palmer *et al.* (1999) found HUI2 to be highly responsive in a prospective study of hearing-impaired patients receiving cochlear implants (see also Krabbe *et al.* 2000). Grossman *et al.* 1998 and Torrance *et al.* 1999 found HUI2 and the St. George's Respiratory Questionnaire to be similarly responsive in detecting changes in chronic bronchitis patients treated with antibiotics. Suarez-Almazor *et al.* (2000) found HUI2 and EQ-5D to be responsive in a cohort of patients being treated for lower back pain. Comerota *et al.* (2000) found HUI2 to be responsive in a study of treatment alternatives for deep venous thrombosis. Raynauld *et al.* (2002) and Torrance, Raynauld *et al.* (2002) found HUI3 to be responsive in treatments of osteoarthritis of the knee. Blanchard *et al.* (2003) provide evidence that HUI3 was among the most responsive of the generic measured used in a study of elective total hip arthroplasty for osteoarthritis. The effect size for overall HUI3 scores was 1.2 (Blanchard *et al.* 2003). Several disease-specific measures were more responsive than the generic ones with effect sizes of 3.3 and 2.9 (Blanchard *et al.* 2003).

Like other multi-attribute preference-based measures, HUI is subject to ceiling effect problems. Given that HUI2 includes 6 attributes and HUI3 includes 8, ceiling effect problems are less frequent than with the EQ-5D.

Clinically Important Differences/Change. Changes or differences in overall HUI2 or HUI3 scores of 0.03 or more are regarded as clinically important (Grootendorst *et al.* 2000; Drummond 2001; see also Samsa *et al.* 1999). Smaller differences may well also be important. Tentatively differences of 0.05 or more in single-attribute HUI2 or HUI3 utility scores are likely to be important.

Practical Aspects, HUI. Standard questionnaires that include HUI2 and HUI3 typically require five to ten minutes for completion. Typically there are fewer problems and missing values than with the SF-36 questionnaire. In a pretest of the NPHS using computer-assisted telephone interviews, Statistics Canada (Houle and Berthelot 2000) found that completion of the HUI3 questionnaire took an average of 2.0 minutes with a 0.3% non-response rate (any item missing).

The Quality of Well Being Scale (QWB). The QWB is oldest of the multi-attribute systems (Patrick *et al.* 1973; Kaplan and Anderson 1996). The original systems included 3 dimensions of health status and a problem/symptom complex: mobility (5 levels), physical activity (4 levels), social activity (5 levels), and symptom/problem (35 items) and described 3500 health states. The newer version has 3 levels for mobility, 3 for physical activity, 5 for social activity, and 27 items in the problem/symptom complex and describes 1215 health states.

The scoring function is linear additive, based on VAS scores obtained from a random sample of the general population in San Diego, California. Only the worst symptom or problem is scored.

Measurement Properties, Content Validity, QWB. The mobility, physical activity, and social activity domains are of clear relevance in virtually all settings. Symptoms cover a wide range of problems and complaints, including trouble learning and remembering, pain, fatigue, difficult sleeping, problems with sexual interest or performance, and excessive worry or anxiety.

Construct Validity, QWB. Kaplan and Anderson (1996) summarize evidence on the ability of the QWB to distinguish among known groups in a wide variety of population health and clinical studies including cystic fibrosis, diabetes, Alzheimer Disease, chronic obstructive pulmonary disease, arthritis, and AIDS.

Reliability, QWB. Frosch *et al.* (2001) report reliability of 0.90 or more in most populations.

Responsiveness, QWB. Kaplan and Anderson (1996) and Bombardier *et al.* (1986) provide evidence on the responsiveness of the QWB.

Clinically Important Differences/Change. The developers of the QWB typically use 0.03 as the clinically important difference in scores. This guideline comes from the preference studies done on the QWB and is the smallest difference that external judges can perceive.

Practical Aspects, QWB. The original version of the QWB required interviewer administration. The newer version provides both self and interviewer-administered versions.

Short Form-6D (SF-6D). SF-6D includes seven of the eight dimensions of health status from the SF-36: physical functioning, role limitations (a combination of role emotional and role physical), social functioning, pain, mental health, and vitality (Brazier *et al.* 2002). There are four to six levels per attribute; SF-6D describes 18,000 health states. A modified linear additive scoring function was estimated using SG scores obtained from a random sample of the population in the United Kingdom.

Measurement Properties, SF-6D. While there is abundant evidence on the content and construct validity, responsiveness, and reliability of the SF-36, there is as yet relatively little evidence on the SF-6D. Several studies indicate that SF-6D, like SF-36, seems to be vulnerable to both floor and ceiling effects. The distribution of SF-6D scores has been observed to be more narrow and compact than the distributions of scores from other multi-attribute measures (Hollingworth *et al.* 2002; Longworth and Bryan 2003; O'Brien *et al.* 2003; see also Kopec and Willison 2003). Preliminary evidence indicates that the responsiveness of the SF-6D is of the same order of magnitude as other multi-attribute measures. Walters and Brazier (2003) provide estimates of the minimum important difference in SF-6D scores ranging from 0.01 to 0.05 with a weighted mean estimate of 0.033.

Decision Analyses, Cost-Effectiveness and Cost-Utility Analyses, Quality-Adjusted Life Years (QALYs), and Quality-Adjusted Time Without Symptoms or Toxicity (Q-TWiST). A major application of preference-based measures is as quality-adjustment weights in various types of analyses designed to assist in the formulation of policy or decisions concerning resource allocation. Clearly survival is important. The quality of that survival is also important. Preference scores are a prominent approach to quantifying the quality of survival.

QALYs are estimated by multiplying the utility weight for a health state by its duration. QALYs provide a convenient index number that summarizes mortality and morbidity effects – the quality-adjusted area under the curve. Thus QALYs are attractive for comparing relevant alternative interventions.

A closely related approach is Q-TWiST (see for instance, Gelber *et al.* 1996). In a number of Q-TWiST studies a finite set of health states is identified (partial response; a partial response and severe peripheral edema; stable disease; etc.) and health-state descriptions are developed for each. Preference scores for these hypothetical health states are then obtained. Sometimes the informants are healthcare professionals (see for instance, Hutton *et al.* 1996; Launois *et al.* 1996; and Brown *et al.* 2001). In some studies patients are asked to evaluate the hypothetical health states (see for instance, Goodwin *et al.* 1988; Leung *et al.* 1999). In early applications of the technique, values for the utility scores were assumed.

Applications. Preference-based measures provide comprehensive information on the value of health outcomes. However, the usefulness of preference-based measures goes beyond their useful as outcome measures. Because preference-based measures can integrate mortality and morbidity and are consistent with the underlying conceptual foundations of economic evaluation, these measures are uniquely suited for estimating QALYs and for use in cost-effectiveness and cost-utility analyses.

An example of a cost-utility analysis based on a preference-based measure is provided by Raynauld *et al.* 2002 and Torrance, Raynauld *et al.* 2002. Patients with osteoarthritis in the knee were randomized to standard care or standard care plus injections of Hylan G-F 20. Cost estimates from the societal viewpoint for each treatment approach were obtained. Outcomes were assessed using the Western Ontario McMaster Osteoarthritis Index (WOMAC), a disease-specific measure, the SF-36, and HUI3. Patients were followed for one year. According to all three HRQoL measures, HRQoL was higher in the treatment than in the control arm. Using HUI3, the incremental QALYs were 0.071; incremental cost was 710. The incremental cost per QALY in 1999 Canadian $ was 10,000.

Strengths and Weakness of Preference-Based Measures. The direct measures have the advantage that each patient can define their own health state and provide a valuation of it. That subjects define their own subjective state may overcome limitations associated with generic and even disease-specific multi-attribute systems. This advantage of the direct approach is particularly important in contexts in which patients have concerns about dimensions of health status that are entirely omitted or given little coverage in multi-attribute systems. The advantages come, however, at a cost. Direct assessments of preferences for health states are more burdensome, both for respondents and investigators.

Both direct and generic multi-attribute systems provide single summary scores. These scores can be used to integrate mortality and morbidity, an exercise of clear importance and relevance. These scores can be used in QALY analyses and in cost-effectiveness and cost-utility analyses.

A key advantage of the preference-based multi-attribute measures is that they impose relatively small burdens on respondents and investigators. They can readily be used serially in prospective studies. Generic multi-attribute systems permit broad comparisons among health problems. HUI3 and EQ-5D have been or are being included in major U.S., Canadian, and United Kingdom population health surveys, providing abundant data on population norms. Multi-attribute systems can also be useful in identifying unanticipated problems or the side effects of treatment that may not be covered adequately by disease-specific measures. For instance, using HUI2 and HUI3, Whitton *et al.* (1997) identified an under recognized burden of pain in survivors of brain tumors and Barr *et al.* (2003) identified problems with cognition among female patients with von Willebrand disease.

The preference-based generic systems such as the HUI, EQ-5D, QWB, and SF-6D may not, however, capture all of the important dimensions of health status. The generic multi-attribute systems are subject to ceiling effect problems.

Preference-Based Measures Complement other Approaches. A number of guidelines for the assessment of healthcare technologies (CCOHTA 1997; Gold *et al.* 1996) recommend the use of preference-based measures alongside of generic-profile and disease-specific measures. This is sound advice. Information from each type of measure can help in the interpretation of results from other measures. Given the coarseness of the generic multi-attribute systems, there is reason to suspect that important aspects of HRQoL may not be captured by these measures. Concurrent use of disease-specific measures with more targeted coverage of HRQoL aspects important in that context will permit an assessment of the quantitative importance of this potential problem.

Conclusions

Preference-based measures, both direct and multi-attribute, have a number of characteristics that make their use highly relevant and important in a wide variety of applications and useful as a comprehensive measure of outcome. Preference-based measures reflect what is important to patients. Preference-based measures capture the value that patients (or the community) place on health states and survival. Preference-based measures can also explore the tradeoffs among different types of morbidity (chemotherapy versus radiation).

Acknowledgments

The author acknowledges the helpful comments and suggestions made by Ron D. Hays on an earlier draft. The paper draws on Feeny 2002a, 2002b, and forthcoming. The author acknowledges the assistance of Janice Varney in searching and retrieving relevant literature.

References

Albertsen, P. C., Nease, R. F., and Potosky, A. L. (1998). Assessment of patient preferences among men with prostate cancer. *Journal of Urology*, **159**, 158–163.

Ashby, J., O'Hanlon, M., and Buxton, M. J. (1994). The time tradeoff technique: how do the valuations of breast cancer patients compare to those of other groups? *Quality of Life Research*, **3**, 257–265.

Barr, R. D., Furlong, W., Dawson, S., and Whitton, A. C., *et al.* (1993). An assessment of global health status in survivors of acute lymphoblastic leukemia in childhood. *American Journal of Pediatric Hematology/Oncology*, **15**, 284–290.

Barr, R. D., Petrie, C., Furlong, W., Rothney, M., and Feeny, D. (1997). Health-related quality of life during post-induction chemotherapy in children with acute lymphoblastic leukemia in remission: an influence of corticosteroid therapy. *International Journal of Oncology*, **11**, 333–339.

Barr, R. D., Simpson, T., Whitton, A., Rush, B., Furlong, W., and Feeny, D. H. (1999). Health-related quality of life in survivors of tumours of the central nervous system in childhood – a preference-based approach to measurement in a cross-sectional study. *European Journal of Cancer*, **35**, 248–255.

Barr, R. D., Sek, J., and Horsman, J., *et al.* (2003). Health status and health-related quality of life associated with van Willebrand disease. *American Journal of Hematology*, **73**, 108–114.

Bayoumi, A. M. and Redelmeier, D. A. (1999). Economic methods for measuring the quality of life associated with HIV infection. *Quality of Life Research*, **8**, 471–480.

Becker, G. S. (1965). A theory of the allocation of time. *Economic Journal*, **75**, 493–517.

Bennett, K. J. and Torrance, G. W. (1996). Measuring health state preferences and utilities: Rating scale, time trade-off, and standard gamble techniques. In B. Spilker (ed.) *Quality of Life and Pharmacoeconomics in Clinical Trials*, 2nd edn, pp 253–265. Philadelphia: Lippincott-Raven Press.

Blanchard, C., Feeny, D., and Mahon, J. L., *et al.* (2003). Is the health utilities index responsive in total hip arthroplasty patients? *Journal of Clinical Epidemiology*, **56**, 1046–1054.

Bombardier, C., Ware, J., and Russell, I. J., *et al.* (1986). Auranofin therapy and quality of life in patients with rheumatoid arthritis: results of a multicenter trial. *American Journal of Medicine*, **81**, 565–578.

Boyle, M. H., Furlong, W., Feeny, D., Torrance, G., and Hatcher, J. (1995). Reliability of the Health Utilities Index – Mark III used in the 1991 Cycle 6 General Social Survey Health Questionnaire. *Quality of Life Research*, **4**, 249–257.

Brazier, J., Jones, N., and Kind, P. (1993). Testing the validity of the EuroQol and comparing it with the SF-36 Health Survey Questionnaire. *Quality of Life Research*, **2**, 167–168.

Brazier, J. E., Walters, S. J., Nicholl, J. P., and Kohler, B. (1996). Using the SF-36 and EuroQol on an elderly population. *Quality of Life Research*, **5**, 195–204.

Brazier, J. E., Harper, R., Munro, J., Walters, S. J., and Snaith, M. L. (1999). Generic and condition-specific outcome measures for people with osteoarthritis of the knee. *Rheumatology*, **38**, 870–877.

Brazier, J., Roberts, J., and Deverill, M. (2002). The estimation of a preference-based measure of health status from the SF-36. *Journal of Health Economics*, **21**, 271–292.

Brown, R. E., Hutton, J., and Burrell, A. (2001). Cost-effectiveness of treatment options in advanced breast cancer in the UK. *Pharmacoeconomics*, **19**, 1091–1102.

Canadian Coordinating Office for Health Technology Assessment (1997). *Guidelines for Economic Evaluation of Pharmaceuticals: Canada*, 2nd edn. Ottawa: Canadian Coordinating Office for Health Technology Assessment.

Carter, W. B., Beach, L. B., and Inui, T. S., *et al.* (1986). Developing and testing a decision model for predicting influenza vaccination compliance. *Health Services Research*, **20**, 897–932.

Chapman, G. B., Elstein, A. S., and Kuzel, T. M., *et al.* (1998). Prostate cancer patients' utilities for health states: how it looks depends on where you stand. *Medical Decision Making*, **18**, 278–286.

Chapman, G. B., Elstein, A. S., Kuzel, T. M., Nadler, R. B., Sharifi, R., and Bennett, C. L. (1999). A multi-attribute model of prostate cancer patients' preferences for health states. *Quality of Life Research*, **8**, 171–180.

Comerota, A., Richard, J., Throm, C., Mathias, S. D., Haughton, S., and Mewissen, M. (2000). Catheter-directed thrombolysis for iliofemoral deep vein thrombosis improves health-related quality of life. *Journal of Vascular Surgery*, **32**, 130–137.

Coons, S. J., Rao, S., Keininger, D. L., and Hays, R. D. (2000). A comparative review of generic quality-of-life instruments. *Pharmacoeconomics*, **17**, 13–35.

Dolan, P. (1997). Modeling valuations for EuroQol health states. *Medical Care*, **35**, 1095–1108.

Dorman, P., Slattery, J., and Farrell, B. (1998). Qualitative comparison of the reliability of health status assessments with the EuroQol and the SF-36 questionnaires after stroke. *Stroke*, **29**, 63–68.

Drummond, M. (2001). Introducing economic and quality of life measurements into clinical studies. *Annals of Medicine*, **33**, 344–349.

Drummond, M. F., O'Brien, B., Stoddart, G., and Torrance, G. W. (1997). *Methods for the Economic Evaluation of Health Care Programmes*, 2nd edn. Oxford: Oxford University Press.

Essink-Bot, M. L., Stouthard, M. E. A., and Bonsel, G. J. (1993). Generalizability of valuations on health states collected with the EuroQol questionnaire. *Health Economics*, **2**, 237–246.

Essink-Bot, M. L., Krabbe, P. F. M., Bonsel, G. J., and Aaronson, N. K. (1997). An empirical comparison of four generic health status measures: the Nottingham Health Profile, the Medical Outcome Study 36-Item Short-Form Health Survey, the COOP/WONCA Charts, and the EuroQol Instrument. *Medical Care*, **35**, 522–537.

Essink-Bot, M. L., De Koning, H. J., Nijs, H. G. T., Kirkels, W. J., van der Maas, P. J., and Schroder, F. H. (1998). Short-term effects of population-based screening for prostate cancer on health-related quality of life. *Journal of the National Cancer Institute*, **90**, 925–931.

EuroQol Group. (1990). EuroQol: A new facility for the measurement of health-related quality of life. *Health Policy*, **16**, 199–208.

Feeny, D. (2000). A utility approach to assessing health-related quality of life. *Medical Care,* **38,** II-151–II-154.

Feeny, D., Furlong, W., and Torrance, G. W., *et al.* (2002). Multi-attribute and single-attribute utility functions for the Health Utilities Index Mark 3 system. *Medical Care,* **40,** 113–128.

Feeny, D. (2002a). Health-status classification systems for summary measures of population health. In C. J. L. Murray, J. A. Salomon, C. D. Mathers, A. D. Lopez (eds) *Summary Measures of Population Health: Concepts, Ethics, Measurement and Applications,* pp 329–341. Geneva: World Health Organization.

Feeny, D. (2002b). The utility approach to assessing population health. In C. J. L. Murray, J. A. Salomon, C. D. Mathers, A. D. Lopez (eds) *Summary Measures of Population Health: Concepts, Ethics, Measurement and Applications,* pp 515–528. Geneva: World Health Organization.

Feeny, D. (forthcoming). The roles for preference-based measures in support of cancer research and policy. In J. Lipscomb, C. C. Gotay, C. Snyder (eds) *Outcomes Assessment in Cancer: Findings and Recommendations of the Cancer Outcomes Measurement Working Group.* New York: Cambridge University Press.

Feeny, D. and Torrance, G. W. (1989). Incorporating utility-based quality-of-life assessments in clinical trials: Two examples. *Medical Care,* **27,** S190–S204.

Feeny, D., Furlong, W., Barr, R. D., Torrance, G. W., Rosenbaum, P., and Weitzman, S. (1992). A comprehensive multiattribute system for classifying the health status of survivors of childhood cancer. *Journal of Clinical Oncology,* **10,** 923–928.

Feeny, D., Furlong, W., Boyle, M., and Torrance, G. W. (1995). Multi-attribute health status classification systems: Health utilities index. *PharmacoEconomics,* **7,** 490–502.

Feeny, D. H., Torrance, G. W., and Furlong, W. J. (1996). Health utilities index. In B. Spilker (ed.) *Quality of Life and Pharmacoeconomics in Clinical Trials,* 2nd edn, pp 239–252. Philadelphia: Lippincott-Raven Press.

Feeny, D., Juniper, E. F., Ferrie, P. J., Griffith, L. E., and Guyatt, G. H. (1998). Why not just ask the kids? Health-related quality of life in children with asthma. In D. Drotar (ed.) *Measuring Health-Related Quality of Life in Children and Adolescents: Implications for Research, Practice, and Policy,* pp 171–185. Mahwah, NJ: Lawrence Erlbaum Associates Publishers.

Feeny, D., Blanchard, C., and Mahon, J. L., *et al.* (2003). Comparing community-preference based and direct standard gamble utility scores: Evidence from elective total hip arthroplasty. *International Journal of Technology Assessment in Health Care,* **19,** 362–372.

Feeny, D., Blanchard, C. M., and Mahon, J. L., *et al.* (2004a). The stability of utility scores: Test–retest reliability and the interpretation of utility scores in elective total hip arthroplasty. *Quality of Life Research,* **12, 13,** 15–22.

Feeny, D., Furlong, W., Saigal, S., and Sun, J. (2004b). Comparing directly measured standard gamble scores to HUI2 and HUI3 Utility Scores: Group and individual-level comparisons. *Social Science & Medicine,* **58,** 799–809.

Frosch, D., Porzsolt, F., and Heicappell, R., *et al.* (2001). Comparison of German language versions of the QWB-SA and SF-36 evaluating outcomes for patients with prostate disease. *Quality of Life Research,* **10,** 165–173.

Furlong, W., Feeny, D., Torrance, G. W., Barr, R., and Horsman, J. (1990). Guide to design and development of health-state utility instrumentation. *McMaster University Centre for Health Economics and Policy Analysis Working Paper* No 90–9.

Furlong, W., Feeny, D., and Torrance, G. W., *et al.* (1998). Multiplicative multi-attribute utility function for the Health Utilities Index Mark 3 (HUI3) system: A technical report. *McMaster University Centre for Health Economics and Policy Analysis Working Paper* No. 98–11.

Furlong, W. J., Feeny, D. H., Torrance, G. W., and Barr, R. D. (2001). The Health Utilities Index (HUI) system for assessing health-related quality of life in clinical studies. *Annals of Medicine*, **33**, 375–384.

Gabriel, S. E., Kneeland, T. S., Melton, L. J., Moncur, M. M., Ettinger, B., and Tosteson, A. N. A. (1999). Health-related quality of life in economic evaluations for osteoporosis: Whose values should we use? *Medical Decision Making*, **19**, 141–148.

Gelber, R. D., Cole, B. F., and Goldhirsh, A. *et al.* (1996). Adjuvant chemotherapy plus tamoxifen compared with tamoxifen alone for postmenopausal breast cancer: Meta-analysis of quality-adjusted survival. *Lancet*, **347**, 1066–1071.

Giesler, R. B., Ashton, C. M., and Brody, B. (1999). Assessing the performance of utility techniques in the absence of a gold standard. *Medical Care*, **37**, 580–598.

Gold, M. R., Siegel, J. E., Russell, L. B., and Weinstein, M. C. (eds) (1996). *Cost-Effectiveness in Health and Medicine*. New York: Oxford University Press.

Goodwin, P. J., Feld, R., Evans, W. K., and Pater, J. (1998). Cost-effectiveness of cancer chemotherapy: An economic evaluation of a randomized trial in small-cell lung cancer. *Journal of Clinical Oncology*, **6**, 1537–1547.

Grann, V. R., Panageas, K. S., Whang, W., Antman, K. H., and Neugut, A. I. (1998). Decision analysis of prophylactic masectomy and oophorectomy in BRCA1-Positive or BRCA-2 positive patients. *Journal of Clinical Oncology*, **16**, 979–985.

Grann, V. R., Jacobson, J. S., Sundarajan, V., Alberta, S. M., Troxel, A. B., and Neugut, A. I. (1999). The quality of life associated with prophylatic treatments for women with BRCA1/2 mutations. *Cancer Journal from Scientific American*, **5**, 283–292.

Green, C., Brazier, J., and Deverill, M. (2000). Valuing health-related quality of life: A review of health state valuation techniques. *Pharmacoeconomics*, **17**, 151–165.

Grima, D. T., Torrance, G. W., Francis, G., Rice, G., Rosner, A. J., and LaFortune, L. (2000). Cost and health related quality of life consequences of multiple sclerosis. *Multiple Sclerosis*, **6**, 91–98.

Grootendorst, P., Feeny, D., and Furlong, W. (2000). Health Utilities Index Mark 3: Evidence of construct validity for stroke and arthritis in a population health survey. *Medical Care*, **38**, 290–299.

Grossman, M. (1972). On the concept of health capital and the demand for health. *Journal of Political Economy*, **80**, 223–255.

Grossman, R., Mukherjee, J., and Vaughan, D., *et al.* (1998). A one-year community-based health economic study of ciprofloxacin versus usual antibiotic treatment in acute exacerbations of chronic bronchities. *Chest*, **113**, 131–141.

Guyatt, G. H., Feeny, D. H., and Patrick, D. L. (1993) Measuring health-related quality of life. *Annals of Internal Medicine*, **118**, 622–629.

Hall, J., Gerard, K., Salkeld, G., and Richardson, J. (1992). A cost utility analysis of mammography screening in Australia. *Social Science & Medicine*, **34**, 993–1004.

Hayman, J. A., Fairclough, D. L., Harris, J. R., and Weeks, J. C. (1997). Patient preferences concerning the trade-off between the risks and benefits of routine radiation therapy after conservative surgery for early-stage breast cancer. *Journal of Clinical Oncology*, **15**, 1252–1260.

Hays, R. D. and Morales, L. S. (2001). The Rand-36 measure of health-related quality of life. *Annals of Medicine*, **33**, 350–357.

Hays, R. D., Anderson, R., and Revicki, D. (1993). Psychometric considerations in evaluating health-related quality of life measures. *Quality of Life Research*, **2**, 441–449.

Heckerling, P. S., Verp, M. S., and Hadro, T. A. (1994) Preferences of pregnant women for amniocentesis or chorionic villus sampling for prenatal testing: Comparison of patient choices and those of a decision-analytic model. *Journal of Clinical Epidemiology*, 47,1215–1228.

Hollingworth, W., Deyo, R. A., Sullivan, S. D., Emerson, S. S., Gray, D. T., and Jarvik, J. G. (2002). The practicality and validity of directly elicited and sf-36 derived health state preferences in patients with low back pain. *Health Economics*, 11, 71–85.

Houle, C. and Berthelot, J. M. (2000). A head-to-head comparison of the Health Utilities Mark 3 and the EQ-5D for the population living in private households in Canada. *Quality of Life Newsletter*, 24, 5–6.

Hutton, J., Brown, R., Borowitz, M., Abrams, K., Rothman, M., and Shakespeare, A. (1996). A new decision model for cost-utility comparisons of chemotherapy in recurrent metastatic Breast cancer. *Pharmacoeconomics*, 9, 8–22.

Jansen, S. T., Stiggelbout, A. M., Wakker, P. P., Nooij, M. A., Noordijk, E. M., and Kievit, J. (2000). Unstable preferences: A shift in valuation or an effect of the elicitation procedure? *Medical Decision Making*, 20, 62–71.

Johnston, K., Brown, J., Gerard, K., O'Hanlon, M., and Morton, A. (1998). Valuing temporary and chronic health states associated with breast screening. *Social Science & Medicine*, 47, 213–222.

Juniper, E. F., Guyatt, G. H., Feeny, D. H., Griffith, L. E., and Ferrie, P. J., (1997). Minimum skills required by children to complete health-related quality of life instruments for asthma: Comparison of measurement properties. *European Respiratory Journal*, 10, 2285–2294.

Kaplan, R. M. and Anderson, J. P. (1996). The general health policy model: An integrated approach. In B. Spilker (ed.) *Quality of Life and Pharmacoeconomics in Clinical Trials* 2nd edn, pp 309–322. Philadelphia: Lippincott-Raven Publishers.

Kind, P. (1996). The EuroQol Instrument: An index of health-related quality of life. In B. Spilker (ed.) *Quality of Life and Pharmacoeconomics in Clinical Trials* 2nd edn, pp 191–201. Philadelphia: Lippincott-Raven Publishers.

Kopec, J. A. and Willison, K. D. (2003). A comparative review of four preference-weighted measures of health-related quality of life. *Journal of Clinical Epidemiology*, 56, 317–325.

Krabbe, P. F., Stouthard, M. E., Essink-Bot, M. L., and Bonsel, G. J. (1999). The effect of adding a cognitive dimension to the EuroQol multiattribute health-status classification system. *Journal of Clinical Epidemiology*, 52, 293–301.

Krabbe, P. F. M., Hinderink, J. B., and van den Broek, P. (2000). The effect of cochlear implant use in postlingually deaf adults. *International Journal of Technology Assessment in Health Care*, 16, 864–873.

Kuppermann, M., Shiboski, S., Feeny, D., Elkin, E., and Washington, A. E. (1997). Can preference scores for discrete states be used to derive preference scores for an entire path of events? AN application to prenatal diagnosis. *Medical Decision Making*, 17, 42–55.

Launois, R., Reboul-Marty, J., Henry, B., and Bonneterre, J. (1996). A cost-utility analysis of second-line chemotherapy in metastatic breast cancer: Docetaxel versus paclitaxel versus vinorelbine. *Pharmacoeconomics*, 10, 504–521.

Laupacis, A., Bourne, R., and Rorabeck, C., *et al.* (1993). The effect of elective total hip replacement upon health-related quality of life. *Journal of Bone and Joint Surgery*, 75-A, 1619–1626.

Lenert, L. and Kaplan, R. M. (2000). Validity and interpretation of preference-based measures of health-related quality of life. *Medical Care*, 38, II-138–II-150.

Leung, P. P., Tannock, I. F., Oza, A. M., Puodziuas, A., and Dranitsaris, G. (1999). Cost-utility analysis of chemotherapy using paclitaxel, docetaxel, or vinorelbine for patients with anthracycline-resistant breast cancer. *Journal of Clinical Oncology*, 17, 3082–3090.

Llewellyn-Thomas, H. A., Sutherland, H. J., and Thiel, E. C. (1993). Do patients' evaluations of a future health state change when they actually enter that state? *Medical Care*, **31**, 1002–1012.

Longworth, L. and Bryan, S. (2003). An empirical comparison of EQ-5D and SF-6D in liver transplant patients. *Health Economics*, **12**, 1061–1067.

Lydick, E. (2000). Approaches to the interpretation of quality-of-life scales. *Medical Care*, **38**, II-180–II-183.

Macran, S. (2003). Test-retest performance of EQ-5D. In R. Brooks, R. Rabin, and F. de Charro, eds., *The Measurment and Valuation of Health Status Using EQ-5D: A European Perspective*, pp 43–54. Dordrecht: Kluwer Academic Publishers.

Macran, S., Weatherly, H., and Kind, P. (2003). Measuring population health: A comparison of three generic health status measures. *Medical Care*, **41**, 218–231.

McDowell, I. and Newell, C. (1996). *Measuring Health: A Guide to Rating Scales and Questionnaires*, 2nd edn. New York: Oxford University Press.

Moore, A. D., Clarke, A. E., and Danoff, D. S., *et al.* (1999). Can health utility measures be used in lupus research? A comparative validation and reliability study of 4 utility indices. *Journal of Rheumatology*, **26**, 1285–1290.

Ness, R. M., Holmes, A. M., Klein, R., and Dittus, R. (1999). Utility valuations for outcome states of colorectal cancer. *American Journal of Gastroenterology*, **94**, 1650–1657.

Neumann, P. J., Kuntz, K. M., and Leon, J., *et al.* (1999). Health utilities and health status in alzheimer's disease: a cross-sectional study of subjects and caregivers. *Medical Care*, **37**, 27–32.

Neumann, P. J., Sandberg, E. A., Araki, S. S., Kuntz, K. M., Feeny, D., and Weinstein, M. C. (2000). A comparison of HUI2 and HUI3 utility scores in Alzheimer's disease. *Medical Decision Making*, **20**, 413–422.

O'Brien, B. J. and Viramontes, J. L. (1994). Willingness to pay: A valid and reliable measure of health state preference? *Medical Decision Making*, **14**, 289–297.

O'Brien, B. J., Spath, M., Blackhouse, G., Severens, J. L., Dorian, P., and Brazier, J. (2003). A view from the bridge: agreement between the SF-6D utility algorithm and the Health Utilities Index. *Health Economics*, **12**(11), 975–981.

O'Connor, A., Boyd, N. F., Warde, P., Stolbach, L., and Till, J. E. (1987). Eliciting preferences for alternative drug therapies in oncology: Influence of treatment outcome description, elicitation technique and treatment experience on preferences. *Journal of Chronic Disease*, **40**, 811–818.

Palmer, C. S., Niparko, J. K., Wyatt, R., Rothman, M., and de Lissovoy, G. (1998). A prospective study of the cost-utility of the multichannel cochlear implant. *Archives of Otolaryngology – Head and Neck Surgery*, **125**, 1221–1228.

Patrick, D. L. and Erickson, P. (1993). *Health Status and Health Policy: Quality of life in health care evaluation and resource allocation*. New York: Oxford University Press.

Patrick, D. L., Bush, J. W., and Chen, M. M. (1973). Methods for measuring levels of well-being for a health status index. *Health Services Research*, **8**, 228–245.

Patrick, D. L., Starks, H. E., Cain, K. C., Uhlmann, R. F., and Pearlman, R. A. (1994). Measuring preferences for health states worse than death. *Medical Decision Making*, **14**, 9–18.

Pickard, A. S., Topfer, L. A., and Feeny, D. H. (2003 in press). A structured review of studies on health-related quality of life and economic evaluation in pediatric acute lymphoblastic leukemia. *Journal of the National Cancer Institute Monographs*, in press.

Rabin, R. and de Charro, F. (2001). EQ-5D: A measure of health status from the EuroQol Group. *Annals of Medicine*, **33**, 337–343.

Ramsey, S. D., Andersen, M. R., and Etzioni, R., *et al.* (2000). Quality of life in survivors of colorectal carcinoma. *Cancer*, **88**, 1294–1303.

Raynauld, J. P., Torrance, G. W., and Band, P. A., *et al.* (2002). A prospective randomized, pragmatic, health outcomes trial evaluating the incorporation of hylan G-F 20 into the treatment paradigm for patients with knee osteoarthritis (part 1 or 2): Clinical results. *Osteoarthritis and Cartilage*, **10**, 506–517.

Revicki, D. A., Osoba, D., and Fairclough, D., *et al.* (2000). Recommendations on health-related quality of life research to support labeling and promotional claims in the United States. *Quality of Life Research*, **9**, 887–900.

Saigal, C. S., Gornbein, J., Nease, R., and Litwin, M. S. (2001). Predictors of utilities for health states in early stage prostate cancer. *Journal of Urology*, **166**, 942–946.

Saigal, S., Stoskopf, B. L., Burrows, E., Streiner, D. L., and Rosenbaum, P. L. (2003). Stability of maternal preferences for pediatric health states in the perinatal period and 1 year later. *Archives in Pediatric and Adolescent Medicine*, **157**, 261–269.

Samsa, G., Edelman, D., Rothman, M., Williams, G. R., Lipscomb, J., and Matchar, D. (1999). Determining clinically important differences in health status measures: A general approach with illustration using the Health Utilities Index Mark II. *PharmacoEconomics*, **15**, 141–155.

Shiell, A., Seymour, J., Hawe, P., and Cameron, S. (2000). Are preferences over health states complete? *Health Economics*, **9**, 47–55.

Singer, L. G., Theodore, J., and Gould, M. K. (2003). Validity of standard gamble utilities as measured by transplant readiness in lung transplant candidates. *Medical Decision Making*, **23**, 435–440.

Stiggelbout, A. M., Kiebert, G. M., Kievit, J., Leer, W. H., Habbema, J. D. F., and de Haes, C. J. M. (1995). The 'utility' of the time trade-off method in cancer patients: feasibility and proportional trade-off. *Journal of Clinical Epidemiology*, **48**, 1207–1214.

Streiner, D. L. and Norman, G. R. (1995). *Health Measurement Scales. A practical guide to their development and use,* 2nd edn. Oxford: Oxford University Press.

Suarez-Almazor, M. E., Kendall, C., Johnson, J. A., Skeith, K., and Vincent, D. (2000). Use of health status measures in patients with low back pain in clinical settings. Comparison of specific, generic, and preference-based instruments. *Rheumatology*, **39**, 783–790.

Suarez-Almazor, M. E. and Conner-Spady, B. (2001). Ratings of arthritis health states by patients, physicians, and the general public. Implications for cost-utility analysis. *Journal of Rheumatology*, **28**, 648–656.

Torrance, G. W. (1976). Social preferences for health states: An empirical evaluation of three measurement techniques. *Socio-Economic Planning Sciences*, **10**, 129–136.

Torrance, G. W. (1986). Measurement of health state utilities for economic appraisal – a review. *Journal of Health Economics*, **5**, 1–30.

Torrance, G. W. and Feeny, D. (1989). Utilities and quality-adjusted life years. *International Journal of Technology Assessment in Health Care*, **5**, 559–575.

Torrance, G. W., Thomas, W. H., and Sackett, D. L. (1972). A utility maximization model for evaluation of health care programs. *Health Services Research*, **7**, 118–133.

Torrance, G. W., Boyle, M. H., and Horwood, S. P. (1982). Application of multi-attribute utility theory to measure social preferences for health states. *Operations Research*, **30**, 1042–1069.

Torrance, G. W., Furlong, W., Feeny, D., and Boyle, M. (1995). Multi-attribute preference functions: Health utilities index. *PharmacoEconomics*, **7**, 503–520.

Torrance, G. W., Feeny, D. H., Furlong, W. J., Barr, R. D., Zhang, Y., and Wang, Q. (1996). Multi-attribute preference functions for a comprehensive health status classification system: Health Utilities Index Mark 2. *Medical Care*, **34**, 702–722.

Torrance, G. W., Walker, V., and Grossman, R., *et al.* (1999). Economic evaluation of ciprofloxacin compared with usual antibacterial care for the treatment of acute exacerbations of chronic bronchitis in patients followed for 1 year. *PharmacoEconomics*, **16**, 499–520.

Torrance, G. W., Feeny, D., and Furlong, W. (2001). Visual analogue scales: Do they have a role in the measurement of preferences for health states? *Medical Decision Making*, **21**, 329–334.

Torrance, G. W., Raynauld, J. P., and Walker, V., *et al.* (2002). A prospective randomized, pragmatic, health outcomes trial evaluating the incorporation of hylan G-F 20 into the treatment paradigm for patients with knee osteoarthritis (part 2 or 2): Economic results. *Osteoarthritis and Cartilage*, **10**, 518–527.

Trippoli, S., Vaiani, M., Lucioni, C., and Messori, A. (2001). Quality of life and utility in patients with non-small cell lung cancer. *Pharmacoeconomics*, **19**, 855–863.

von Neumann, J. and Morgenstern, O. (1944). *Theory of Games and Economic Behavior*. Princeton, NJ: Princeton University Press.

Walters, S. F. and Brazier, J. E. (2003). What is the relationship between the minimally clinically important difference and health statue utility values? The case of the SF-6D. *Health and Quality of Life Outcomes*, **1**, 4.

Ware, J. E. (1996). The SF-36 Health Survey. In B. Spilker (ed.) *Quality of Life and Pharmacoeconomics in Clinical Trials*, 2nd edn, pp 337–345. Philadelphia: Lippincott-Raven Press.

Ware, J. E. and Sherbourne, C. D. (1992). The MOS 36-Item Short-Form Health Status Survey (SF-36): I. Conceptual framework and item selection. *Medical Care*, **30**, 473–483.

Whitton, A. C., Rhydderch, H., Furlong, W., Feeny, D., and Barr, R. D. (1997). Self-reported comprehensive health status of adult brain tumor patients using the health utilities index. *Cancer*, **80**, 258–265.

Younossi, Z., Boparai, N., McCormick, M., Price, L. L., and Guyatt, G. (2001). Assessment of utilities and health-related quality of life in patients with chronic liver disease. *American Journal of Gastroenterology*, **96**, 579–583.

Discrete choice experiments

Mandy Ryan and Karen Gerard

Introduction

One of the greatest challenges facing health economists is the identification and valuation of benefits from health care interventions. Until the 1990s benefit assessment in health economics was dominated by an assumption that health was the only important outcome from health care. This is evidenced by the large amount of research devoted to valuing health outcomes using quality adjusted life years (QALYs). The 1990s saw a challenge to this assumption. It was recognized by *some* health economists that concentration on health outcome fails to allow for the possibility that individuals derive benefit from what were being called non-health outcomes and process attributes. Non-health outcomes refer to sources of benefit such as the provision of information, reassurance, autonomy and dignity in the provision of care. Process attributes include such aspects of care as waiting time, location of treatment, continuity of care and staff attitudes. The debate about going beyond health outcomes led to the question of how we can value such attributes. It became clear that the standard approaches to benefit assessment in health economics, standard gamble and time-trade off, would not be appropriate for valuing non-health outcome and process attributes. For example, it would not be realistic to ask individuals how many years at the end of their life they would be willing to give up to have waiting time reduced by three months! This led to the development and application of another stated preference elicitation technique, discrete choice experiments (DCE), in health economics.

In what follows we describe the various stages of conducting a DCE in health economics, consider some of the pragmatic and emerging methodological issues that may be faced at each stage and suggest some topics for future research. We also give specific consideration to the issue of validity. Finally, the potential for using DCEs to estimate preferences for HRQoL will be considered, before conclusions are drawn. An appendix provides more detail on a study concerned with patient preferences in the treatment of menorrhagia.

Discrete choice experiments

Discrete choice experiments (DCE), as described in Ryan and Gerard (2003), are being increasingly used in health economics. The technique is an attribute-based stated preference valuation technique. In other words it is a way to quantify preferences (utilities) for commodities such as health care by analysing the responses provided by subjects in surveys about how they would behave in hypothetical situations. Subjects choose their preferred alternative from a series of hypothetical choices, each alternative being uniquely described by a combination of attribute levels. Certain economic theories of consumer behaviour underlie the technique: Lancaster's theory of value – essentially, that commodities are consumed for their attributes rather than for their own sake; and random utility theory – essentially, that preference or utility is regarded as a latent concept which can be observed from choosing and is a function of deterministic and stochastic elements. Using these theories, the total satisfaction (or utility) that an individual subject derives from the commodity is determined by the utility to the individual of each of the attributes.

There are a number of key stages to follow when designing and implementing a DCE. The attributes of the commodity being valued are first defined and then levels assigned to them. For example, alternative treatments for menorrhagia can be considered as comprising a number of underlying health, non-health and process attributes, each one differing by its combination of attribute levels. Experimental design theory is used to sample combinations (often referred to as scenarios). These scenarios are set in a choice context familiar to the subject and constitute statistically efficient 'choice sets'. Subjects are then asked to choose between the scenarios. Analysis of the choice data allows estimation of the relative importance of the individual attributes and the 'marginal rates of substitution' (MRS) between attributes (a term used by economists to quantify how individuals trade between attributes). A *price* attribute is often included in a DCE exercise so that a monetary measure of benefit, willingness to pay (WTP), can be indirectly estimated. WTP values can be estimated for both changes in individual attributes and changes in any combination of attributes. DCEs potentially provide richer information than direct WTP estimates by taking account of how component attributes impact on utility, and use a less restrictive utility framework than the quality adjusted life year (QALY) paradigm, thereby allowing for consideration of attributes beyond health.

Identifying the attributes

The first stage of a DCE is for the analyst to define the relevant decision-making situation and the likely factors affecting choices of relevance to the commodity being valued. These factors form the basis for identifying key attributes. Attributes may be determined in a number of ways. If a particular policy question is being addressed then the attributes will be predefined. For example, a health care provider may be concerned with the trade-offs that individuals are willing to make between the location of a clinic and the waiting time. Where the attributes are not predefined, preliminary investigations using literature reviews, group discussions, individual interviews and/or direct questioning of individual subjects will be necessary.

One potential strength of the DCE approach, although yet to be demonstrated empirically, is that using a price attribute to estimate indirect WTP values may mitigate or avoid a number of problems associated with direct WTP estimates – see Ryan *et al.* (2001a) and Hanley *et al.* (2001) for further details.

A number of DCEs in health economics have included risk as an attribute, such as risk of complication or recurrence (Ryan and Gerard 2003). The value of reductions in risk is something that has long been a concern of economists. There is an implicit assumption here that subjects understand the way the risk attribute is defined. However, findings from the psychological literature challenge this assumption. It is argued that individuals view events as more likely if they are familiar; view hazards as more risky for other people than themselves; respond to risk information differently if presented in terms of either gains or losses or as a relative risk compared to an absolute risk; and code risk data in a categorical manner i.e. 'low' or 'high' (Lloyd 2001). Wider literature ought to be considered when incorporating and defining risk into DCEs.

Two further issues when deciding on attributes are how many can be reliably evaluated in a DCE, and what effect the number of attributes has on respondent's ability to complete the choice task. Louviere *et al.* (1997) argue that increasing the number of attributes will not significantly affect results, although there is a consensus of opinion that DCEs should not be too 'complex' (Hensher *et al.* 2001). More research is needed to clarify what is a manageable number of attributes, particularly as applications in health economics to date have included anywhere between 2 and 24, with a mode of six.

Assigning levels to the attributes

Once attributes have been determined, two or more levels must be assigned to them in order to introduce necessary variability for parameter estimation. These levels may be numerical units (*cardinal*), such as cost, time, distance, or number of visits, in which case they are relatively straightforward to convey. However, conveying other attribute levels can be more complicated. For example, when an attribute such as pain is described, it is possible to say that 'severe pain' is worse than 'moderate pain' but not that it is twice as bad. In such instances levels may be naturally *ordered* in some way. When levels are described qualitatively it is important to minimize the ambiguity with which the levels are perceived, e.g. 'severe pain' should have similar meaning for all respondents. Attribute levels may also be *categorical*. Then there is no a priori assumption about which level is preferred to another. For instance, it may not be clear, a priori, whether users of a service would prefer to consult a specialist nurse, a general practitioner or consultant. Pragmatically, the levels must be plausible and actionable, enabling the respondents to give the survey questions due consideration and avoiding the raising of unrealistic expectations. They must also be sufficiently variable to estimate the parameters efficiently, which can mean levels set beyond current policy or practice level.

An important question when including price as an attribute is the appropriate payment vehicle to use in collectively funded health care systems. Most studies in health economics have used payment at the point of consumption. Other alternatives include willingness to accept (WTA) compensation, travel costs and taxation (Ryan and Gerard 2003). Better understanding of the appropriateness of these alternative payment vehicles is needed for applications of DCEs to collectively funded health care interventions.

A number of studies in health care have included time as an attribute, defining it in a number of different contexts such as: waiting time, travel time, time to return to normal activities, duration of illness and preference for present or future time (*time preference*). Interestingly, whilst most studies use a price proxy when estimating the overall value of health care, Ryan *et al.* (2001b) and Gerard *et al.* (2004) estimated value in terms of time. Given that time is a commodity that individuals are used to trading in a publicly provided health care system and it is measured on an interval scale, its potential use within the framework of an economic evaluation should be explored further. In the former study, a monetary measure of the value of time was estimated using the value of waiting time for public transport (Department of Environment, Transport and Region Highways 1997). This method assumes that the value of time when waiting for public transport is the same as waiting time in a health care setting. Such an assumption should be tested empirically, and consideration should also be given to the relative value of the different types of time included in DCEs.

An important question when defining attribute levels is the sensitivity of the parameter estimates to the number and range of levels. Ryan and Wordsworth (2000) conducted an experiment to look at the sensitivity of the coefficients to the level of attributes. They found that whilst estimated coefficients were not significantly different across five of the six attributes included in the experiment, mean WTP estimates were significantly different for four of the five welfare estimates. Within the marketing literature Ohler *et al.* (2000) found that whilst attribute range influences main effects to a small degree, substantial effects were found on attribute interactions and model goodness of fit. Ratcliffe and Longworth (2002) varied the number of attribute levels within a choice experiment and found that the relative importance of the attributes whose levels were varied increased as the number of levels increased, whilst remaining stable for those attributes whose levels did not vary. Future work should investigate this issue in more detail.

Asking the question

Once the attributes and levels have been defined, the respondent is presented with a number of alternative scenarios that describe the commodity being valued in terms of different combinations of attribute levels. A number of different preference elicitation formats may be used – rating, ranking and choice-based exercises – but not all are consistent with an economic framework. Also, although ranking exercises can be analysed in a manner consistent with economic theory, they have not proved popular with health economists. Therefore our interest in this chapter lies only with choice-based exercises.

The choice-based approach requires respondents to choose their preferred scenarios from a series of choices and the question can be posed in a variety of ways. If the *single binary choice approach* is used, it involves presenting individuals with a number of scenarios described in terms of the alternative attribute levels and for each scenario asking them if they would take it up, with possible responses being 'yes' or 'no'. An extension to this format, *best attribute scaling,* involves asking respondents, in addition to making a choice, to indicate which attribute they most and least prefer (Szeinbach *et al.* 1999). This additional information allows attributes to be anchored by the least and most preferred choices, and circumvents the problem of interpreting marginal utilities for attribute levels measured on different scales. It also avoids dependency of overall effect on individual attribute level scale values. A third approach is to present individuals with *multiple choice options,* in which they have to choose between a number of scenarios that constitute a 'choice set'. Once again there are a number of ways of asking the question. Individuals may be *forced* to choose between two or more options (would you choose A, B, ... N), or they may be given an *opt-out* (the opportunity to say they would choose none of the options on offer or defer their decision). Alternatively they may be given the option to state their *strength of preference* for the alternatives posed (on a scale ranging from strongly prefer B to strongly prefer A).

There has been very little research comparing these different approaches and more research in this area should be encouraged. A single best approach is not anticipated; rather better understanding is needed of the conditions under which different types of questions perform better. For example, best attribute scaling questions may be particularly germane for studies that do not incorporate a common valuation scale such as money, risk or time.

Experimental design

A central part of DCEs is deciding what scenarios to present to respondents. The number of possible scenarios multiplies factorially with the number of attributes and levels. Rarely can all the scenarios generated be included in the set of choices presented to respondents. Experimental designs are purposeful samples of scenarios from the full factorial number and are used to reduce scenarios presented in the questionnaire to a manageable number. The sample of scenarios is sufficient to estimate a utility model of a given form (usually additive linear, see below). Catalogues, computer software or experts may be used to identify optimal designs.

The application of experimental design will be a function of how the DCE question is posed. If the single binary choice approach is adopted then all scenarios derived from the experimental design can be presented to individuals. When the multiple scenarios approach is used, scenarios obtained from experimental designs must be grouped into choice sets. This step raises the important question of how these choice sets should be constructed. Important principles in the design of choice sets include orthogonality, balanced design and minimum overlap. A number of methods may be adopted to help meet these, including randomly allocating scenarios from experimental designs to choice sets, fold-over designs, using one scenario as the constant comparator (could be the status quo) and pairing all others to it, or constructing choice sets that are orthogonal in differences between attribute levels (Louviere *et al.* 2000; Ryan and Gerard 2003). It is very difficult to create a DCE that satisfies all design principles simultaneously. Nor can the principles be applied in an unambiguous manner as there is no consensus for how to do this. Rather, the researcher needs to generate a number of choice set designs, check their properties with respect to these principles and select one, preferably with the most favourable properties. It is important at this stage to take account of realism as well as statistical properties of the design, and the researcher may forgo some level of orthogonality to select choices that are realistic.

Analysis of data

The choice data are analysed within a 'random utility' framework, using discrete choice analysis (a number of readily available econometric and statistical software packages, such as Limdep (Greene 1998) and STATA (Intercooled Stata 2002), allow for such analysis). Random utility theory states that whilst the individual knows the nature of their utility function, this is not observable. Utilities are therefore 'latent', and can be decomposed into a *systematic* measurable component and a *random* component. The systematic component includes the attributes of the commodity being valued (as well as other socio-economic factors that may be argued to influence choice). This is shown by:

$$U_{iq}(A) = vi_q(A) + e_{iq} \qquad (1)$$

where $U_{iq}(A)$ represents the latent utility of individual q for good i with attributes A, $vi_q(A)$ represents the measurable component of utility estimated empirically, with i, q and A as defined above, and e reflects the unobservable factors. Given that the researcher cannot observe $U_{iq}(A)$, but only $vi_q(A)$, the researcher can only predict the probability that individual q will choose good i from the total choice set. Assuming a choice between i and j:

$$P(i_q|A,C) = P[(vi_q + e_{iq}) > (vj_q + e_{jq})] \qquad (2)$$

where P represents the probability, C the total choice set (i and j in this example), and all other terms are defined above. For purposes of empirical measurement, a probability distribution is assumed for e_{jq} and e_{iq}, the random component.

When analysing the data, assumptions must be made about the functional form of the observable indirect utility function (vi_q). Most applications assume an additive linear relationship between choice and the attributes included in the study. The additive assumption implies that there are no significant interactions between attributes and that the effects of the attributes on choice do not change as the level of that attribute changes, i.e. each unit change in an attribute has a constant marginal effect on choice. Despite evidence from outside health economics that main effects explain over 80 per cent of the preference structure (Pearmain *et al.* 1991), the problem with (health) economic theory is that very often there is little a priori guidance for researchers on what interactions or higher order effects should be considered in a design. Selected two-way interactions, in particular, may be sufficiently important to be included if they are expected to be as, or more, significant than an individual main effect in explaining model variance. To ignore these effects or pay insufficient attention to them will undermine the model. Focus on main effects plans mirrors past practice in the environmental economics literature, but here the view is changing and it would be apposite for health economists to keep apace of these developments (Adamowicz 2001). Such modelling needs to be built into the experimental design of the study, and requires data to be collected on a larger choice set.

Having decided the functional form of the utility function, the response data is analysed. The appropriate technique will depend on what method was used to collect the data (Ryan and Gerard, 2003) and the following utility function will be estimated (assuming a linear utility function as is most commonly done):

$$v = c_0 + \Sigma c_n X_n + \cdots + dP + \in \qquad (3)$$

where c_0, c_n, and d are the parameters of the model to be estimated, X_n's represent the levels of the n attributes of the commodity being valued (n-1,2,...,k), $\Sigma c_n X_n$'s represents the summation of all the model effect coefficients, P the price level (or some proxy for price), and $\in$ the unobservable error term for the model. c_0 reflects the subject's preferences for one commodity over another when all attributes in the model are the same – referred to in the literature as the alternative specific constant (ASC) most likely to be important in 'labelled' DCEs. The c parameters are equal to the marginal utilities of the given attributes (i.e. $\partial v / \partial X_k = c_k$), and the ratio of any two parameters show the marginal rates of substitution between attributes. Following on from this, the ratio of any given attribute to the absolute parameter on the price attribute shows how much money an individual is willing to pay for a unit change in that attribute (i.e. c_n/d). From this it is possible to estimate overall WTP for a change in the provision of a service by summing the product of attribute coefficients and their independent variables (i.e. $\Sigma c_n X_n$) and dividing by the absolute parameter on the price – the measure commonly used to estimate the welfare impact of a change in policy is given by:

$$WTP = \{(\Sigma c_n X_n)/d\}. \qquad (4)$$

Validity of responses

It is important to include tests of validity, i.e. to test the extent to which individuals behave in real settings as they state they would. Given that many of the applications of

DCEs have taken place in countries with a publicly provided health care system, where secondary data sets are unavailable to compare real with stated behaviour, a number of alternative validity tests have been applied. Current practice indicates that the most commonly considered notion is theoretical (internal) validity. This involves checking that model coefficients have the signs expected given theory or previous evidence. The evidence on the theoretical validity of DCEs is generally encouraging (Ryan and Gerard 2003). More recently assessments of validity have tested the underlying axioms of DCEs. In what follows we consider this growing literature. Finally we comment on the importance of conducting tests of external validity.

Testing the underlying axioms

The application of DCEs, as with any method of preference elicitation, assumes that individual have *complete*, *rational* and *continuous* preferences. In brief, completeness refers to the notion that individuals are able to form and express a complete order of preferences, being rational refers to the notion that an individual should prefer more of a good thing rather than less, and continuous preferences to the notion of unlimited substitutability between attributes (i.e. an individual evaluates all the alternatives in a choice set simultaneously, considering trade-offs among all attributes, selecting the one with the highest utility, also referred to as compensatory decision-making). Evidence has been found of both complete and rational responses to DCEs (Ryan and Gerard 2003). The axiom of continuity has received considerable attention. Evidence from health care suggests that this assumption may be violated, although testing of the axiom is limited (Ryan and Gerard 2003). Interestingly, there has been little debate regarding the relationship between adherence to economic axioms and complexity of the DCE design. Whilst a limited number of economists have discussed this (De Palma *et al.* 1994; Heiner 1983; Scott 2002), more extensive literature from psychology has argued that as complexity of tasks increase, so would reliance on simple decision-making strategies (Payne *et al.* 1993; Gigerenzer and Todd 1999). This may lead to violations of the assumptions of compensatory decision-making (and rationality) and is an essential area for future research. Further, if non-compensatory decision making is identified, questions are raised concerning the analysis of response data. Recently Swait (2001) has developed a formal model for analysing a wide range of decision strategies that relax the assumption of compensatory decision-making. Future work should consider the application of this model in health care.

External validity

The preferred test of validity is whether individuals behave in the real world as they state in the DCE. Thus far no studies have tested this in health economics. The environmental economics literature has also focused on internal validity, with only one study carrying out a direct comparison of stated and actual WTP (Carlsson and Martinnsson 2002). They found that DCE estimates of values for wildlife protection were insignificantly different from actual payment. Health economists clearly need to apply tests of external validity, as they are attempting to do in the direct willingness to pay literature, see Blumenschein *et al.* (2001) and Clark (2002). Consideration should be given here to setting up an experiment to compare real and stated behaviour, or identifying secondary data sets where information on actual behaviour exists. Possibilities in predominantly publicly funded health services include those parts of the health care system that require co-payment, such as in the UK the demand for pre-scriptions, dental care or assisted reproductive techniques. An alternative would be to go back to respondents with the results from a DCE, and ask them if the results are consistent with their preferences. Future work should also explore the fusion of stated preference and revealed preference data (Tami and Swait 2004).

Using DCEs to estimate HRQoL utilities

As noted by Feeny in Chapter 6.2, preference-based measures are playing an increas-ingly important role in the assessment of health-related quality of life. Feeny intro-duced three methods that have been commonly used to estimate preferences – visual analogue scale (VAS), standard gamble (SG) and time trade-off (TTO). As well as being used to value specific health states, these techniques have also been used to estimate quality weights with the development of generic QALYs. Whilst DCEs were developed to go beyond health outcomes, they could equally be used to estimate pref-erence weights within HRQoL preference measures. This would involve presenting individuals with a number of choices where the attributes and levels were the dimen-sions of health outcome instrument. There are a number of potential advantages of using DCEs over SG and TTO to elicit preferences for HRQoL.[1]

- An attractive feature of DCEs is their ability to take account of risk in a potentially less complicated manner than SG-type questions (though this is ultimately an empirical question). SG has been proposed as the gold standard to estimate utilities under uncertainty. However, it is well recognized that individuals find such ques-tions difficult to answer, resulting in internally inconsistent responses (Llewellyn *et al.* 1982; Rosser and Kind 1978). The TTO technique has been developed to over-come such problems. However, this technique is not rooted in economic theory. DCEs have the advantage that risk can be incorporated into the decision-making process by including it as an attribute, and that, following this, the type of question posed to the individual more accurately reflects the type of decision they face every day. It is also rooted in economic theory.

- In everyday life individuals often choose between several options. However, they very rarely consider their probability indifference level, or the number of years at

---

[1] VAS is not liked by economists because it does not embody the concept of opportunity cost and has no theoretical basis.

the end of their life they are willing to give up for a good or service. Thus, the DCE approach may be argued to resemble more accurately the type of decisions individuals make on a daily basis.

♦ There is some evidence that, when asking individuals to trade between attributes, the attribute that is being traded off becomes salient. That is, people give more importance to this attribute (Maas and Stalpers 1992). This has been shown within SG experiments in which individuals are first asked their probability indifference point between a gamble and certain outcome and are then presented with a pairwise comparison between these two scenarios (i.e. the certainty equivalent and the gamble to which individuals said they were indifferent). In such choice experiments the certainty equivalent is usually preferred to the gamble (Von Winderfelt 1980; Tversky *et al.* 1988). One possible explanation for this is that the attribute that is traded (risk in this example) is weighted more highly than in a situation where a choice is made. This would manifest itself by individuals saying in a TTO setting that they were not willing to trade *any* number of years for a better quality of life, but choosing a scenario that gave a better quality of life with fewer years to live in a choice question. DCEs would potentially overcome this problem.

Conclusions

This chapter has discussed the role of the DCE technique in producing valid and versatile measures of benefit in health economics, particularly for health economic evaluation but also for other uses. It is expected that DCEs will be used more. However, a number of key methodological concerns remain. Some of these have been highlighted and serve as a useful agenda for future research in this area. These relate to: having a better understanding of how respondents interpret price and risk attributes; comparing direct willingness to pay and DCEs in empirical studies; understanding the most appropriate way to ask the question; strengthening analysis; investigating decision-making heuristics employed when completing DCEs, and the extent these are related to the complexity of the task and external validity. Collaborative work with experimental design experts, psychologists, sociologists and qualitative researchers should prove useful when investigating these issues. It is clearly also necessary to link this research agenda to work being carried out in other economic areas (such as environmental economics) and to health economics benefit assessment more generally.

References

Adamowicz, W. (2001). *Personal Communication*, International Health Economic Conference, University of York.

Blumenschein. K., Johannesson, M., Yokoyama, K., and Freeman, P. (2001). Hypothetical versus real willingness to pay in the health care sector. *Journal of Health Economics*, **20**, 441–457.

Bradley, M. (1991). *User's Manual for the Speed Version 2.1 Stated Preference Experimenter Editor and Designer.* Hague: Hague Consulting Group.

Carlsson, F. and Martinnsson, P. (2002). Do hypothetical and actual marginal willingness to pay differ in choice experiments? *Journal of Environmental Economics and Management,* **41,** 179–192.

Clark, P. (2002). Testing the convergent validity of the contingent valuation and travel cost methods in valuing the benefits of health care. *Health Economics,* **11,** 117–127.

Department of the Environment, Transport and the Regions Highways. (1997). Economics Note **2,** November 1997. In *Design Manuals for Roads and Bridges, Volume 13.* London: HMSO.

De Palma, A., Myers, G., and Papageorgious, Y. (1994). Rational choice under an imperfect ability to choose. *American Economic Review,* **84,** 419–440.

Gerard, K., Lattimer, V., Turnbull, J., Smith, H., George, S., Bailsford, S., and Maslin-Prothero, S. (2004). Reviewing emergency care system 2: measuring patient preferences using a discrete choice experiment. *Emergency Medicine Journal,* in press.

Gigerenzer, G. and Todd, P. (1999). For The ABC Research Group. *Simple Heuristics that make us Smart.* New York: Oxford University Press.

Greene, W. (1998). *Limdep Version 7.0: User's manual.* Plainview, NY: Econometric Software Inc.

Hanley, N., Mourato, S., and Wright, R. (2001). Choice modelling: a superior alternative for environmental valuation? *Journal of Economic Surveys,* **15,** 435–462.

Heiner, R. (1983). The origin of predictable behaviour. *American Economic Review,* **73,** 560–595.

Hensher, D., Stopher, P., and Louviere, J. (2001). An exploratory analysis of the effect of numbers of choices sets in designed choice experiments: an airline choice application. *Journal of Air Transport Management,* **2,** 373–370.

Intercooled Stata 7.0 for Windows 98/95/NT (2002). College Station, Texas: Stata Corporation.

Lloyd, A. (2001). The extent of patients' understanding of the risk of treatments. *Quality in Health Care,* **10,** (Suppl. I), i14–i18.

Louviere, J., Oppewal, H., Timmermans, H., and Thomas, T. (1997). Handling large numbers of attributes in conjoint applications: Who says existing techniques can't be applied? But if you want an alternative, how about hierarchical choice experiments? *Mimeograph.*

Louviere, J. J., Hensher, D. A., and Swait, J. D. (2000). *Stated Choice Methods. Analysis and Application.* Cambridge: Cambridge University Press.

sLlewellyn, T., Sutherland, S., Tobshirani, R., Ciampi, A., Till, J., and Boyd, N. (1982). The measurement of patients' values in medicine. *Medical Decision Making,* **2,** 449–462.

Maas, A. and Stalpers, L. (1992). Assessing utilities by means of conjoint measurement: An application in medical decision analysis. *Medical Decision Making,* **12,** 288–297.

Ohler, T., Le, A., Louviere, J., and Swait, J. (2000). Attribute range effects in binary response tasks. *Marketing Letters,* **11,** 249–260.

Payne, J., Bettman, J., and Johnson, E. (1993). *The Adaptive decision-maker.* New York: Cambridge University Press.

Pearmain, D., Swanson, J., Kroes, E., and Bradley, M. (1991). *Stated Preference Techniques: A guide to practice.* Hague: Steer Davis Gleave and Hague Consulting Group.

Ratcliffe, J. and Longworth, L. (2002). Investigating structural reliability within health technology assessment: a discrete choice experiment. *International Journal of Technology Assessment,* **18,** (1), 139–144.

Rosser, R. and Kind, P. (1978). A scale of valuations of states of illness: is there a social consensus? *International Journal of Epidemiology,* **7,** 347–358.

Ryan, M. and Gerard, K. (2003). Using discrete choice experiments to value health care: current practice and future prospects. *Applied Health Economics and Policy Analysis*, **2**, 55–64.

Ryan, M. and Wordsworth, S. (2000). Sensitivity of willingness to pay estimates to the level of attributes in discrete choice experiments. *Scottish Journal of Political Economy*, **47**, (5), 504–524.

Ryan, M., Scott, D. A., Reeves, C., Bate, A., van Teijlingen, E., Russell, E., Napper, M., and Robb, C. (2001a). Eliciting public preferences for health care: a systematic review of techniques. *Health Technology Assessment*, **5**, (5), 1–170.

Ryan, M., Bate, A., Eastmond, C., and Ludbrook, A. (2001b). Using discrete choice experiments to elicit preferences. *Quality in Health Care*, **10**, 155–160.

San Miguel, F., Ryan, M., and McIntosh, E. (2000). Demonstrating the use of conjoint analysis in health economics: an application to menorrhagia. *Applied Economics*, **32**, 823–833.

Scott, A. (2002). Identifying and analysing dominant preferences in discrete choice experiments: An application in health care. *Journal of Economic Psychology*, **23**, 383–398.

Swait, J. (2001). A non-compensatory choice model incorporating attribute cut-offs. *Transportation Research*, **35**, 903–928.

Szeinbach, S. L., Barnes, J. H., McGhan, W. F., Murawski, M. M., and Corey, R. (1999). Using conjoint analysis to evaluate health state preferences. *Drug Information Journal*, **33**, 849–858.

Tami, M. and Swait, J. (2004). Using stated preferences and revealed preference modeling to evaluate prescribing decisions. *Health Economics*, **13**, 563–573.

Tversky, A. Sattath, S., and Slovic, P. (1988). Contingent weighting in the judgement of choice. *Psychological Review*, **95**, 371–384.

Von Winterfeldt, D. (1980). Additivity and expected utility in risky multiattribute preferences. *Journal of Mathematical Psychology*, **21**, 66–82.

Example: applying DCEs to assess preferences for the treatment of menorrhagia

In this appendix we demonstrate the application of the DCE approach within the context of a study concerned with women's preferences for treatment for menorrhagia (excessive menstrual bleeding). Menorrhagia affects approximately 22 per cent of healthy women. Treatment options include hysterectomy or minimal access surgical alternatives to hysterectomy, known as conservative treatments. Randomized trials have shown reduced post-operative morbidity, reduced operative complications and shorter stay in hospital following conservative surgery. However, hysterectomy shows greater effectiveness in terms of the relief of symptoms since two-thirds of women who have conservative treatment will require re-treatment (either hysterectomy or conservative) within four years.

A DCE was used to assess the value of these different attributes of care (San Miguel *et al.* 2000). Six attributes were included in the experiment: number of nights in hospital after operation; time to return to normal activity; chance of complications following operation; chance of re-treatment with conservative treatment; chance of conservative re-treatment and chance of hysterectomy re-treatment. In addition, a price proxy was included so that WTP could be estimated indirectly. Realistic levels were assigned. The attributes and levels resulted in 1296 possible scenarios ($3^4 \times 4^2$). These were reduced to 25 scenarios using experimental design software (Bradley 1991). These 25 scenarios were randomly split into two groups of 12 and 13 scenarios and two versions of DCE were produced. In both questionnaires all scenarios were compared with the current situation of hysterectomy. Women were randomly allocated to one of the two questionnaires. An example of one of the discrete choices is shown in Figure 6.3.1. A random effects probit model was used to analyse responses and the following utility equation estimated:

$$\Delta V_{(C-H)} = c_0 + c_1 \text{Nights} + c_2 \text{Time} + c_3 \text{Comp} + c_4 \text{ReCon} + c_5 \text{ReHys} + d\text{Cost} + \in$$

	Hysterectomy	Conservative
Number of nights in hospital after operation	7	0
Time to return to normal activity (weeks)	11	2
Chance of complications following operation	45%	20%
Chance of re-treatment with Conservative	0%	15%
Chance of re-treatment with Hysterectomy	0%	30%
Cost of the treatment (£)	1,400	5,000
	Prefer hysterectomy	Prefer conservative
Which treatment would you prefer? (*tick one box only*)	☐	☐

Fig. 6.3.1 Example of discrete choice in questionnaire.

$\Delta U_{(C-H)}$ is the change in utility in moving from hysterectomy to conservative surgery, c_0 represents the constant term, 'Nights' is the difference in the nights stay in hospital after the intervention for both types of treatment, 'Time' is the difference in time to return to normal activities, 'Comp' is the difference in complications following both types of interventions, 'ReCon' is the difference in the chance of having a re-treatment with conservative surgery, 'ReHys' is the difference in the chance of having a re-treatment with hysterectomy and 'Cost' is the difference in cost between hysterectomy and conservative surgery. c_i are the parameters of the model to be estimated and $\in$ is the error term.

The results are shown in Table 6.3.1. Three of the six attributes were significant at the 1 per cent level. These attributes all have the expected negative sign, indicating that the lower the level of these attributes in the conservative treatment compared with hysterectomy, the more likely the individual is to choose conservative treatment. The positive constant implies a general preference for conservative treatment over hysterectomy when all attributes are the same in the two treatment regimes. This shows the value of the process of treatment. Women were willing to pay £220 for a 1 per cent reduction in the chance of re-treatment with hysterectomy and £149 for a 1 per cent reduction in the chance of complications.

Table 6.3.1 Results from regression model

Attribute	General Model		Specific Model*		Marginal WTP (£)
	Coefficient	P Value	Coefficient	P Value	
Constant (c_0)	1.6216	0.2355	2.2841	0.0009	7,613
Nights in hospital (c_1)	−0.0272	0.6792	–	–	–
Time to return to activity (c_2)	−0.1109	0.3834	–	–	–
Chance of complications (c_3)	−0.0496	0.0038	−0.0446	0.006	149
Chance of re-treatment with conservative surgery (c_4)	−0.0342	0.1143	–	–	–
Chance of re-treatment with hysterectomy (c_5)	−0.0671	0.0000	−0.0659	0.0000	220
Cost (d)	−0.0003	0.0000	−0.0003	0.0000	n/a
N	907		907		
Log-likelihood	−252.79		−255.01		
Mc Fadden R^2	0.53		0.53		
Chi-squared	580.72		577.08		
Individual predictions	68.9%		68.9%		

* Model after dropping those variables non–significant at the 5% level. Source: San Miguel *et al.* (2000)

Table 6.3.2 Utility scores and WTP measures

Attributes	Attribute coefficient	Hysterectomy attributes levels	Conservative attributes levels	Difference in attribute levels	Attribute Score	Marginal WTP (£)
Constant (c_0)	2.2841	–	–	–	2.2841	7,613
Chance of complications (c_3)	−0.0446	45	15	−30	1.338	4,440
Chance of re-treatment with hysterectomy (c_5)	−0.0659	0	20	20	−1.318	−4,460
Cost (d)	−0.0003	1,400	1,200	−200	0.066	–
Utility score					2.3701	
Total WTP						7,593

Source: San Miguel *et al.* (2000).

Overall utility scores and WTP measures (following a change from conservative surgery to hysterectomy) are shown in Table 6.3.2. A 30 per cent decrease in the chance of complications following conservative surgery increases utility by 1.338, a reduction in cost of £200 increases utility by 0.066 and increase in the chance of re-treatment with hysterectomy of 20 per cent decreases utility by 1.318. The overall effect of these changes (when moving from hysterectomy to conservative surgery) is an increase in utility of 2.37. The results from the utility score estimates are supported by the WTP estimates. Respondents were willing to pay £4,440 for a 30 per cent reduction in the chance of complications and they should be compensated with £4,460 for a 20 per cent increase in the chance of re-treatment with hysterectomy. If there were no differences in the attributes between hysterectomy and conservative surgery (which in this particular case is unrealistic) women are willing to pay £7,613 to have conservative surgery. Thus, total WTP for changing from hysterectomy to conservative surgery is £7,593 i.e. women prefer conservative surgery to hysterectomy as indicated also by the positive utility score obtained.

Combining clinical trials: meta-analyses

Peter Fayers and Neil Scott

Summary

Patient-reported outcomes are becoming more frequently reported as the primary end points in randomized clinical trials, and this has led to the emergence of systematic reviews and meta-analyses of health-related quality of life (HRQoL) outcomes. In the past, meta-analyses have been most commonly used for specific dimensions of HRQoL, principally pain and depression. One reason for this may be the apparent complexity of combining results from diverse HRQoL instruments: to many investigators, it may seem impossible to combine the disparate scales that are reported. In this chapter we will explain, with examples from published literature, the main issues involved and some of the decisions that must be taken when planning and carrying out meta-analysis of HRQoL outcomes.

Introduction

The modern trend towards evidence-based medicine has led to the acceptance that meta-analyses are the best means of summarizing the results from a number of randomized controlled trials (RCTs) (or other studies) that address similar treatment objectives. Much of the success in gaining this recognition is due to the efforts of the Cochrane Collaboration, which is an international organisation that started up in 1993 as a response to Archie Cochrane's call for systematic, up-to-date reviews in health care. Cochrane was an epidemiologist who observed that, first, health care practice is not always based on good evidence; secondly, there is too much information for any individual clinician to access and use; and thirdly, resources are always limited, so it is all the more important to know which interventions work. Although conscientious clinicians may regularly and informally review the literature in their field, systematic reviews are far more reliable. Since its inception, the Cochrane Collaboration has promoted systematic reviews of clinical trials in all disease and treatment areas.

Literature reviews and meta-analyses are also increasingly undertaken before initiating new primary research into the impact of interventions, as a means of determining what work has already been done in the topic area and to inform decisions about the need for, and the design of, a new clinical trial.

However, until recently only a minority of clinical trials have had HRQoL end points as the major outcome of interest, and there have been few instances of meta-analyses involving HRQoL outcomes. In principle it should be possible to combine HRQoL data, and carry out the same statistical summarization and meta-analysis in a similar manner to any other quantitative measurements. However, HRQoL data has a number of distinct properties that introduce greater complexities than are normally encountered. For example, when a clinical trial measures survival benefits from a new treatment, there is one clearly and uniquely defined outcome – survival. That outcome should normally be obtainable for all patients in the clinical trial, even though there may be differences in the way that individual studies report the survival outcomes. A similar situation arises when outcomes such as blood pressure or haemoglobin levels are being analysed; trials are expected to have data for most patients, and the reporting of these outcomes is fairly well standardized. In both these situations it becomes in principle relatively straightforward to combine the endpoints from the different studies to obtain an overall estimate of treatment benefits.

In contrast, when dealing with HRQoL outcomes, there are particular problems in carrying out meta-analysis. First, there may be a whole range of different outcomes and scales reported. A few examples are that some studies might report a single global question about overall health using a visual analogue scale (VAS); other studies might use a question about overall quality of life using five or more response categories; others might use a summated score derived from items and scales on a lengthier instrument, possibly with unequal weightings or with utility weights; and yet others might report transition ratings in the form of the number of patients reporting a 'moderate' improvement in health, in quality of life, or in some other beneficial outcome. How can such a variety of outcomes be combined into a meaningful analysis?

Secondly, another common feature of HRQoL studies is that there may be extensive attrition problems due to compliance issues, and in many trials there may also be attrition due to death; furthermore, both of these may occur at unequal rates in the randomized treatment arms. In many disease areas some trials may report results when fewer than 60 per cent of assessable patients complete and return a valid HRQoL assessment. Can we trust such trials? How should we synthesize data from different trials when some have far superior compliance than others?

Meta-analyses and systematic reviews

'Meta-analysis' may be regarded as the formal quantitative analysis, by statistical methods, of a systematic review. One of the primary objectives of a meta-analysis is to increase the probability of detecting a significant effect – that is, to increase the power – because individual trials may be too small and lack power to detect worthwhile treatment effects with reasonable certainty. The other major objective is to increase the precision of the estimated effect size. In addition, meta-analyses that include independent trials from several countries can also serve to confirm the generalizability of the conclusions, and provide more convincing evidence regarding treatment effects. It is worth noting, however, that it may not always be possible or appropriate to conduct a meta-analysis as part of a systematic review.

Most commonly, the review and meta-analysis may be based entirely upon results such as means, percentages and other summary statistics, abstracted from published reports. However, some have argued that it may be beneficial to obtain individual patient data (IPD) from the clinical trial investigators, and that all analyses should be based upon IPD (Stewart and Clarke 1995). Clearly, IPD allows more refined analysis and permits the quality of the trials to be explored more comprehensively. It may also overcome the problem of different publications presenting different statistics. However, contacting trial coordinators, collecting IPD and analysing it is considerably more expensive and time-consuming than using summaries from publications. Although systematic reviews using IPD are still relatively rare, they are becoming more frequent.

Definition of target population and treatment

The assumption in meta-analysis is that the trials and end points being combined are all assessing broadly the same scientific question, and that observed treatment differences vary from trial to trial through chance. The aim of meta-analysis is to amalgamate results across treatments, target populations and events. This is both its strength and weakness. For homogeneity one might be tempted to be very restrictive about the treatments that are being compared (e.g. precise specification of therapy and dosage) and the type/condition/severity of disease; then there may be few studies eligible for inclusion, and critics of the meta-analysis may also claim that it cannot be generalized to other settings. On the other hand, if the therapy is too loosely defined, or if too wide a range of disease types or severities are included, critics may protest that the data are too heterogeneous, that any treatment effect has consequently been diluted, and that the review is questionable. Thus it is essential to define in advance exactly what range of treatment options are permissible, the target disease group and disease severity that are being assessed, and the outcomes or events to be evaluated. A balance must be struck between being restrictive or permissive.

Example: postoperative pain after hernia surgery

We will illustrate different methods of meta-analysis using data from a review of postoperative pain after groin hernia surgery.

These data came from reanalysis of patient level data supplied by the trial authors through the framework of an international collaborative group (EU Hernia Trialists

Collaboration 1999). This group aimed to address a number of questions, but in this chapter we use one particular comparison, namely mesh (whether placed laparoscopically or through an open operation) versus non-mesh repair for groin hernia. Where individual patient data (IPD) could not be obtained from the trial authors, published data were used where possible.

Example: impact of problem-solving treatments on depression

Townsend *et al.* (2001) published a meta-analysis of the impact of problem-solving treatments on depression, hopelessness and improvement in problems. We use the depression data to illustrate methods.

Identification of studies

The aim is to identify all relevant randomized trials. Because of publication bias (trials with 'positive' results are more readily published than negative ones), it is important to identify non-published trials, too. Searching can be surprisingly difficult and labour intensive; yet ensuring comprehensive identification of *all published trials and non-published trials* is one of the most important aspects of carrying out a systematic review. A balance needs to be struck, however, as the effort in terms of time and resources required for identifying a small proportion of the published studies may be considerable and may not be worthwhile. Identification of unpublished trials is also extremely difficult. The Cochrane Collaboration has a wealth of experience in searching techniques, and organizes training courses for beginners. Cochrane reviewers not only make use of registers of trials, but also rely on several means of searching for relevant reports, including both electronic and manual methods. Search strategies have been developed for use with the major online bibliographic databases such as Medline and Embase. For complete identification of published reports, there may be no alternative to a page-by-page search of the literature. Care must also be taken to avoid including trials with duplicate publications more than once.

Quality of studies

The quality of a published study depends on the study's design, methods of sample recruitment, completeness of data, and the analysis and reporting of the outcomes. Any study that might be subject to bias, or does not meet other criteria for quality, should be excluded from the analysis. Although a number of checklists have been proposed for assessing study quality, it may be better to examine specific components of study quality individually instead.

Most meta-analyses are restricted to systematic reviews of *randomized* clinical trials. It has long been recognized that the most important aspect of study quality is adequate concealment of the random allocation, and that trials of lower quality tend to show larger – and biased – treatment effects (e.g., Schulz *et al.* 1995). Publications of trials should have provided evidence that the concealment of allocation and randomization were adequate, and that blinding was effected when feasible. Sensitivity analyses, excluding poorer quality studies, can then be conducted.

An additional aspect to consider for meta-analyses of HRQoL outcomes is whether the instruments (questionnaires, scales or single-item questions) have been adequately validated, and shown to be sensitive and reliable. If ad hoc instruments were used in a study, a decision must be made whether data from that study can be regarded as valid and reliable.

Example: postoperative pain after hernia surgery

Abstracts of the references retrieved by the search were evaluated and those that were clearly not eligible were discarded. Two reviewers studied the full text of the remaining references for quality of design, assessment of outcomes and completion rate, and they independently extracted data from the studies that were selected for inclusion. If no agreement could be reached a third person acted as arbiter.

Example: impact of problem-solving treatments on depression

Each trial was rated for quality, using the recommended Cochrane assessment criteria. Each trial was rated by two independent reviewers who were blind to its authorship.

Compliance and attrition

Compliance can be a major problem in some disease areas. As noted in Chapter 3.2, this particularly applies to chronic diseases and cancer, where some clinical trials report that 50 per cent or fewer of the anticipated (i.e. from living patients) questionnaires were received. Many investigators have found that poor compliance is frequently associated with less well patients who have a poorer HRQoL, and so trials with high levels of missing data are susceptible to bias and are of low validity. Although there is no consensus as to what is an acceptable level of compliance, consideration should be given to excluding from the meta-analysis all trials that fall below some pre-specified minimum threshold (although they may be retained in the systematic review).

Increasingly, 'imputation' is used when analysing trials with missing data (see Chapter 3.3). If published reports of trials are used for the meta-analysis there may be little control over whether or not imputed results are used – one is at the mercy of the publications – but if individual patient data is available there is more flexibility over the decision about whether to impute or not.

Of course in many cases HRQoL meta-analyses may be carried out for diseases where improving HRQoL is the principal objective of treatment – for example, relief of back pain or treatment of depression. Then compliance with assessment is likely to be high. One such example is palliative care, where HRQoL is by definition the aim of management and therapy. However, two particular problems arise in this setting.

First, when patients deteriorate it may be regarded as unethical to risk further stress by asking them to complete questionnaires, and many patients also refuse during their final months. Secondly, a substantial proportion of patients may die before the target time point for assessment. This 'attrition' can raise problems of interpretation. At the very least, it is essential to report the levels of attrition observed in the various trials.

Definition of outcome

One very important step in any systematic review is to agree precise definitions for the outcomes to be examined. Thus if overall HRQoL is the outcome of interest, should the meta-analysis only include studies that used global questions about 'your overall quality of life'? Or are questions about 'your overall health' or, for example, 'well-being' acceptable? Some instruments advocate multi-item scales that focus on physical aspects, others may emphasize mental well-being – can all these be included? Where several suitable outcomes are available in a trial, criteria must be specified for determining the most appropriate ones. Similar decisions are also needed when a particular dimension of HRQoL is the primary outcome of interest – such as (in our examples) pain and depression.

Other aspects needing definition include specification of the assessment time point. In randomized trials this will usually be HRQoL assessed at a fixed time after randomization, although (as in explanatory analyses of clinical trials) additional analyses may explore assessments at other time points, such as three months after the end of a course of chemotherapy. Individual trials that include multiple assessments may report other measures, such as area under the curve or scores from longitudinal analysis, but it is improbable that there will be sufficient consistency in design and reporting across the trials to make the use of such summary measures a feasible option for most meta-analyses. However, although detailed longitudinal analysis may not be feasible, some reviews focus on change from baseline – i.e. whether patients have improved or deteriorated from before the intervention.

Having determined a suitable time point, consideration must also be given to defining the maximum acceptable window. For example, if the target time point is three months after randomization, will trials be accepted if they only provide a 10-week assessment? Or only a four-month assessment? Or a six-month assessment?

When using reports from trials the reviewer is limited to the published data, but IPD analyses offer greater opportunities for flexibility extraction of data and the use of longitudinal summaries.

Example: postoperative pain after hernia surgery

The endpoint was 'short term pain', which was defined as pain measured at seven days after surgery. However, not all trials had collected information on pain at this particular time point. Therefore to increase the amount of included data it was decided that, when no seven-day data were available, information for days 5–10 could be used instead. In each case the closest time point to seven days was used.

Forty-one trials comparing mesh versus non-mesh repair were identified. Of these only 15 had collected information on short-term pain according to our definition. Two could not be included because they compared laparoscopic mesh repair against a mixture of open mesh and non-mesh repairs and it was not possible to separate out a subset of mesh versus non-mesh surgeons or centres, even using IPD.

Of the remaining 13 studies, ten had measured short-term pain using a VAS, or ordered categorical scale which could be treated as a continuous outcome. The other three studies had used a categorical measure of pain. Separate meta-analyses were conducted based on treating pain as both binary and continuous data.

Measures of treatment effect

The main outcomes of interest are usually the assessment at a pre-specified time point and/or the change from baseline until that time. The most usual method of meta-analysis, the 'effect size' method, involves representing each study with a single figure summary measuring the size of effect for each study. Examples of effect sizes measures include odds ratios and differences in means. The effect size for each study can be thought of as an estimate of the 'true' effect of the treatment being studied. The uncertainty surrounding each effect size can be represented by calculating its standard deviation (SD) or variance, and constructing a 95 per cent confidence interval for each study's effect size.

Meta-analyses are fairly straightforward in the situation where the included studies use the same outcome measures. However, in practice it is likely that a variety of HRQoL instruments will have been used, and it may then be necessary first to standardize the measure used for assessing the treatment effect in each study; for example, it would not make sense to combine and average the mean scores from, say, a numerical rating scale and a VAS scale if they were coded 0 – 7 and 0 – 100 respectively.

For continuous data, provided the same instrument was used in all studies, the mean difference can be used as the measure of effect size. When different scales are used in the studies – as is frequently the case in HRQoL meta-analyses – the method of standardized mean difference (SMD) may instead be used, as shown in Table 6.4.1; this represents treatment effects as the number of SDs between the treatments. For carrying out the meta-analysis, we ideally require an estimate of the mean treatment effect in each group, the corresponding SD, and the number of patients. This can of course be calculated for IPD, but when extracting data from published sources not all of this information may be available explicitly. The *Cochrane Reviewers' Handbook* (Deeks *et al.* 2004) explains methods for imputing the necessary values from other information – for example, if *t*-statistics or confidence intervals are presented, the standard error (SE) and SD can usually be estimated.

Table 6.4.1 Effect size measures for continuous and binary outcomes

	Effect size	Standard error
Continuous outcomes		
Mean difference	$T_{MD} = \bar{x}_t - \bar{x}_c$	$SE_{MD} = SD_{MD}\left(\dfrac{1}{n_t} + \dfrac{1}{n_c}\right),$ where $SD_{MD} = \sqrt{\dfrac{(n_t - 1)s_t^2 + (n_c - 1)s_c^2}{n_t + n_c - 2}}$
Standardized mean difference	$T_{SMD} = \dfrac{\bar{x}_t - \bar{x}_c}{SD_{MD}}$	$SE_{SMD} = \sqrt{\dfrac{n_t + n_c}{n_t n_c} + \dfrac{T_{SMD}^2}{2(n_t + n_c)}}$
Binary outcomes		
Odds ratio*	$OR = \dfrac{ad}{bc}$	$SE_{Ln(OR)} = \sqrt{\dfrac{1}{a} + \dfrac{1}{b} + \dfrac{1}{c} + \dfrac{1}{d}}$
Relative risk*	$RR = \dfrac{a/(a + b)}{c/(c + d)}$	$SE_{Ln(RR)} = \sqrt{\dfrac{1}{a} - \dfrac{1}{a + b} + \dfrac{1}{c} - \dfrac{1}{c + d}}$
Risk difference (Risk reduction)	$RD = \dfrac{a}{a + b} - \dfrac{c}{c + d}$	$SE_{RD} = \sqrt{\dfrac{(a/(a + b))(1 - (a/(a + b)))}{a + b}} + \sqrt{\dfrac{(c/(c + d))(1 - (c/(c + d)))}{c + d}}$

* The SE of Log(OR) and Log(RR) are given; the calculation of the confidence interval is carried out using Log values which are then exponentiated to convert back into normal units.

Confidence interval $100(1 - \alpha)$% CI is calculated as (Effect size) $\pm Z_{\alpha/2}$ (Standard error).

Notation:

Continuous outcomes				Binary outcomes		
	number	mean	standard deviation		"no"/ failure/ dead	"yes"/ success/ alive
New/experimental treatment	n_t	$\bar{x}_t$	s_t	New/experimental treatment	a	b
Control	n_c	$\bar{x}_c$	s_c	Control	c	d

In principle, change scores (i.e. change in HRQoL from baseline) can be treated exactly the same way as other continuous variables, and combined with them by using the method of SMDs. In practice, however, many published reports fail to supply the SD or SE of the change scores, and these can be difficult to estimate from the more commonly cited SD of the baseline or final score. In such cases it may be preferable to use the after-treatment time point rather than the change-score.

For binary data three effect size measures are commonly used: the odds ratio, relative risk and risk difference, each with certain advantages and disadvantages (Table 6.4.1). The relative risk represents the ratio of the risks of having the event of interest. The odds ratio has no specific clinical interpretation although it does approximate the relative risk when the event rate is low. Its main advantage is its good statistical properties. The risk difference is probably the easiest effect size measure to interpret, but has the least desirable statistical properties and tends to give the least consistent results when the event rate is varied. When using the odds ratio or relative risk (in each case a value of one represents no difference between the study groups) it is common to take a logarithmic transformation before conducting meta-analysis. The new log transformed effect size is symmetrical about zero and therefore has more desirable statistical properties. Such a transformation is unnecessary for the risk difference because zero already represents no difference between the groups.

For ordinal variables the choice is between assuming they can be treated as if they were continuous variables, converting to binary data by introducing a cut-point, or using more complex analytical methods (see below).

Example: postoperative pain after hernia surgery

Information about mean pain scores at seven days was available from continuous scales for 13 trials; for 10 trials IPD was available permitting reanalysis, and for three trials the SD was not available and had to be estimated from a graph in a published article. For one of these trials the SE of the mean was reported instead of the SD, but this was converted to an SD by multiplying by the square root of the total number of patients included. For a second trial, although a mean for pain at seven days was reported, only SDs for pain at ten days and for days one to seven combined were given, so the average of these two values was used. The third trial gave only error bars without making it clear if these represented ranges, SDs or confidence intervals. As the meaning was unclear it was decided to use the mean of the SDs of the other trials in the review as the best estimate of the SD of this trial.

As the majority of trials used a scale from 0 (no pain) to 10 (maximum pain) it was decided to use this scale as the standard and for VAS using other ranges the mean and SD were rescaled appropriately. One study reported pain on a 1–100 scale and therefore the scores were divided by 10. Another study used a 1–10 scale where no pain was indicated by a score of 1; the scores were converted to 0–10 using an appropriate rescaling formula.

Three trials used a categorical measure of pain. Two of these used a four-point scale (no pain, mild, moderate, severe) and one a five-point scale (no pain, very mild, mild, moderate, severe, very severe). In such a situation a decision must be made as to whether it will be possible to use the categorical information as continuous. Based on the work of Collins *et al.* (1997) who compared descriptive pain categories and a VAS, moderate pain was assigned a value of 4.9 and severe pain assigned 7.5. No information about mild pain was available, but it was decided to assume a score of 0 represented no pain and 2.5 mild pain as these were the midpoint values for no and moderate pain. For the study using the six-point categorical pain measure values of 0, 1.6, 3.3, 4.9, 6.6 and 8.3 were assigned to the categories using similar reasoning.

Example: impact of problem-solving treatments on depression

Much of the data needed to perform meta-analyses on these outcomes were missing from the reports (e.g. means and SDs. Only one author was able to provide the original trial data. For the other trials missing data were imputed from information that was reported. Specifically in two trials mean scores on some skills at follow-up were reported in graph format only. Two reviewers estimated means independently from the graphs. Where there was disagreement, consensus was reached with a third member of the review group.

Four of the reports had not included SDs associated with mean test scores at follow-up. For one trial the SDs associated with the mean scores at follow-up were imputed from t-test statistics by rearranging the equation used to derive the value of t, and for another trial the reported F-test statistics were used. One study only gave means and SDs of change scores, so these were used instead in the analysis.

Combining studies

There are a number of different methods for combining effect sizes. For continuous variables, the simplest method of meta-analysis is known as the 'inverse variance weighted' or 'weighted mean difference' method. For this the average mean difference is calculated, giving more 'weight' to estimates from larger studies. The weights are the inverse variances of the means from each study, that is, $1/(SE)^2$. This means that studies with the least variability, usually the largest studies, will receive the highest weighting in determining the overall combined result. A 95 per cent confidence interval for the combined effect size can then be calculated. This is usually much narrower than those for the individual study estimates.

Although the inverse variance method may be used to combine binary data too, it is more common to use one of two similar methods instead. The first of these is the Mantel–Haenszel method. Research has shown that this method is especially beneficial when trials are small or when there are only a small number of trials in the review. The other method (Peto's odds ratio) involves using Peto's estimate of the log odds ratio defined as (O-E)/V where O and E are the observed and expected events in the treatment group and V is the variance of O-E (Yusuf *et al.* 1985). This estimate has excellent statistical properties and is combined using the inverse variance weighted method. Peto's method is particularly useful when some trials have no events or when events are rare, but does not perform well when treatment effects are large.

For ordinal variables, which are commonly encountered in HRQoL assessments, there are two possible approaches. If ordinal scale data appear to be approximately normally distributed, or if the analyses reported by the investigators suggest that parametric methods and a normal approximation are appropriate, then the outcome measures can be treated as continuous variables. The second approach is to concatenate the data into two categories which best represent the contrasting states of interest, and to treat the outcome measure as binary.

Often in HRQoL meta-analyses there will be a combination of dichotomous and continuous data (also including ordinal scales). It may be useful to present separate tables for the continuous data and dichotomous data, while also combining all data for a statistical analysis. There are statistical approaches available which will re-express odds ratios as SMDs (and vice versa), which allow dichotomous and continuous data to be pooled together, subject to the assumption that the underlying distribution of the continuous measurements follows a logistic distribution (roughly similar in shape to the normal distribution). Then the odds ratios can be re-expressed as a standardized mean difference according to the simple formula SMD = $(\sqrt{3}/\pi)$ log OR (Deeks *et al.* 2004), or alternatively SMDs can be converted to log ORs. The SE of the log odds ratio can be converted to the SE of an SMD by multiplying by the same constant (0.5513). After this, an inverse variance weighted analysis can be carried out as usual.

Heterogeneity

A further complication in meta-analysis is the issue of heterogeneity. All the methods mentioned so far have been fixed-effect methods which make the assumption that the true effect sizes for each study are the same, i.e. if all studies enrolled huge numbers of patients they would all have the same effect size. This may not be a reasonable assumption, especially when studies have varying entry criteria, for example in age or stage of disease. Homogeneity between studies can be assessed either by a statistical test (although this may lack power) or by visual inspection of the results. If significant heterogeneity is identified then there are a number of options available. One is to use the fixed-effect method possibly with exploration of the reasons for the heterogeneity, one is not to perform meta-analysis at all, and another is to use a 'random effects' model instead. Random effects methods do not assume the same underlying effect size for each study, but allow random study-to-study variability. Although often the results from both methods may be similar, in practice the random effects method will tend to give more weight to smaller studies and result in wider confidence intervals than the fixed effect method. There is no consensus as to which is the best approach to use when heterogeneity is present.

Example: impact of problem-solving treatments on depression

SMDs were calculated for the depression scores. Using a fixed effects model, the overall results were SMD = −0.36; 95 per cent confidence interval −0.61 to −0.11. A random effects model gave estimates SMD = −0.49; confidence interval −0.89 to −0.08. The SMD for these trials indicated a significantly lower depression score of about one third of an SD in the group of patients who were offered problem-solving treatment.

Forest plot

The results from a meta-analysis are frequently summarized as a 'forest plot'. Figure 6.4.1 shows a forest plot, based on the results reported for the problem-solving example. Each of the four trials that was included is shown on a separate line, together with the SMD, the corresponding 95 per cent confidence interval, and the inverse-variance weight applied to the trial (as a percentage). These results are also shown graphically as a black box whose area indicates the weight assigned to that study in the meta-analysis, with a horizontal line depicting the 95 per cent confidence interval. Thus the confidence interval indicates the range of treatment effects compatible with the trial's result and indicates whether it was statistically significant. The pooled result is also shown, with a diamond indicating the overall estimate and the overall confidence interval.

Conclusions and further reading

Now that an increasing number of clinical trials include HRQoL end points we can expect to see a corresponding increase in the number of meta-analyses of such

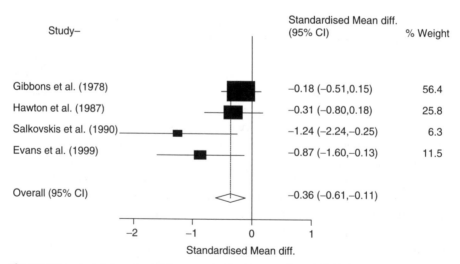

Fig. 6.4.1 Forest plot, based on data presented by Townsend *et al.* (2001).

outcomes that are carried out and published. Although meta-analysis for HRQoL may seem to be, and in some ways is, more complicated than analyses of other end points, there are no fundamental reasons why it cannot be carried out in exactly the same way.

This chapter can only superficially address the issues. Anyone contemplating performing a systematic review is strongly urged to contact the Cochrane Collaboration (or relevant Cochrane review group) for more detailed advice (http://www.cochrane.org/), and we gratefully acknowledge the *Cochrane Reviewers' Handbook* (Alderson *et al.* 2004), which we have consulted extensively when writing this chapter. The *Handbook* contains advice on all aspects of systematic reviews and meta-analyses.

There are also a number of useful books that cover the general issues of systematic reviews and meta-analysis, including Egger *et al.* (2001), Hedges and Olkin (1985) and Sutton *et al.* (2000).

This chapter has discussed and illustrated the particular issues involved in carrying out meta-analyses of HRQoL end points, illustrating some specific problems that arise in this setting and showing how they may be resolved. However, it is also important to emphasize that carrying out a systematic review is a major exercise that calls for appreciable investment of time and resources.

References

Alderson, P., Green, S., and Higgins, J. P. T. (eds) (2004). *Cochrane Reviewers' Handbook 4.2.1,* updated December 2003. In The Cochrane Library, Issue **1**, 2004. Chichester, UK: John Wiley and Sons, Ltd; also available online at http://www.cochrane.dk/cochrane/handbook/handbook.htm. (Updated at intervals).

Collins, S. L., Moore, R. A., and McQuay, H. J. (1997). The visual analogue pain intensity scale: what is moderate pain in millimetres? *Pain,* **72,** 95–97.

Deeks, J., Higgins, J., and Altman, D. (eds) (2004). Analysing and presenting results. In P. Alderson, S. Green, J. P. T. Higgins (eds) *Cochrane Reviewers' Handbook 4.2.1, Section 8,* updated December 2003. In The Cochrane Library, Issue **1,** 2004. Chichester, UK: John Wiley and Sons, Ltd.

Egger, M., Davey Smith, G., and Altman, D. G. (eds) (2001). *Systematic Reviews in Health Care: Meta-analysis in Context.* London: BMJ Books.

EU Hernia Trialists Collaboration. (1999). Overview of randomised trials of inguinal hernia repair – a European Union Concerted Action. *Surgical Endoscopy,* **13,** 1030–1031.

Hedges, L. V. and Olkin, I. (1985). *Statistical Methods in Meta-analysis.* Orlando, FL: Academic Press.

Schulz, K. F., Chalmers, I., Hayes, R. J., and Altman, D. (1995). Empirical evidence of bias. Dimensions of methodological quality associated with estimates of treatment effects in controlled trials. *Journal of the American Medical Association,* 273, 408–412.

Stewart, L. and Clarke, M. (1995). Practical methodology of meta-analyses (overviews) using updated individual patient data. *Statistics in Medicine,* **14,** 1057–1079.

Sutton, A. J., Abrams, K. R., Jones, D. R., Sheldon, T. A., and Song, F. (2000). *Methods for Meta-analysis in Medical Research.* Chichester: John Wiley and Sons Ltd.

Townsend, E., Hawton, K., Altman, D. G., Arensman, E., Gunnell, D., Hazell, P., House, A., and van Heeringen, K. (2001). The efficacy of problem-solving treatments after deliberate self-harm: meta-analysis of randomised controlled trials with respect to depression, hopelessness and improvement in problems. *Psychological Medicine*, **31**, 979–988.

Yusuf, S., Peto, R., Lewis, J., Collins, R., and Sleight, P. (1985). Beta blockade during and after myocardial infarction: an overview of the randomized trials. *Progress in Cardiovascular Diseases*, **27**, 335–271.

Index

Page numbers in *italic* indicate boxes and tables.